Health and Welfare in St. Petersburg, 1900–1941

W0113169

In the first book to chart late Imperial and Soviet health policy and its impact on the health of the collective in Russia's former capital and second 'regime' city, Christopher Williams argues that in pre-revolutionary St. Petersburg radical sections of the medical profession and the Bolsheviks highlighted the local and Tsarist government's failure to protect the health of poor peasants and the working class due to conflicts over the priority and direction of health policy, budget constraints and political division amongst doctors. They sought to forge alliances to change the law on social insurance and to prioritise the health of the collective. Situating pre- and post-revolutionary health policies in the context of revolutions, civil war, market transition and Stalin's rise to power, Williams shows how attempts were made to protect the Body Russian/Soviet and to create a healthier lifestyle and environment for key members of the new Soviet state. This failed due to shortages of money, ideology and Soviet medical and cultural norms. It resulted in ad hoc interventions into people's lives and the promotion of medical professionalization, and then the imposition of restrictions resulting from changes in the Party line. Williams shows that when the health of the collective was threatened and created medical disorder, it led to state coercion.

Christopher Williams is former head of the Department of History and Politics and Professor of Modern History at Liverpool Hope University, UK.

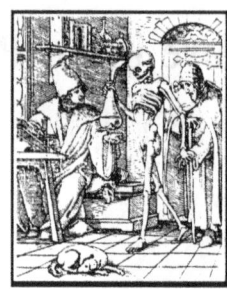

The History of Medicine in Context

Series Editors: Andrew Cunningham (Department of History and Philosophy of Science, University of Cambridge) and Ole Peter Grell (Department of History, Open University)

For more information about this series, please visit: https://www.routledge.com/The-History-of-Medicine-in-Context/book-series/HMC

Health and Welfare in St. Petersburg, 1900–1941

Protecting the Collective

Christopher Williams

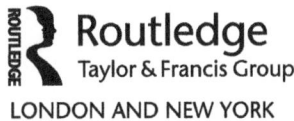
Routledge
Taylor & Francis Group

LONDON AND NEW YORK

First published 2018
by Routledge
2 Park Square, Milton Park, Abingdon, Oxon OX14 4RN

and by Routledge
605 Third Avenue, New York, NY 10017

First issued in paperback 2021

Routledge is an imprint of the Taylor & Francis Group, an informa business

British Library Cataloguing-in-Publication Data
A catalogue record for this book is available from the British Library

Library of Congress Cataloging-in-Publication Data
Names: Williams, Christopher, 1959- author.
Title: Health and welfare in St. Petersburg, 1900–1941 : protecting the collective / by Christopher Williams.
Description: New York : Routledge, 2018. | Series: History of medicine in context | Includes bibliographical references and index.
Identifiers: LCCN 2017060791 (print) | LCCN 2018000393 (ebook) | ISBN 9780429507205 (ebook) | ISBN 9780754655343 (hbk : alk. paper) | ISBN 9780429507205 (ebk)
Subjects: | MESH: Public Health—history | Social Welfare—history | History, 20th Century | Russia (Pre-1917) | Soviet Union
Classification: LCC RA395.R9 (ebook) | LCC RA395.R9 (print) | NLM WA 11 GR9 | DDC 362.10947/21—dc23
LC record available at https://lccn.loc.gov/2017060791

Typeset in Sabon LT Std
by diacriTech, Chennai

ISBN 13: 978-1-03-209522-6 (pbk)
ISBN 13: 978-0-7546-5534-3 (hbk)

This book is dedicated to my son, Michael Alexander

Table of contents

List of posters

List of tables

Preface and acknowledgements

My own interest in the question of Russian, then Soviet, public health goes back to my days as an undergraduate of Russian & Soviet Studies at the University of Portsmouth in the late 1970s–early 1980s where Dr. Frances Millard (now at the University of Essex) first encouraged me to embark upon historical research on Soviet public health for my BA Dissertation. The late Dr. Michael Ryan and Prof. Roger Pethybridge of Swansea University, then enabled me through a Welsh scholarship, to carry out two years valuable Masters research under their valuable guidance in the early to mid-80s on health care under Brezhnev, which formed the basis of my MSc (Economics).

My greatest debt of gratitude however must go to Professor Stephen A. Smith of the Department of History, University of Essex (now of All Souls College, Oxford), who was extremely generous with his time advice and support when I undertook my UK Economic and Social Research Council funded PhD on 'Soviet Public health: A Case study of Leningrad, 1917–32' at the University of Essex 1985–89 under his guidance. Dr. Christopher Davies of CREES, Birmingham (now of Nuffield College, Oxford) as my PhD external examiner also supported and encouraged me. Both have continued encouraging me over the last two decades.

This 1989 PhD was written and completed before widespread access to newly opened Russian archives was possible. The original PhD explored the relationship between the one-party state and Soviet health care professionals based upon an extensive reading of Soviet newspapers, medical and other journals and official documents covering the period from the start of the October Revolution until the end of the First five-year plan.

Now nearly 20 years after its completion, some of the questions posed have changed, as the debate moved on and as our knowledge and interest in Soviet health care increased. More importantly the source base for this work has been significantly expanded to include Moscow and St. Petersburg based archives. This has enabled not just greater insights into Soviet thinking and the expansion of the time frame to 1941, but also a change of focus onto three main areas: state, medical profession and the collective (*kollektiv*) in Petrograd/Leningrad.

I am grateful to Prof. David Goldfield, Editor, *Journal of Urban History*; Conny Opitz, President of IARCEES; Matthew Rendle and Aaron Retish, editors of *Revolutionary Russia* and SKS in Helsinki for their kind permission to refer and use some previously published material in a revised form here.

Beyond academic mentors and past publishers, I would also like to express my gratitude to the British Academy for awarding me a grant for my research project 'Politics and Health care in the Soviet workers state under Lenin and Stalin' which enabled me to consult Russian Ministry of Public Health RSFSR declassified material in GARF (State Archive of the Russian Federation) archives in Moscow between 2003–05. Second, Liverpool Hope University awarded me a Professorial grant in 2013–14 that enabled me to employ Yury Basilov, European University St. Petersburg, as Research Assistant to carry out research on my behalf in TsGAIPD, TsGA SPb, TsGANTD and the Russian National Library (RNB) in St. Petersburg. Third, I would like to express thanks to inter library loan staff at Essex, Swansea, Cork, University of Central Lancashire and now Liverpool Hope and to librarians in the UK at the following institutions: Aleksandr Baykov library, former CREES, University of Birmingham (in particular Jenny Brine and Jackie Johnson); The British library; the SSEES, University of London; the London School of Hygiene and Tropical medicine; the Wellcome units for the History of Medicine, London and Oxford (in the latter Prof. Paul Weindling, deserves a special mention). Finally, beyond the UK, the following staff and librarians deserve special mention: staff at the Lenin library and RNB in Moscow; the RNB in St. Petersburg; the University of Amsterdam and the International institute of Social History, Nederlands; The Department of Economic and Social History and Renvall Institute of Historical Research, University of Helsinki and the Slaavilianen Kirjasto, University of Helsinki, Finland. These trips to Holland and Finland where kindly funded by Dutch and Finnish Ministries of Education grants in 1988–89 and by the British Academy, 2003–05. I would like to thank the University of Central Lancashire, my former institution until the summer of 2013, for a period of research leave in 2007–08, which made trips to the USA possible. In this regard, I would like to thank staff of the European Reading Room, Library of Congress, Washington DC for their help in locating some of the sources used here.

Particular thanks go to the RNB, to Philippa Morton at the Wellcome Trust; Hazel Stewart, Diarmid Ross and Dr. Emily Goetsch at the National Library of Scotland; Kate Higgins at the LSE; Mary Beth Sigado and Wendy Chmielewski, Curator, of the Soviet poster collection at Swarthmore College, USA and Ginny Roth of the United States National Library of Medicine, for their help in locating and permission to use visual images (health posters and propaganda) from their collections in this book. I would like to acknowledge my gratitude to the Scouloudi Foundation in association with the Institute of Historical Research for funding in 2016 to purchase some of the visual images used.

I would like to thank Dr. Georg Wiessala for his help proofreading this book which is much appreciated.

Unfortunately my late partner, Agueda Pons Pons, lost her battle against lung cancer in January 2014 and did not live long enough to see this book published. Ague was always there with a lovely smile and lots of encouragement for my love of Russia's history, as we went on our travels and spent many happy times in Ferreries, Menorca enjoying the forests, mountains, pale blue seas, beaches and most of all family meals and festivals, with Tomeu and the wonderfully warm and welcoming, Pons Pons family. Molt d'amor a tots.

It is no exaggeration to say that without the support of my son, Mike, after Ague's passing this book would never have been finished.

I am dedicating this book to Mike, now a father himself, with a wonderful son of his own, Tom. Mike, you make me so proud.

I would also like to thank the former Dean of the Faculty of Arts & Humanities at Liverpool Hope University, Prof. Nick Rees, and Dr Guy Cuthbertson, former chair of the Faculty Research Committee, and now Head of the Department of English at Liverpool Hope University for the award of a period of research leave in July 2016 do the final research necessary to complete this book and my colleagues in the Department of History and Politics, at Liverpool Hope for their support and encouragement between October 2013 and the end of September 2017, when I retired.

Finally, I would like to thank the series editors, my Routledge History editors, Jennifer Morrow and Max Novick, Jonathan Merrett and Gillian Steadman for their assistance at all stages of production.

Liverpool, UK.

Abbreviations and glossary

Agitprop	Agitation and propaganda
Aktiv	Activists in the Party and other organisations
AMA	American Medical Association
Arkhiv sudebnoi meditsiny i obshchestbennoi gigieny	Archive of forensic medicine and social hygiene
babka (pl. babki)	uneducated midwives performing illegal abortions
BCG	Bacillus Calmette-Gurein vaccinations
besprizornye	homeless children
BMA	British Medical Association
Bol'nichnaia komissiia	Hospital commission
Bol'nichnyi sbor	Hospital fund
byt	way of life
byvshie	'former people'
Cheka	All-Russian commission for the Struggle against counter-revolution, sabotage and speculation
chinovnik	Tsarist official
d.	delo (files, in archive)
detskie konsultatsii	children's outpatient consultancies
detskiie polikliniki	children's clinics
detskikh profilakticheskikh ambulatorii	children's prophylactic units
Duma	Parliament

Ezhovshchina	Campaign of mass terror in 1937–38 (named after NKVD head, Ezhov)
f.	fond (collection, in archives)
Fabrichno-zavodskaia kommissii	Factory Commission
feldsher	doctor's assistant
fund meditsinskoi pomoshchi (FMP)	medical assistance fund
FYP, FYPs	Five-year plan, five-year plans
g.	grams
GARF	State Archive of the Russian Federation
golod	hunger, famine
Gorkom	City committee (of Party)
Gosplan	State planning commission
Gosstrakh	State insurance agencies
GPU	State political directorate (secret police, successor to Cheka)
guberniia	province
Gubispolkom	Executive Committee (of regional Party organisation)
Gubkom	Party Regional Committee
Gulag	Chief Administration of Camps
IMR	Infant mortality rate
individual'nost'	individuality
k	kopeck
kadrovye rabochie	cadre workers
kartochki ob aborte	abortion record cards
kassa obezpecheniia	welfare funds
kassy	medical insurance funds
kg	kilogram
khozraschet	Cost accounting
klassovost'	class restrictiveness
kolkhoz, kolkhozy	collective farm, collective farms
kollektiv	collective
Komitet obshchestvennogo zdraviia	Public Health Committee

Kommissariata zdravookhraneniia Petrogradskoi trudovoi kommuny	Petrograd Health Service
Komsomol (YCL)	All-Union Leninist Communist League of Youth
kontrol'no-inspektsionnaia komissiia	control-inspection commission
kulak	wealthy peasant
kul'turnost'	cultured approach
l., ll.	list, listy (page, pages, in archive files)
lichnaia zhizn'	private life
Meditsinskii otdel, Ministerstvo Vnutrennykh del	Medical Department of the Ministry of the Interior
Meditsinskii Vestnik	Medical Herald
Medsantrud	medical employees trade union
medtekhnikum	medical training college
meshchanin	petty bourgeois
militsia	police
Ministerstvo Vnutrennykh del	Ministry of Internal affairs or Home Office
MMA	Military Medical Academy (St. Petersburg)
nalog	tax
Narkomiust' (NKiu)	People's Commissariat of Justice
Narkompros	People's Commissariat of Enlightenment (Education)
Narkomtrud (NKT)	People's Commissariat of Labour
Narkomzdrav (NKZ)	People's Commissariat of Health
narod	the people
nekul'turnye rabochie	uncultured workers
NEP	New Economic Policy
nepmen	Small traders (beneficiaries of NEP)
nizy	lower classes, those at the bottom
NKSO	People's Commissariat of Social Security
NKVD	People's Commissariat for Internal Affairs (political police, successor to the OGPU)

ob	reverse (in archive reference)
oblast'	administrative region
Obshchestvo okraneniia narodnogo zdraviia	Society Protecting People's Health
OGPU	Unified State Political Directorate (political police, successor to the GPU)
okrug	administrative region
op.	opis' (inventory, in archives)
Otdel meditsinskoi ekspertizy	Medical Experts' Department
Otdel okhrany materinstva i mladenchestva	Mothers and Infants' Department
otkhodniki	seasonal workers
Partiimost'	Party spirit
Petrogradskaia gorodskaia duma	Petrograd City Duma
Petrogradskii gubzdravotdel	Petrograd Provincial Regional Public Health Department
Peterburgskoe oshchestvo zavodchikov i fabrikantov	St Petersburg Society of Mill and Factory owners
Petrogradskoi gorodskoi otdel zdravookhraneniia	City of Petrograd Public Health Department
Petersburgskoi uezdnoi sanitarnoi kommissii	District Level Sanitary Commission in St. Petersburg
Politburo	Political Bureau of the Central Committee of the Party
potomstvennye rabochie	hereditary workers
Prikazy	Committees of Public Assistance
profsoiuzy	trade unions
propiska	residence permit
punkty kvartirnoi pomoshchi	housing based medical points
r	rouble
Rabfak	Workers' Faculties of Universities, Institutes and Colleges
Rabkin	People's Commissariat of Workers' and Peasants' Inspection
Rabmedy	Workers' Medical Departments

rabochii	worker (industrial)
rabochii vopros	workers' question
raz"ednaia sistema	circuit system of medical provision
RNB	Russian National Library
RSDLP	Russian Social Democratic Workers (Labour) Party
RSFSR	Russian Soviet Federative Socialist Republic
samogon	moonshine
Sankt-Peterburgskoe obshchestvo popecheniia o narodnom zdraviia	St Petersburg Society for the Protection of Public Health
Sanktpeterburgskogo obshchestva russkikh vrachei	Society of Russian Doctors in St Petersburg
statsionaia sistema	stationery system of medical provision
Soiuz aptechnykh rabotnikov	Union of Pharmaceutical Workers
Soiuz medrabotnikov	Union of Medical Workers
Soiuza sluzhaschikh v aptekakh	Pharmacy Employees Union
sotsial'naia gigiena	social hygiene
Sovet	Councils of Workers, Peasants and Soldiers deputies
Sovet okrany materinstva i mladenchestva	Council for the Protection of Mothers and Infants
Sovet po delam strakhovaniia rabochikh	The Council of Workers' Insurance
Sovet s"ezdov prestavitel promyshlennosti i Torgovli	Association of Trade and Industry
Sovet vrachebnykh kollegii	Council of Medical Boards
Sovnarkom	Council of People's Commissars
spetseedstvo	specialist baiting/harassment
Spetsial'naia komissiia po bor'be s detskim tuberkulezom	Special Commission to Combat Children's TB
spetsy	specialists
SRs	Social Revolutionaries
strakhovaia meditsina	insurance medicine
sudebnoi vrachei	judicial doctors

TB	tuberculosis
TFR	Total fertility rate
TsGA SPb	Central State Archive in St. Petersburg
TsGAIPD SPb	Central State Archive of Historical and Political Documents in St. Petersburg
TsGANTD	Central State Archive of Scientific-Technical Documents in St. Petersburg
TsSU	Central Statistical Administration
uchastok	sub-district
uezd	district
USSR	Union of Soviet Socialist Republics
vaktsino-syvorotchnaia komissiia	vaccine serum commission
VD	venereal disease
verkhi	upper classes, those at the top
VKK – vrachebno- kontrol'nye komissii	Medical Control Commission
Voprosy Strakhovaniia	Questions of Insurance
VTEK	Medical Labour Expert Commissions
VTsIK	Central Executive Committee of the Soviet
VUZ	Higher educational institutions
vydvizhentsy	upwardly mobile cadres (usually proletarian)
zavodskaia meditsina	factory medicine
zemshchina	proponents of zemstvo medicine
zemstvo	institutions of local government in Russia, 1864–17
zhakty	housing co-operatives
Zhenotdel	Women's Department (of Party)

Introduction

Despite the existence of community medicine before the Russian Revolution, levels of disease, illness, hygiene, cleanliness and housing, the tsarist regime, as typified by the situation in the capital St. Petersburg, was woeful. By 1900 widespread epidemics, high infant mortality and death rates, heavy drinking, prostitution, social diseases (VD, tuberculosis) and serious overcrowding showed that the tsarist state and municipal government had failed in its duty to protect the poorest members of society. Doctors and other staff were employed by the state but no centralised health system was put in place. Furthermore, although the medical profession was valued it was not professionalised, and over time some physicians became increasingly politicised. For Marxists, this unhealthy environment, facing children and adults alike, were symbols of oppression and an indication that Russian capitalists and landowners put profit before the health of its citizens. For a variety of reasons to be explored in the first chapter, the central and municipal governments realised that the health and sanitation had reached crisis point, especially after the 1905 Revolution, but their reactions and responses were divided, a consensus on the best way forward was hard to achieve, and the desire, in certain quarters to create a central, Ministry of Public health to address these health crises came very late (1910) and progress towards this goal was interrupted by the outbreak of the First World War and by the fact that certain sections of the Russian medical profession, primarily Pirogov Society doctors, and other socially conscious organisations, though in favour of public health and sanitary reform and their professionalization, opposed such a move because it threatened all the gains made in zemstvo medicine since the mid-1860s.

Lenin and the Bolsheviks argued, as this book will demonstrate, that a fundamental reconfiguration of health and welfare was required to address these problems and that a new, modern form of health governance was needed to eradicate the 'ills' and adverse impact of Russia's industrial capitalism and urbanisation on the population, especially the poorest classes of peasants and industrial workers, in St Petersburg. This led, after 1917, to Soviet state intervention, through a Ministry of Public Health, which originated in Petrograd, and was later expanded to all the regions and cities of the Soviet state. This goal was driven by a desire to create and use the new socialist health care system to protect the collective health, hygiene and lifestyle of the citizens of the new Workers' State.

Bolshevik health care discourse after 1903 increasingly constructed a view that, in the tsarist era, cities (such as St Petersburg) were polluted, unhealthy and activists held the government, industrialists and landowners responsible. The Bolsheviks sought to move the capital from its backward, unhealthy state to a more pure, hygienic and healthy condition. This is shown by their social insurance campaign after the introduction of the 1912 insurance law and the fight to get medical funds for industrial workers. The reforms and changes fought for were geared towards improving the health and welfare of the people (*narod*) and to protect the collective *(kollektiv)* because the tsarist regime had failed to generate the conditions essential for a healthy population at city and regional level in St. Petersburg. Later, once in power, Lenin and the Bolsheviks relied upon the primacy of medical science as a means of social engineering and the reorganisation of health care, along socialist lines, to resolve the lack of clean water and sewage system problems, create cleaner streets, a more enlightened population (overcoming ignorance through the use of health education and propaganda campaigns) and most of all, through the emergence of a more active state that put prophylaxis and the collective at the forefront of its health policy. Thus health can be used as a lens through which historians can assess how the Soviet state sought to redefine attitudes to disease and health and to forge a new collectivist way of delivering and thinking about health and welfare between the October Revolution of 1917 and the siege of Leningrad in 1941–42.

Health and Welfare in St Petersburg argues that, by analysing trends in the former capital of the Russian Empire, it is possible to assess first, how the Soviet regime understood the sources of various illnesses; second, how official discourse and health officials promoted certain attitudes towards health; third, how Lenin and Stalin defined health norms and the responsibilities of individuals about what was deemed 'normal' and 'acceptable' in terms of health and hygiene in order to protect the collective health of the nation; fourth, how the early Soviet state and its later Stalinist counterparts recorded, reported and interpreted health conditions and trends; and finally, and most importantly, how they managed changes in the population and health status.

Most books analysing Soviet Russia from the October Revolution to the German invasion of the Soviet Union have naturally focused upon economic and political changes. Social changes, in particular the health and welfare needs of the new Soviet regime, were for many years a neglected field of Soviet history and politics. There is now a growing interest in this area. A number of ground-breaking overviews of Russian and Soviet Public Health now exist.[1] Other recent studies have analysed the role of specific groups such as pharmacists[2] or assessed certain policy areas such as alcohol[3] or particular areas of concern such as prostitution,[4] sex,[5] homosexuality[6] and suicide;[7] or finally, historians have analysed the nature of the Soviet health and welfare project in general in particular periods.[8] These excellent studies show how Bolshevik and Stalinist thinking in a number of health and welfare areas, drawing upon faith in the humanities and social sciences, as Pinnow and Daniel Beer[9] emphasise, helped over time to create what Tricia Starks terms the 'body Soviet' in her 2008 seminal work.[10]

Health and Welfare in St. Petersburg, 1900–1941 explores how such public health anxieties played out at a local level in one major city. In particular we analyse how the new Soviet state sought to create a new way of life (*byt*) amongst the collective in Leningrad. This book shows that the local population had had to endure major changes in their health ever since pre-revolutionary times, not just during the Leningrad siege[11] and the famine that followed it, and this book puts these events in a broader long-term historical and public health context complementing earlier contributions on this topic.

Using declassified documents from the State Archive of the Russian Federation (GARF) relating to the RSFSR Ministry of Public health as well as materials from the St. Petersburg city historical and other archives (Central State Archive of St. Petersburg (TsGIA SPb) the Central State Archive of Historical-Political Documents (TsGAIPD SPb), the former party archive) and the Central State Archive of Scientific-Technical Documents (TsGANTD), together with Russian newspapers and medical journals, this book argues that in philosophical terms there was a break with zemstvo medicine after the October Revolution of 1917, but at the same time Lenin and the Bolsheviks, whilst having their own Marxist approach, also drew upon certain progressive traditions among the medical profession from the pre-revolutionary era, to eventually create a welfare state, albeit one based upon socialist principles.

We assess developments in the period 1900–41 from three perspectives: first, policy making on health and welfare by the Russian/Soviet state in Moscow and at a local level in Petrograd/Leningrad; second, the role of the Party and different parts of the medical profession in implementing health and welfare policies; and third, the impact of these new collectivist policies on different sections of society, especially workers and peasants.

More specifically, this book charts the organisation and development of health and welfare in one city – St. Petersburg, the former capital of the Russian Empire, later renamed Petrograd and Leningrad. This city was a major industrial and commercial part of European Russia, a significant port, with a mix of peasants, workers and other social classes and groups at the start of the Twentieth century. The focus is on exploring how the Tsarist and Soviet systems of health and welfare were shaped by continuity and change, as determined by the common legacies of Empire, revolution, civil war, the death of Lenin and the rise of Stalin, and the latter's time in power from 1928–41.

We examine how far Russian and Soviet science and medicine, progressive thinking, ideology and Marxist thinking all blended together in giving new meanings to health and welfare in the newly created Soviet socialist medicine. David Priestland argues that the Bolshevism of Lenin and Stalin can be characterised as revivalist, technicist or neo-traditionalist throughout the period under discussion. The revivalist strategy was common in the civil war and, according to Priestland, focused on the power of ideas, the proletariat and the use of popular mass mobilisation to build a new socialist state and health and welfare system. The technicist trend in Bolshevism was more prevalent under the New Economic Policy (NEP) and emphasised the importance of economic progress following the end of the civil war, the greater use of technology, achieving greater efficiencies and establishing a scientific medical order. At this time, liberalism, trade and the market impacted upon trends in the health care sphere. By the late 1920s, the revivalism of War Communism had returned and in the 1930s this gradually gave way to neo-traditionalism as Stalin used popular mobilisation strategies against enemies as he intensified the class struggle against the bourgeois medical profession and other groups.[12]

We will trace Lenin and Stalin's plans for health and welfare, their policy and decision-making processes, the response of the medical profession (hostility and cooperation, their relationship to the old Russian and new Soviet regime) and the impact of these changes for the average Soviet citizen at home, in the workplace and with regard to age, gender, class and place of residence (city district or remote parts of St. Petersburg/Leningrad Province/Oblast).

The actions, aspirations and voices of some of those participating in the Soviet health experiment in this one city will be heard and interpreted using official documents, party debates and practices, press reports, medical journal discussions and through the use of local and central archival materials, all of which now reveal the public, and private, hitherto secret thinking, of the leaders, political and medical elites, the institutions and networks to which they belonged as well as the opinions of workers, peasants and other Soviet citizens, which allow us as medical and social historians to determine official and popular beliefs about Russian and Soviet health and welfare since 1900 and up to the outbreak of war with Nazi Germany in Leningrad.

A key component of our analysis is the Tsarist medical profession which now served the new Soviet state, and we will examine how far doctors and other medical staff learnt to navigate the enormous changes after 1917, out of mere pragmatism or for professionalization reasons, and in the process how they helped, wherever possible, to fulfil in challenging circumstances, the promises made to transform health and welfare.

This work also explores the relationship between disease, patient, doctor and state in St. Petersburg, Petrograd and Leningrad. This involves not just the development and implementation of a new philosophy of medicine but the application of the latest technology to deliver health care and the use of propaganda to carry out health enlightenment and surveillance of the population.

The city of St. Petersburg's doctors and other medical staff as the experts, dealing on a daily basis with the 'body Russian' and 'Soviet', were constrained by the constantly fluctuating Party line, but acted as in pre-revolutionary times, as servants of the state, this time in the new Soviet, communist regime. Those not opposing the Bolsheviks, sought to assist in the regulation of population behaviour and beliefs on health and hygiene, using the emergence and state sponsorship of relatively new disciplines, such as public, social and labour hygiene, and various government institutions, to carry out their jobs and to try and adapt to the new situation. The medical profession provided this support to the Soviet state in the hope of gaining greater autonomy, professionalization and because of certain shared attitudes on sexuality, birth and reproduction, drinking, eating and so forth. These former tsarist doctors, such as bacteriologists, social hygienists, industrial hygienists and feldshers, had reconfigured themselves, and with their new 'Soviet' colleagues helped push through laws and policies to medicalise Soviet society. Both sides sought to improve the urban environment of the city by purifying water, redesigning housing, cleaning the streets, modernising sewage systems and by promoting healthy communal hygiene and new ways of living. This book argues that there was more to unite than divide them from a public health perspective.

The collective is at the centre of this book as it 'became the defining characteristic of the new regime'[13] and shaped Soviet health policy. The Soviet state wanted the collective to become a form/way of life and both Lenin and Stalin sought to protect the health of the collective – society, and its key members, the industrial working class and peasants. The aim was to 'reject the private realm as a legitimate space'[14] and achieve self-realisation via membership of the collective, a community of individuals. This situation in Pinnow's view 'forced the Soviets to confront the individual'.[15] This raises the question of what was the mandate of the state in relation to the collective and what constituted the authentic collective? As Soviet public health policy emerged, it will become clear that the difference between the private and collective aspects of the population's lives in Petrograd and Leningrad were blurred and there was no clear boundary between the two. Oleg Khorkhardin argues that the Soviet regime sought to develop a collectivist lifestyle, in this context in relation to health and welfare, with a search for self-perfection evident, among Party members and the general public. Lenin and Stalin wanted to eradicate individualist attitudes and to replace them with a collective identity and new vision of people's way of life. As a result, the collective eclipsed the individual as a centre of attention.[16] In relation to this book, the goal was to refashion individual health practices and so there was a strong relationship between the latter and the content of public health discourse and propaganda as the Soviet regime sought to cultivate a group self and a collective *mentalité*.

This book explores how this impacted upon the question of one's health identity, with the emphasis being less on the personal or individual and more on the collective. This led to a conflict between the individual and the collective and between public and private self.[17] In Kenneth Pinnow's view, '[t]o be alone and outside the collective risked a loss of purpose and meaning'.[18]

The Soviet government sought to create a new socialist collective purified of individualistic, bourgeois and harmful influences on the population's health and to eliminate other weaknesses attacking the body Soviet and the socialist cause. In this context, other sections of the collective (state and medical profession) acted as an agency of medical socialisation for the population of Petrograd/Leningrad. This was deemed necessary in order to reframe public health values and attitudes and to provide the health security of all. Soviet health posters were part of the collectivist approach and represented a collective ideal scenario and painted images of particular individuals, diseases or of urban and rural health as positive or negative. The medical profession and the state used health propaganda to establish models of self and individual behaviour and set moral and public health codes for everyone to follow as individuals were 'central to maintaining the health of the kollektiv'.[19] This involved the promotion of moral purity, mutual respect, love of family, children and so forth to ensure that all citizens promoted and pursued goals that met the collective purpose in general and in relation to public health in particular. The idea was to unite individual practice and the new Soviet collective tradition and to create a sense of collective ethics with regards to health attitudes and practice. According to Pinnow, the desire was 'to create a citizenry that was healthy in a physical, mental and political sense'.[20]

This was important as the Soviet state wished individuals to recognise that they were part of a group and so the emphasis was on 'We' rather than 'I'. This stress on human agency effectively absolved 'Soviet society of responsibility' for 'the vagaries and uncertainties (of) modern life' in health and welfare terms Petrograd and Leningrad.[21] Thus the health education and enlightenment campaigns discussed in this book were geared towards ensuring people of the city maintained their personal health and monitored with the help of medical professionals their health behaviour. These campaigns 'assumed the internalization of certain values and beliefs'[22] but as we see they were not always successful and this situation led to the medicalisation of health deviance for those seen as threatening the health of the collectivist social order. So health became 'public property'. There was an expectation that all members of the collective would be involved in building socialism and a socialist health care system and that they would in the process create a collective healthy space at home and at work and obey Soviet health norms and responsibilities. This was part of the new collectivist thinking and communist upbringing. The aim was to create a sense of collective belonging and consciousness and thus citizens of Petrograd/Leningrad were expected to give up their self for the benefit of the collective. Thus any changes in government policy were seen as part of guaranteeing the collective good and as evidence of collective success, if achieved. The state believed that such positive changes would only occur through collective mobilisation. The Party wished everyone to produce better health care and facilities for all and to improve the overall well-being of the collective society so their lives and bodies were not 'their own' instead the 'Soviet regime had a claim on the individual' and their health.[23] In turn, the population was expected to make sacrifices to meet the needs of the collective. This strategy, in turn, drew the population into the collective project of building socialism and a socialist health care system. It was hoped that this would motivate people and shape the collective imagination and consciousness. However, it also increased the level of pressure on those deemed to be ruining the collective. They were to be exposed and punished not just in the health posters featured in this book (which told people what to think and how to behave) but via self-criticism and later via court appearances. To do this there was a need for collective supervision of health service leaders and rank and file to see how far Party targets were achieved and to impose the necessary corrections if required. This involved the use of negative collective opinion to change individual attitudes and to ensure that citizens of Petrograd/Leningrad worked collectively and in the interests of the collective. The aim was to ensure that individuals were fully integrated into the collective, had the correct political consciousness, spirit of collectivism and did not show old bourgeois health values. This led to a shift of emphasis onto individuals as part of the collective in order to maintain the collective order, ensure a good quality collective experience of health care and to prevent any enemies threatening the collective by breaching health norms. Public health crises required collective responses and actions. This gave rise to the idea of collective responsibility so in the case of alleged abuse of power in the health sphere, the collective had the right to appeal to higher authorities.[24] Pinnow argues that Party members were meant to be a good example to others by leading healthy lives so were advised against drinking and mixing with hostile elements.[25]

The aim was to connect one's own interests to that of the national collective. During the terror of the 1930s, this led to collective responses to perceived public health problems or people were able to express their collective outrage in the cases of perceived failures which in turn produced a process of collective shaming and unmasking of the 'guilty'. As Pinnow notes, any unhealthy parts of the population or body politic were attributed to the existence of 'class enemies or residual social elements that resisted the progressive developments of socialism'.[26] The collective may have had responsibility to prevent illness and disease but this book shows, however, that the collectivist health approaches adopted were not as totalising and controlling as totalitarian scholars of Stalinist Russia would have us believe. As a result, public health surveillance of the population was deemed necessary to align the actions and behaviour of the individual with that of the collective. This sometimes involved medicalisation of illness and at other times criminalisation of disease, such as suicide or a combination of the two, as in the case of abortion. The Soviet regime used its health policies or changes in the law to manage and shape the population.

Soviet historiography has promoted a highly positive view of Soviet health and welfare. Whilst some of the achievements highlighted in this book were genuine, the reality as a whole was generally very different. The official Soviet discourse has argued that any failures were the result of medical opposition to the regime, and this book challenges that assumption and argues that there are other more compelling reasons why the class basis of medicine was ineffective and inefficient as access to health facilities was not offered to all on an equal basis. Also, some groups (the insured for instance) were prioritised over others. Furthermore, eligibility criteria to access health care shifted over time. National (Tsarist and Narkomzdrav) and local health leaders in affecting the above collectivist-oriented changes in policy also sometimes clashed and we will also assess the attempts made at a local level to influence the direction of health and welfare policies coming from above. We will analyse municipal responses to key changes, how they coped with change – such as the arrival of the revolution and its new philosophy of medicine or central planning – and what strategies were used in St. Petersburg (and its successors) to ease pressure on staff, services and patients.

This book assesses the 'contested meanings' given to selected health issues discussed here – baby and maternal care, infectious diseases, abortions, alcohol, venereal diseases, industrial injuries and accidents – by government and Party officials, medical professionals and by the insured and non-insured members of the general public, all members of the collective. Such an approach enables us as historians to analyse shifting perceptions of key health crises or perceived problems across time (1900–17, 1918–20, 1921–27, 1928–41) and space (Russian/Soviet; tsarist/Soviet) as well as the impact of social, cultural, economic and political changes on the fate of health and welfare in the USSR's second city.

These issues are explored through a series of key questions: Did a change of regime or ruler make a difference? What motivated state/party officials' attitudes to health and welfare? How did the Russian/Soviet state react to perceived cooperation and/or opposition from the medical profession? How did central authorities impact upon local public health decision and policy making? Did local state/Party officials or medical professionals try to retain local autonomy or just push central health and welfare reforms through? Finally, in what way did the market under NEP or Stalin's victory influence the nature and direction of public health policy? Such questions will enable us to assess the level of continuity and change in health care from tsarist to Soviet periods/eras or between Soviet leaders (Lenin and Stalin), the degree of central–local conflict over medicine, the impact of other changes on health policy, such as the civil war, NEP and Stalin's 'great break' (rapid industrialisation, forced collection, central planning, the cultural revolution), and the impact of the Great and mass Terrors and the run up to the Great Patriotic War, on trends in one city – St. Petersburg (1900–14, later renamed Petrograd, 1914–24 then Leningrad, 1924–41).

Health and Welfare in St. Petersburg, 1900–1941 explores a number of key themes:

First, the development of public health and in particular the physicians and other medical personnel's professional aspirations, sense of community and work. Particular emphasis is put upon the degree of professional autonomy or lack of it.

Second, the relationship of different sections of the medical profession to the Tsarist and Soviet regimes is analysed. This requires an examination of the degree of dependence of doctors and other health service personnel on the tsarist state, later the Soviet party-state bureaucracy, and in particular how far and in what way the medical profession supported or opposed government goals before and after 1917, especially collectivist policies. It also involves assessing trends in health care by exploring organisational and professional structures, disciplinary agendas, the role of interest groups, the relationship between medico-politics and patronage and different cultures and forms of practice in the health service. The aim is to show how different actors and groups interacted and also to place developments in health and welfare within the broader political and economic context of the collapse of the tsarist regime and trends during the Lenin and Stalin eras.

Third, an assessment will be provided of the way in which trends in the health service and the medical profession became subject to the ever changing economic and political agenda, ranging from the changes after the Crimean War and the outbreak of the Bolshevik Revolution to War Communism, the shift to the market during the New Economic Policy era in the 1920s and then onto Stalin's revolution from above and below in the 1930s and beyond.

Fourth, the book assesses the relationship between health policy and high politics, in particular that of Russian/Soviet patron (state) and client (medical profession and health service personnel) relationships. This involves an analysis of the tactics adopted by both sides, whereby the state sought to control the medical community (via the allocation of wages, research funds, resources and the replacement of medical professionals by party hacks) whilst the medical profession and health service personnel sought prestige and legitimacy by demonstrating their usefulness to the state as a means of fulfilling key priorities, such as monitoring changes in illness and disease at a time of hunger, industrialisation, collectivisation and the purges, and attempting to meet the needs of the collective. Particular emphasis is placed on fate of the medical profession – shortages of finance, structural reorganisation, pressure once five-year plans were introduced, the impact of Stalin's Cultural Revolution (the popularisation of medical sciences, a desire to reach the masses in order not to be accused of 'bourgeois idealism') – and the degree to which, if any, Soviet state bureaucrats and the Party needed to or was successful in establishing a system of control over the medical profession in the 1930s and on the ways in which medical scientists and health service professionals sought to avoid and exploit this situation to serve their self or professional interests. We will analyse how far their independence was eroded how successful both parties were in achieving these goals.

Fifth, an analysis will be carried out on whether or not existing views of the Soviet health service and its employees as simply 'agents' of the state are accurate and the degree to which the situation was much more complex than previously assumed because neither the state nor medical professionals and health service workers were monolithic, and the boundaries between them were often blurred. This book embarks upon an examination of how medical personnel tried to shape their own fate in the Soviet period.

The sixth theme involves an analysis of the extent to which, if any, the medical community and party-state apparatus had merged by the late 1930s and early 1940s due to the class war against tsarist trained staff, the rise of proletarian medicine and Communist Party infiltration and subjugation of public health and medical science. We will explore the consequences, in particular the need to conform to a materialist point of view, a class line in medicine and above all through adopting a 'correct' medical position on illness and health and how far former tsarist staff actually resisted these policies or were perceived to do so.

Finally, this study analyses how the party-state bureaucracy from the civil war period onwards tried to define patterns of health behaviour and medical science rituals and we will assess if it succeeded or not.

This book seeks to add to our understanding of the complexities of Soviet Russia by assessing how far the 'collective' ideal drove these trends in public health and welfare.

At this point, it is important to point out that this work seeks to challenge the assumption that so-called 'tsarist' ideas and beliefs about health and welfare at all levels were simply replaced by Soviet worldviews in a sequential pattern. This book argues instead that Soviet health and welfare policy, at least on the basis of this case study, was in fact more of a hybrid of old and new, a fact underplayed by Soviet historiography primarily due to the desire to promote Soviet exceptionalism and its distinctiveness. The reason for this was that both the Soviet government and its medical practitioners, old and new, sought to prevent disease, carry out health surveys and collect statistics, promote a healthy population and regulate the so-called 'social' (later 'socialist') order in the process. It will be also become clear that both groups, operating in different states and contexts, believed in the power of medical science and wanted to create an active state that sought to transform medicine, and the health and welfare of citizens for the better.

What distinguished Tsarist and Soviet approaches to health and welfare was the way in which they governed; both carried out health enlightenment to encourage a healthy, modern lifestyle but the degree to which they intervened, at city and national level, through health surveillance of the individual and the collective differed. This notion of the 'collective' was one of the defining features of the new Soviet welfare state. The individual existed, but only in the context of, or in relation to, the broader collective. The aim of the Soviet welfare state was to protect its citizens and 'the body politic' from a range of possible health corruptors or pollutants – vestiges of the old bourgeois order, alcoholics, prostitutes, those having illegal abortions, sexual deviants, those endangering others in the factory, class enemies etc. – and to remove any obstacles (non-communist party members, bourgeois tsarist trained staff) and others who all endangered the state and the health of its citizens. It was the responsibility of the state and everyone else within it, including the Party and medical profession, as well as the members of the population, to help build a socialist society and health care system, which in turn sought to provide comprehensive health care for those from the collective who aided the socialist cause and system.

This book utilises the disciplines of social history, and the history of medicine, to analyse how different social classes and groups accessed Tsarist/Soviet medicine; the role of medical disciplines and the corresponding institutions which evolved from and in response to changes in tsarist and Soviet social, economic and political trends and the history of health and attitudes to disease from 1900 to 1941. What will become clear in this book is the leading role played by the zemstvo and the public health movement staff and its locally administered health measures which were used to combat the environmental and social hazards facing the citizens of St Petersburg. The Bolsheviks, prior to and after the October Revolution, developed an alternative, Marxist model, which did not seek to use the welfare state to contain the threat posed by the working class, but to serve its interests. It was the continuity of staff that partly enabled this collectivist strategy to be implemented.

Health and Welfare in St. Petersburg, 1900–1941 consists of the following chapters:

Chapter 1 looks at health conditions and medical care in St. Petersburg, 1900–17, with regard to industrial workers and peasants focusing on birth and death rates trends, the widespread existence of infectious diseases, famines, a high death rate and a low birth rate, on the one hand, and the poor housing, sanitation, food and provision on the other. The chapter examines how the state and medical profession responded to these issues and also assesses the drawbacks of having a fragmented system with no direct control at the centre. Finally, it analyses the emergence of future Bolshevik policy on health and welfare via a case study of social insurance. It argues that Tsarism failed to protect the 'body Russian' and some members of the medical profession allied themselves with the Bolsheviks to produce change.

The second chapter analyses the Bolshevik vision of health and welfare after October 1917 until the end of the civil war (1920) and explores the new Leninist principles of health and welfare including state responsibility for public health; attempts to centralise health care; the notion of free and comprehensive medical aid; the emphasis on preventive medicine; and the unity of theory and practice. We consider the way in which the external environment (hostility, isolation, economic blockade) as well as internal difficulties (opposition, shortages of food, housing, doctors, epidemics of infectious diseases and rapidly changing health conditions and status) created problems in putting the above principles into practice.

Chapter 3 goes on to assess health conditions and medical care in Petrograd/Leningrad under the market economy of the New Economic policy, 1921–27. It focuses on birth and death rates trends, the reasons behind the decline in infectious diseases, hunger, and high death rates, and focuses upon the challenge of social diseases and why the birth rate and population recovered in the 1920s. Although the situation with regards to housing, sanitation, food and health service development improved, the chapter examines how the local authorities and medical profession responded to cuts in health financing, the rising importance of insurance medicine, the market and what the start of an attack on the so-called 'bourgeois specialists' and growing party penetration of the health service from 1926 meant for tsarist doctors and other medical personnel and students. Finally, we end by looking at what the abandonment of NEP meant for health and welfare in Leningrad by 1927.

Chapter 4 assesses health conditions and medical care in Leningrad during the Stalinist era, focusing in depth on trends during the first, second and third five-year health plans, 1928–32, 1933–37 and 1938–41 respectively. The goals and targets set and the ability of the Leningrad health service to fulfil them will be considered. This chapter shows how Stalin's welfare modernisation in some respects marked a continuation with earlier strategy whilst in other regards constituted a fundamental break with the past. The abandonment of NEP, the introduction of central planning and the pursuit of rapid industrialisation and forced collectivisation, all had an adverse effect upon health service development and health conditions generally. This led to unrealistic FYP health targets and to plan non-fulfilment generating shortages of food, housing, doctors and to a declining standard of living which affected people's health. Infectious diseases, influenza, alcoholism, VD and TB all rose. These problems were then compounded by the purges in the mid-late 1930s. The medical profession was attacked mainly because it allegedly failed to prevent medical disorder. There was also a 'retreat' in other areas, as abortion was banned in 1936 and draconian labour laws were introduced in the late 1930s early 1940s.It is shown that the greater emphasis on heavy industry and defence rather than health and welfare had an adverse effect on the population of Leningrad.

The conclusion summarises and ties the arguments of the book together. It emphasises how and in what way an in-depth, wide ranging analysis of life and death in one of Russia's major cities can help throw new light on the Bolshevik welfare modernisation project and Bolshevik approaches to health enlightenment and surveillance. The contribution which this book seeks to make to debates in social and medical history is through its focus on the degree of continuity in personnel and financial constraints and the way in which shared Tsarist/Soviet concepts and goals on the need for a welfare state and a state that strongly supports the latter and professionalisation, enabled tsarist medical profession cooperation with the new Soviet state, at least until the Terror started to erode that process. The book's biggest contribution is in showing the relationship between public health and the collective and finally in detailing the rise and fall of St. Petersburg/Petrograd and especially Leningrad as a public health centre (following the move of Narkomzdrav and the Academy of Sciences to Moscow) and the impact which the perception of Leningrad as a centre of counter-revolutionary activity had on the fate of the medical profession and its ability to deal with declining health conditions and medical disorder in the 1930s.

Finally, a word should be said about terminology. The capital of Russia was called St Petersburg before 18 August 1914 and after that date until Lenin's death in January 1924 its name changed to Petrograd. When referring to the period 1924 until 1941, the city will be referred to by its Soviet name Leningrad. This book uses old style dates until 14 February 1918, all dates thereafter are given in the new style. Except in quotations, measures of weight have been converted into metric units and the currency of roubles and kopecks are abbreviated as 'r' and 'k' respectively. The transliteration system used for Russian into English is that of the Library of Congress. All Russian/Soviet medical terms and concepts have been rendered into their Western equivalents, wherever possible, with definitions and explanations being given in other instances.

Notes

1 John. H. Hutchinson, *Politics and Public Health in Revolutionary Russia, 1890–1918* (The John Hopkins University Press, Baltimore and London 1990); John. H. Hutchinson and Susan Gross Solomon (eds), *Health and Society in Revolutionary Russia* (Indiana University Press, Bloomington and Indianapolis 1990) and Frances L. Bernstein, Christopher Burton and Daniel Healey (eds), *Soviet Medicine: Culture, practice and science* (Northern Illinois University Press, Dekalb 2010).

2 Mary Schaeffer Conroy, *In health and in sickness: Pharmacy, pharmacists and the pharmaceutical industry in late Imperial, early Soviet Russia* (Eastern European monographs, Boulder distributed by Columbia University Press 1994).

3 Patricia Herlihy's, *Alcoholic Empire: Vodka and Politics in Late Imperial Russia* (Oxford University Press, New York 2003), Laura A. Phillips, *Bolsheviks and the Bottle: Drink and Worker Culture in St. Petersburg, 1900–1929* (Northern Illinois University Press, Dekalb 2000); and Kate Transchel, *Under the Influence: Working-class drinking, temperance and the cultural revolution in Russia, 1895–1932* (University of Pittsburgh Press, Pittsburgh 2006).

4 Laurie Bernstein, *Sonja's daughters: Prostitutes and their regulation in Russia,* (University of California Press, Berkeley, Los Angeles, London 1995).

5 Laura Engelstein, *The Keys to happiness: Sex and the search for modernity in fin-de-siecle Russia* (Cornell University Press, Ithaca and London 1992); Frances Lee Bernstein, *The Dictatorship of Sex: Lifestyle advice for the Soviet* Masses (Northern Illinois University Press, Dekalb 2011); Daniel Healey, *Sexual Forensics: Diagnosing sexual disorder in clinic and courtroom, 1917–1939* (Northern Illinois University Press, Dekalb 2009).

6 Daniel Healey, *Homosexual desire in Revolutionary Russia: The regulation of Sexual and Gender Dissent* (University of Chicago Press, 2001).

7 Kenneth M. Pinnow, *Lost to the Collective: Suicide and the promise of Soviet Socialism, 1921–1928* (Cornell University Press, Ithaca and London 2010).

8 See for instance, Eric Naiman, *Sex in Public: The incarnation of early Soviet ideology* (Princeton University Press, Princeton NJ 1997), David L. Hoffman, *The Cultural norms of Soviet Modernity, 1917–1941* (Cornell University Press, Ithaca and London 2003) and David L. Hoffman, *Cultivating the Masses: Modern state practices and Soviet Socialism, 1914–1939* (Cornell University Press, Ithaca and London 2011).

9 Daniel Beer, *Renovating Russia: The human sciences and the fate of liberal modernity in Russia, 1880–1930* (Cornell University Press, Ithaca and London 2008).

10 Tricia Starks, *The Body Soviet: Propaganda, hygiene and the Revolutionary State* (University of Wisconsin Press, London 2008).

11 John Barber and Andrei Dzeniskevich (eds), *Life and death in besieged Leningrad, 1941–44* (Palgrave, London 2004).

12 See David Priestland, *Stalinism and the politics of mobilisation: Ideas, power and terror in inter-war Russia* (Oxford University Press, Oxford 2007).

13 Pinnow, *Lost to the Collective*, 15.

14 Ibid.

15 Ibid.

16 Oleg Khorkhardin, *The collective and the individual in Russia: A study of practises* (University of California Press 1999), 4, 7.

17 Pinnow, *Lost to the Collective*, 16.

18 Ibid., 16.

19 Ibid., 21.

20 Ibid., 55.

21 Ibid., 22.

22 Ibid., 55.

23 Ibid., 69.

24 Khorkhardin, *The collective and the individual in Russia*, 327.

25 Pinnow, *Lost to the Collective*, 75.

26 Ibid., 250.

1 The 'body Russian' in Tsarist St. Petersburg

> Labour unrest, political intrigue, massive demonstrations and ultimately bloody revolutions were all nurtured by the poverty and despair which were as much a part of industrialisation as the factories themselves.[1]

If you ask someone in 2017 to say what they associate most with modern day St. Petersburg, they will probably reply the beautiful palaces, bridges and art galleries. At the start of the twentieth century although some of these symbols of luxury existed, the city also had its underside – factory chimneys, badly lit streets, wooden houses and rubbish piled up and it was generally viewed as an unhealthy place to live. This chapter, which offers radically different interpretations to existing historiography, sets the scene for the central argument that the Tsarist state failed to protect the 'body Russian', in particular poor peasants and the rising industrial working classes. This was because the government management of budgets and public health was seriously flawed. A fundamental change of system was deemed necessary to launch a reorientation of public health, and the Bolsheviks and radicals within the medical profession, were at the forefront of this movement.

This chapter analyses the main trends in public health and sanitation from the mid-1850s until the October Revolution of 1917. Four themes predominate: first, an assessment is made of the patterns of illness and disease in the Russian capital; second, we analyse the municipal authority's response to this situation; and third, the view of the emerging the medical establishment to these issues is outlined. The factors explaining the high levels of disease, illness, poor hygiene, cleanliness and overcrowded housing are discussed, including lack of money, the failure on the part of the municipal authorities to take the necessary initiative, and the Russian elite's poor commitment to the population's needs, and the ineffective management of local health and welfare services. It is also shown that this was also a time of medical professionalization, and the battle with the state over this goal, together with differences between radicals and conservatives within the medical profession, compounded an already difficult public health situation. The final and fourth theme is the role of the Bolsheviks, their assessments of Tsarist policies, connections with radicals within the medical profession and the shared notion that the Tsarist regime and its institutions had failed to protect the health and welfare of poor peasants and rising industrial working class. This point is emphasised through a case study of social insurance. This approach offers us insights about what the main flaws of the tsarist health system were and what the Bolsheviks thought was required to eradicate them.

Life and death in St Petersburg, 1854–1917

The first part of this section analyses changes in demographic, health and sanitation patterns with an emphasis on the impact of industrialisation and urbanisation on public health conditions in the capital and how the municipal authorities and medical profession dealt with the challenges posed by water supply contamination, poor sewage, inadequate housing and the outbreaks of infectious and other diseases that followed. We argue that medical issues increasingly became a political issue and as a result medical students and doctors moved beyond the desire for professionalization to pursue broader political goals.

Population growth was slow between the 1850s and mid-1880s but increased after 1895, due to the arrival of immigrants from the countryside and other cities of the Russian Empire a consequence of the railways, the growth of industry and the development of trade and commerce. James Bater points out that prior to 1890, the annual net increment in St Petersburg averaged about 15,000 people, but thereafter averaged roughly 50,000 in the dozen years up to the First World War.[2] The data furnished in Table 1.1 shows, by 1917 Petrograd had a population of 2.3 million, making it the fifth largest city in Europe.

By December 1912, the city of St Petersburg employed nearly 189,000 industrial workers in its factories and mills,[3] and although this growth is important, for reasons explored below, it is essential to realise that there were more servants that those working in manufacturing or construction according to the 1910 city census, with other people working in catering,

Table 1.1 Population of St Petersburg and Petrograd, 1895–1917

Year	Size of population
1895	1,202,100
1900	1,418,000
1905	1,635,100
1910	1,881,300
1914	2,217,500
1915	2,314,500
1916	2,415,700
1917	2,300,000

Sources: *Obshchii svod' po imperii rezul'tatov razrabotki dannykh perepisi naseleniia, proizvedennoi 28 ianvaria 1897 goda* (St. Petersburg 1905), 2; *XV let diktatory proletariata: Ekonomiko-statisticheskii sbornik po gor. Leningradu i Leningradskoi oblasti* (Leningrad 1932), 135 and S. A. Novosel'skii, *Demografiia i statistika (Izbrannye proizvedeniia)* (Moscow "statistika" 1978), 102.

local government, trade, insurance and transport.[4] Thus what in Soviet parlance was termed the 'collective' was relatively small at this point.

The population of St Petersburg's growth was the product of the arrival of migrants who accounted for more than 80% of the increase in St Petersburg's population between 1870–1914.[5] In 1869, most of these peasant workers came from Iarovslavl and Tver (over 38% between them) and by 1910, nearly 33% of Petersburg migrants still came from these two regions, with the rest coming from Novgorod, Kostroma, Pskov, Riazan, Moscow, Smolensk and Vitebsk.[6] McKean argues that these immigrants came from areas that

> were characterised by a lower soil fertility than average, (had) a higher proportion of the population engaged in secondary industry, and consequently a lower ratio of involvement in traditional agriculture (and) a significant rate of out-migration and (by) the greater literacy of its inhabitants.[7]

The problem was that this urban demographic revolution put extreme pressure on the quality of the environment and space which in turn affected the birth and death rates. Data collected by the Petrograd statistical bureau shows that the birth rate stood at 32 per 1,000 inhabitants in 1850.[8] Table 1.2 indicates that the birth rate remained steady at around 30 until 1910 but then fell until it reached 18.8 by 1917. The death rate was also declining from 30 per 1,000 in 1850 to 23.3 by 1917. In 1913, on the eve of war, St Petersburg's birth rate of 28.7 was slightly higher than that of London, Amsterdam, Milan, Stockholm and Paris whilst St Petersburg's death rate of 26 per 1,000 in 1900 was higher than that of Berlin, London, Paris and Vienna.[9]

One reason for this trend in birth rate in St Petersburg was the increase in the total fertility rate among women aged 15–44 years, which rose from 3.82 in 1900 to 5.23 by 1910. Later marriages and a declining infant mortality rate from 27.0 in 1897 to 23.6 by 1913, undoubtedly helped too, although the First World War, a high level of abortions, unsanitary housing conditions and

Table 1.2 Birth and death rates in St Petersburg and Petrograd, 1895–1917

Year	Number of births	Births per 1,000	Number of deaths	Deaths per 1,000	Rate of natural increase/decrease
1895	35,478	29.5	31,552	26.2	3.3
1900	43,300	30.5	36,520	25.8	4.7
1905	49,177	30.1	42,935	26.3	3.8
1910	56,230	29.9	46,909	25.0	4.9
1914	55,460	25.0	47,597	21.5	3.5
1915	51,956	22.5	52,866	22.8	−0.3
1916	46,188	19.1	55,980	23.2	−4.1
1917	43,109	18.8	52,623	23.3	−4.5

Sources: *Materialy po statistika Leningradu i Leningradskoi gubernii, Vyp. 6* (Leningrad 1925), 202 and S A Novosel'skii, *Demografiia i statistika (Izbrannye proizvedeniia)* (Moscow "statistika" 1978), 102

female unemployment, created a lack of security and caused severe financial hardship affecting people's decisions on whether or not to start a family.[10]

Because of the high level of spatial mobility within St Petersburg, no district of the city of St Petersburg was socially homogeneous and all parts of the city contained a mix of different social classes. Between 1869–1910, the nobility tended to reside in the city centre; merchants and honoured citizens in Vasil'evskii island, near places of commercial activity and the working class in Petersburg side, Moscow and Narva districts of the city.[11] The situation by 1910 is shown in Table 1.3.

Better conditions prevailed in the likes of Admiralty district which had street lighting and stone pavements whereas on the outskirts and were the working class predominated in areas such as Neva, there was a tendency to use kerosene lamps and a few pavements.[12] The poorer classes also tended to occupy the cellars and garrets, while the upper classes lived in better quality accommodation.[13] By 1897, the death rate ranged from 12.0 per 1,000 in Admiralty district compared to 24.7 per 1,000 in Narva, 22.4 per 1,000 in Petersburg side and 18.8 per 1,000 in Moscow district of St Petersburg. Thus although the death rate had been falling since the 1870s, health inequalities still existed according to social class.[14]

The most important reasons for birth and death variations in the city were poverty or standard of living; inadequate housing; a poor water supply and sewage system; an inadequate diet and the existence of widespread environmental pollution, which we shall now analyse.

With regard to housing, demand outstripped supply, which caused high rents. Costs varied from 142–180r per person per room in Admiralty in the city centre to 33–34r in Petersburg side and 22–42r per person per room

Table 1.3 Social composition of different districts of St Petersburg, 1910 (as a percent of total population)

District	Gentry	Bourgeoisie	Peasants	Workers
Admiralty	11.0	19.5	63.5	13.0
Kazan	9.3	25.0	58.1	20.0
Kolomna	9.6	24.8	62.3	22.9
Liteinyi	16.0	21.7	57.4	15.0
Moscow	9.0	23.3	64.4	25.2
Narva	4.7	19.1	73.2	30.3
Neva	1.7	14.6	81.6	36.8
Okhta	2.7	24.4	69.7	27.6
Petersburg side	11.5	23.3	60.1	22.1
Rozhdestvo	9.3	21.5	65.6	25.2
Spasskaia	5.2	18.0	73.6	32.2
Vasilevskii island	8.4	20.5	66.6	24.6
Vyborg	4.1	16.8	72.3	29.0

Source: Robert B. McKean, *St Petersburg between the Revolutions: Workers and Revolutionaries, June 1907-February 1917* (Yale University Press, New Haven and London 1990), 37

in Narva in 1895.[15] The cost of a single room in St Petersburg increased from 300r in 1905 to 480r by 1912.[16] For these sums, people in poorer areas were expected to live in sub-standard accommodation. For example, a survey of 30,000 people living in cellar apartments in the wards of Spasskaia and Moscow and in industrial areas of Narva, Aleksander-Nevskii, Rozhdestvo and the Petersburg side in 1870–71, 40% of dwellings were flooded, few had ventilation, most inadequate lighting and the large majority were cold and damp.[17] By 1904, little had changed – 51,732 people had leased out 'partitioned off corners of rooms', slept on floors, on plank beds or on stoves and in 1910, 63,039 people in St Petersburg were still housed in damp, frequently flooded basements.[18] This put inhabitant's health at risk. The problem was that people needed an annual income of 500r to rent a room or a flat of their own but unfortunately annual income was only 366r in 1904 and 384r by 1913.[19] Wages varied by sector and in 1912 they were highest in the metal industry (519r), followed by woodworkers (420r), print workers (378r) and chemical industry labourers (352r), with the lowest levels in cotton (268r) and food processing (261r), which tended to employ women or the unskilled. The overall average was 375r. These wages were eroded by a high cost of living.[20] Thus there was little opportunity for most people to improve their housing situation. As a result, by 1912, St Petersburg had an average of 8.7 person per apartment compared to 3.6 in Berlin, 4.2 in Vienna and 2.7 in Paris around 1910.[21] The municipal authorities tried to cope by building more accommodation. The number of buildings in the capital increased from 8,242 in 1869 to 9,043 in 1900 whilst the number of apartments contained within them rose from 87,779 to 154,882 over the same period. Despite this rise in housing stock, overcrowding persisted with the number of people per apartment going up slightly from 7.0 to 7.4 in this 30 year period.[22] This situation was made worse by the number of factory workers in St Petersburg which grew from 73,200 in 1890 to 242,600 by 1914.[23] There was not enough housing construction, partly due to the economic downturn, which led to job layoffs, and the failure to resolve the housing crisis meant that the level of illness and death in St Petersburg went on rising. The death rate tended to be greater in densely populated areas ranging from 24.5–27.2 per 1,000 and less in better appointed neighbourhoods where the death rate ranged from 12.6–14.3 per 1,000 between 1909–12.[24] Furthermore, many cellars were also closely located to accumulated excrement and refuse, with over 30,000 tons of filth piled in courtyards in 1869 alone.[25] There was still no underground system of sewage disposal by 1905, and cesspools existed in backyards and rubbish still piled up in the streets.

St. Petersburg had no centralised water supply for its first 150 years and so the availability and quality of the water supply varied according to district of the city. The first water supply station was not set up until 30 November 1863 and it was capable of pumping up 17,000km of River Neva water. The problem was that this water was pumped without prior purification and a filtration system was not introduced until the Autumn of 1889.[26] The problem of water purity and domestic and industrial sewage were linked, as Bater explains:

> The time honoured method of collecting and disposing of waste, while simple, was part of the problem. It was collected from apartments and stored temporarily in the courtyards then … the waste barrels were carried to the nearest stretch of water and the contents tipped in. During the winter months, the problem of disposal was rather greater and the courtyards and alleys were frequently jammed with receptacles of solid waste. Prevailing temperatures deferred the potential hazard to public health but only until the Spring thaw.[27]

The population of St Petersburg also often lived in housing with no water supply. Thus in 1895, the percentage of apartments with water ranged from a high 81.7% in city centre districts, such as first ward of Admiralty, to lower levels of 54.8% in second ward of Narva and 37.8% in first ward of Petersburg side.[28] Hence inhabitants without water ranged from 19% in upper and 46% in poorer areas of the city. In addition, the first plan regarding the development of a proper sewage system in St Petersburg was discussed as early as 1865.[29] Unfortunately, there were no maximum permissible concentrations for pollutants; too few health inspectors and the medical department of the Ministry of the Interior (*Meditsinskii otdel, Ministerstvo Vnutrennykh del*) either lacked the willingness to enforce the violation of laws or the resources and technical know-how to use the proper purification filters. Thus one British official, A. W. Woodhouse, noted: 'Recent analyses have proved that the filters themselves are contaminated by the "cholera vibration" with samples found in the Neva and in house taps in various parts of the city'.[30] The impure water supply was associated with epidemics of infectious diseases such as cholera and typhoid (see below).

St Petersburg experienced rapid industrial expansion. In the period 1866–94 the number of industrial enterprises increased 2.5 times.[31] This led to the development of factories, with belching chimneys creating air pollution, lots of noise and an unhygienic and sometimes dangerous place to work. The city's major industries were metallurgy, textiles, chemicals and printing. Rapid growth in the number of industrial enterprises caused environmental pollution by the 1880s:

> Industrialisation brought change to St Petersburg – there were factories and shops everywhere and streets choked with goods-laden wagons, while even the air and water testified to the transition from a court administrative centre to an industrial commercial complex.[32]

St. Petersburg Industrialists, who exerted significant local power, made little attempt to protect the environment from the gases and smoke emitted from their factories and workshops and the authorities also failed to push through the appropriate anti-pollution legislation or enforce that which existed. The consequences were that the 'lack of ventilation, the overcrowding, the impaired water supply and the generally filthy physical environment assisted in the spreading of disease'.[33] Sysin also notes how the medical professions' hands were tied as well. He concludes:

> The whole past of the history of tsarist sanitation can be outlined in terms of three negative factors: the absence of a strong and authoritative central sanitary authority; the absence of nationwide sanitary and health legislation and the absence of local sanitary organisations organised in a planned and universal basis.[34]

Most police officials and the medical professionals in the capital acknowledged that public health conditions were far from adequate. Thus the Buksgeuden Commission of the 1840s expressed the government's alarm about unhygienic conditions in St Petersburg especially among the lower classes.[35] Of the 1,007 living quarters investigated and inhabited by various occupational groups, 471 were deemed 'good', 428 'adequate' and 238 were said to be in a 'bad condition'. Against this background, a cholera epidemic broke out in St Petersburg in June 1848. Things became so serious that the Cossacks were used to maintain order primarily because it was feared that factory workers were threatening to attack a hospital. To placate the population, a Society for the improvement of lodgings of the labouring population was created, but despite good intentions, it had accomplished little by 1860 completing only three out of a six-floor building and not renting out any rooms.[36]

In the light of growing concern, a public health committee (*Komitet obshchestvennogo zdraviia*) was set up in 1860, under the initial chairmanship of Ignat'ev, the military governor, then Suvorov his replacement, to set standards for and to investigate the cleanliness of workers housing, especially those who lived in the co-operative association of workmen and peasants (*arteli*).[37] This indicated some commitment, but a shortage of funds and resources hampered its efforts and failed to prevent a new typhus epidemic in 1864–65 which helped to push the death rate up to 57 per 1,000 population. A year later the city suffered a cholera epidemic. Commenting on this situation, the medical officer of the Privy Council in London stated:

> The mixed epidemic (of relapsing fever, typhus and cholera) testifies to the miserable state of a starving and overcrowded proletariat and there seems reason to believe that if the St Petersburg epidemic is of more than common severity, this is only the result of extremely aggravated conditions of privation, overcrowding, operating on large masses of the lowest population.[38]

Whilst the police blamed climatic conditions for this situation, members of the medical profession argued instead that social factors were the root causes of these epidemics.[39] General F. F. Trepov, the municipal Chief of Police and head of the new sanitary commission, admitted in 1868 that the measures introduced so far had been inadequate and failed to prevent widespread disease. He attributed this to a lack of doctors.[40] Other reasons highlighted for this deplorable situation was the failure to carry out even superficial health inspections and a lack of suitable medical facilities (despite the epidemics, St Petersburg was short of 5,000 hospital beds).[41] In 1868, the St Petersburg Society for the protection of public health (*Sankt-Peterburgskoe obshchestvo popecheniia o narodnom zdraviia*) was tasked with supervising cleanliness in the city, the delivery of medical aid to the sick and disseminating information about sanitary-hygienic matters to the local population. However, this work was put into practice slowly and had not fully implemented by the end of the 1860s.[42] Although the police and local authorities were slow to act, and shifted blame onto the medical profession, doctors were not the real culprits. Factory owners continued to poison the water supply and/or the atmosphere and landlords still ran unhygienic lodgings. One incident that epitomised the situation occurred at the Egorov tannery on Vasil'evskii island in November 1870. When the police and a private doctor inspected the housing quarters of factory workers, they were filthy, cold and damp, and a decision was made to prosecute Egorov using an 1857 statute that stated manufacturers must provide adequate housing for workers. Although found guilty, Egorov was only fined 50r, a pittance in comparison to the damage done to workers health.[43]

The bad outcome was not lost on the St. Petersburg medical profession and in 1871, several recommendations were in made in the Archive of forensic medicine and social hygiene (*Arkhiv sudebnoi meditsiny i obshchestbennoi gigieny*) including: the need for proper surveillance of industrial establishments; the introduction of effective factory legislation (of the type in existence in Britain since the 1840s) and the training of health personnel capable of carrying out the aforementioned tasks.[44] But before these measures could be put in place, in 1872 there were 9,000 registered cases of cholera resulting in 2,600 deaths as well as an outbreak of 16,000 cases of smallpox, causing 3,000 deaths.[45]

The information provided in Table 1.4 shows that the majority of the illnesses increased with the exception of smallpox, whooping cough, TB of

Table 1.4 Incidence of various types of diseases in St Petersburg, 1866–1897

Type of disease	Absolute number of deaths 1866–95	Absolute number of deaths 1897	Deaths per 10,000 population 1866–95	Deaths per 10,000 population 1897
Typhus	672	1,494	7.1	8.4
Smallpox	112	123	1.2	1.0
Measles	564	810	5.9	7.0

(continued)

Table 1.4 Incidence of various types of diseases in St Petersburg, 1866–1897 (continued)

Type of disease	Absolute number of deaths 1866–95	Absolute number of deaths 1897	Deaths per 10,000 population 1866–95	Deaths per 10,000 population 1897
Diphtheria	426	1,717	4.5	14.8
Whooping cough	224	77	2.3	0.7
Cholera	513	-	5.4	-
TB of lungs	4,225	3,735	44.3	32.2
Influenza	124	207	1.3	1.8
Syphilis	104	71	1.1	0.6
Parasitic diseases	15	12	0.2	0.1
Nutritional diseases	2,985	2,987	31.3	25.7
Suicide	151	150	1.6	1.3
Other infectious diseases	33	28	0.3	0.2
Total deaths	26,601	27,738	268.1	238.9

Source: 'Sankt Peterburg' in Entsiklopedicheskii slovar' (St. Petersburg 1900) tom. XXVIIIa, 317

the lungs, syphilis, parasitic and nutritional diseases from 1866 until 1897. As a result of these trends, one scholar concludes that 'No other city in Russia came close to having as much disease and death as the capital'.[46]

Furthermore, whilst other cities in Russia, such as Moscow, or in Europe (Paris, London, Vienna and Berlin) experienced an improvement in typhus levels from the 1890s onwards,[47] the reverse was true in St Petersburg where the incidence of typhus more than doubled by the end of the nineteenth century.

After the 1905 Revolution, the city's illness and disease pattern varied as Russia headed towards the First World War, with gastric related diseases falling between 1912–14, together with some parasitic diseases (such as typhus), but the large majority of infectious diseases rose in Petrograd as the data contained in Table 1.5 demonstrates. The city also had a high infant mortality rate (hereafter IMR). Thus between 1850–56, there were 31.59 deaths per 100 children aged under one year old and 53.77 deaths per 100 among those aged up to 5 years.[48] The IMR increased to 34.1 between 1867–81. In 1881, doctors in St Petersburg created a Society protecting people's health (Obshchestvo okraneniia narodnogo zdraviia) which established food and milk norms in the hope of reducing the infant mortality rate. But this was not enough so that IMR rose slightly to 34.5 between 1886–97.[49] By 1915, St Petersburg's IMR reached a level of 24.8 per 100 births before falling to 23.7 by 1917.[50] The Society protecting people's health also embarked upon cleanliness programmes in the city, and called for more effective factory legislation to protect industrial workers.[51] This is an issue which we will now discuss.

Table 1.5 Incidence of various types of diseases in Petrograd, 1912–1914

Type of disease	Absolute number of deaths 1912	Absolute number of deaths 1913	Absolute number of deaths 1914
Acute-gastro intestinal	4,605	4,469	3,340
Dysentery	1,151	608	564
Tyhoid fever	9,667	15,448	8,401
Typhus	342	131	216
Relapsing fever	19	14	8
Diphtheria	2,559	2,869	3,497
Measles	2,419	1,951	2,982
Smallpox	649	156	1,474
Influenza	10,497	9,035	7,484
TB	12,754	13,050	13,548
Whooping cough	122	118	158
Other parasitic diseases	23,546	23,048	21,420
Total infectious diseases	77,557	78,889	71,917

Source: Z. I. Frenkel', 'Sanitarnoe blagoustroistvo i vrachebno-sanitarnoe delo' in *Petrogradskaia gorodskaia duma v 1913–1915gg* (Petrograd 1915), 253

Factory medicine in tsarist Russia

The arduous working conditions, along with overall poverty, coupled with the other issues highlighted above, contributed to a low average life expectancy among adults. Commenting upon the problems facing industrial workers, a key component of the collective and the state in the Soviet era, Reginald E. Zelnik argues that in the period 1855–70 nowhere were living conditions 'as bad as they were among the lower class populace in general' as in St Petersburg.[52]As factory workers were a significant group in the city, who served as one of the main source bases for Bolshevik support after 1917, and constituted a key focus of their social insurance campaigns discussed below, it is essential to discuss factory medicine in Russia before 1917. In the following discussion, it is important that we recall our earlier conclusions about the rate of industrial expansion and the growth of the factory workforce as well as the fact that industrial workers lived in cold and damp housing accommodation for which they paid relatively high rents, although some, living near the Lessner, were fortunate enough, as least with regards to commuting to work, to live close to their factories.

In 1859, an official factory observation team was set up in St Petersburg to investigate industrial accidents in relation to existing legislation, the length of the working day, the organisation of female labour, the provision of labour protection and the observation of safety standards in factories. Whilst a useful step forward it had little impact.[53] On 26 August 1866, another law was passed making factories liable for providing sufficient funds for medical facilities especially hospitals. This law set the norm of one hospital bed for every 100 workers. However, factory inspectors and local doctors' reports testify to the fact that this legislation was poorly enforced.[54]

Throughout the 1860s and 1870s discussions of the flaws of factory medicine and health care for workers' issues took place, as shown by the publication of Bervi-Flerovskii's book, *The condition of the working class in Russia* (*Polozhenie rabochego klass v Rossii*) and by debates in the Archive of forensic medicine and social hygiene (*Arkhiv sudebnoi meditsiny i obshchestbennoi gigieny*). This echoed similar discussions, starting with Engels' classic *The Condition of the Working Class in England* (1845) or the first volume of Marx's *Das Capital* (1866). In the *Archive of forensic medicine and social hygiene*, St Petersburg physicians called for the introduction of factory legislation which would provide adequate labour protection and they also advocated the establishment of systematic training programmes for medical personnel intending to work in factories. In addition, physicians demanded educational establishments devise curricula enabling doctors and factory inspectors to conduct research on mechanisation and the harmful impact of chemical and other substances on the health of industrial workers.[55] These early beginnings culminated in the setting up of a district level sanitary commission (*Petersburgskoi uezdnoi sanitarnoi kommissii*) in St Petersburg in 1872 under the chairmanship of the physiologist F. V. Ovsyannikov, to examine labour conditions in the capital and by 1875 zemstvo doctors began systematically studying 'hygiene' at the Medical-Surgical Academy under A. P. Dobroslavin.[56] The Russian Society of Doctors in St Petersburg played a key role here. According to Alekseev, from the early 1870s many Military Medical Academy figures – N. I. Bystrov, V. I. Dobrovol'skii and Professor V. M. Florinskii – dealt with questions of hygiene and sanitation.[57] In 1873, for instance, Dobroslavin highlighted the need to develop an adequate sewage system and discussed this with the St Petersburg engineer Burov and the municipal sanitation commission and in 1877 he chaired two sessions at the Second Sanitary Congress dealing with questions of the water supply, food and the fight against plague.[58] By 27 November 1881, a Factory Commission (*Fabrichno-zavodskaia kommissii*) was set up in Russia composed of representatives from the Ministries of Internal Affairs, Finance and Justice, a police chief, an architect and a doctor. In May 1882, the Factory commission began its investigations of 501 industrial enterprises and factories employing 42,266 workers in St Petersburg. The Commission found that there was a lack of medical aid 'in the majority of enterprises', that only in some did medical aid exist and that there were insufficient medical personnel to treat the sick. It was also discovered that the provision of medical aid varied according to branch of industry. Thus 80.4% of metallurgical enterprises, 78.5% of textiles, 71.7% of chemical, 16.7% of printing, 12.9% of woodworking and 4.9% of food factories had medical aid. On further inspection, the factory commission found that out-patient aid was available for 58.6% of workers. In addition, of those questioned, 8.8% stated that medical examinations were conducted three times a week by a doctor or a feldsher. All in all, a total of 14,268 workers in 14 enterprises had access to medical aid, but some 11,115 workers in 30 enterprises had no such provision. Factory commission officials also found that in 18 factories with a workforce of 2,539 'medical aid only existed on paper'. The level of medical services available included five hospitals with 190 beds; five clinics with 55 beds; 13 casualty wards with 38 beds and 16 wards without beds. Hospital aid was available to 13,484 workers in 18 enterprises. In the Thornton there were 20 beds; in the Nevskii mechanical plant a hospital with 50 beds and in the Putilov, one hospital with 45 beds.[59] In certain cases, workers could receive treatment at the city hospital but in the majority of cases workers were treated in their own factory in out-patient clinics run by a single doctor and up to three feldshers.[60] Some did not get treated due to the absence of sufficient factory medicine facilities and the lack of commitment on the part of some St Petersburg industrialists. Thus in 1885 workers from local factories had insufficient money in the hospital fund (bol'nichnyi sbor) to cover medical costs for their injuries.[61] Less was spent on factory medicine in St Petersburg than in other towns. Thus in 1907 St Petersburg spent one rouble per worker on health care compared to 1 rouble 25 kopecks in Moscow, although both were not sufficient to maintain an adequate factory medicine service in either city.[62]

Although Tsarist employers provided few facilities for their industrial workforces, not all factories were this bad. Smith argues that services in the foreign owned Parvianien and Siemens-Schukkert were decent[63] and the Putilov workers had at their disposal in 1902, a pharmacy, an out patients clinic (open three times a week), two surgical and therapeutic hospital units containing 54 beds and an infection ward with 26 beds run by three doctors.[64] Such a level of provision was excellent, but by no means typical.

Doctors and factory inspector reports suggest that some St Petersburg industrialists had a poor record in terms of safety standards and labour protection. The data in Table 1.6 shows that the number of maimed workers

Table 1.6 The level of industrial injuries in enterprises in Petersburg gubernia, 1901–1904

Year	Number of maimed workers	Number of badly crippled workers	Number of maimed workers as a proportion of all workers receiving treatment (%)
1901	4,683	184	2.3
1902	4,701	114	3.0
1903	4,900	161	3.2
1904	12,734	283	8.3

Source: S N Semenov, 'Zabolevaemost' i travmatizm Peterburgskikh rabochikh v nachale XX veka', Gigiena truda i professional'nye zabolaevaniia 1966, 2, 44

increased from 4,683 to 12,734 cases or by two and a half times between 1901–1904 with only a small proportion of the injured receiving medical treatment.

Petersburg factory inspector reports show that the frequency and level of industrial injuries varied according to branch of industry. Some indication of this, in relation to 1900, is detailed in Table 1.7. This shows that it was metal workers who had the highest level of injuries, followed by those working in textiles, with those working in the paper making industry suffering the lowest levels. Semenov attributes these patterns of injury to the lack of safety precautions for workers, to the employers' failure to provide adequate labour protection, drinking, insufficient visits made by factory inspectors and their lack of power to enforce the existing, albeit inadequate, labour legislation.[65]

The medical profession in St Petersburg voiced their concerns at local level and via national bodies about factory conditions. For example, at the 11th Pirogov Society Congress in 1911, A. N. Vinokurov's paper on 'Sanitary conditions and medical aid in the factories of Peterburg gubernia (1885–1908)' reached the conclusion that the medical provision was 'extremely poor'.[66] Dr. L. P. Nikol'skii added that there were too few health inspections carried out by factory inspectors.[67] Little was done to remedy the situation, so by 1913, according to Smith, there were 14,300 accidents reported to the Petersburg Factory Inspectorate with the highest rates still in metal industry and textiles.[68] As Petrograd industry transferred over to the war effort output, the rate of sickness and injury increased. Thus in the Lassner works alone the number of accidents rose from 180 in 1914 to 312 in 1915.[69] Working conditions in the capital's factories were unhygienic and hazardous to health, and hence Smith concludes: 'Conditions of work in Petrograd's factories before 1917 were exceedingly miserable. Employers paid little heed to standards of safety and hygiene and provided few facilities for their workforces'.[70] One 1912 survey found that there was an absence of ventilation in 42% of metalworking factories, in 70% of print shops and in 75% of textile mills. Furthermore, 44% of metalworking factories, 59% of print shops and in 56% of textile mills were said to be damp

Table 1.7 Variations in the level of industrial injuries, according to branch of industry, in Petersburg, 1900

Maimed workers branch of industry	Absolute total	Percentage of cases
Metallurgy	1,503	49.4
Textiles	767	25.3
Chemicals	241	7.0
Wood	142	4.7
Paper	127	4.2
Other	288	9.4
Total	3,041	100.0

Source: S N Semenov, *Peterburgskie rabochie nakanune pervoi russkoi revolutsii* (Moscow-Leningrad "Nauka" 1966), 129

and in 97% of metalworking factories, in 58% of print shops and in 55% of textile mills, smoke, gas and steam did not disperse due to the failure to install extractors.[71] Industrial workers' health was at risk.

The rapid population increase and the tempo of urbanisation in St Petersburg from the 1880s onwards outstripped the resources of the municipal government. Demand for housing outstripped supply, the death rate was amongst the highest in Europe, the water supply was frequently polluted, there was a lack of suitable sewage disposal facilities and inhabitants of the capital lived with the almost constant threat of illness and disease. By the time of the outbreak of the First World War, Petrograd had a disastrous record with regard to factory conditions. The municipal authority's and factory owners had made few concerted efforts to improve health affairs. The consequence of this poor response was that

> Disease and death were characteristic features which distinguished, if that is the right word, the Russian capital from other major centres in Europe and North America in the early 1900s. Few places were ever so hazardous to live in. Overcrowding had reached levels that had long become a national scandal. In a word, the urban environment was pestilential.[72]

Explaining failures to protect the 'body Russian'

The municipal authority's failure to maintain adequate standards of public health was due first, to a lack of finances; second, a lack of will; third, a poor commitment to public needs; and, finally, to the local authority's inability to manage the challenges facing St Petersburg effectively and efficiently. We will analyse each.

Although Russia as a whole increased the proportion of the zemstvo budget spent on public health from 8.6% in 1868 to 25.1% by 1913 (or in absolute terms from 1.3 million roubles to 63.4 million roubles over the same period),[73] how this health budget was distributed made a big difference. St Petersburg's allocation of funding in Table 1.8, totalled 15.4 million between 1871–1904, and increased over 11-fold in this 30 or so year period.

Table 1.8: Allocation of funds on public health, St Petersburg gubernia, 1871–1904

Year	Absolute total (in roubles)	Per capita expenditure (in kopecks)	Percent of budget
1871	50,600	7.9	9.0
1880	119,200	16.6	17.0
1890	204,800	19.1	22.6
1901	487,300	21.7	-
1904	562,800	47.0	20.2

Source: V. Veselovskii, *Istoriia zemstva za sorok let* (St Petersburg) tom 1, 18, 414–415, 422

In per capita terms, health expenditure per head of the population rose by 600 percent from 7.9 to 49 kopecks.

Screening and strict supervision of the population by physicians was viewed as essential, but this goal was impossible to achieve given the shortage of doctors and medical personnel. The number of zemstvo doctors in St Petersburg increased from 14 in 1870 to 61 in 1905, with the expansion in the number of doctors slow up to the 1880s but speeding up thereafter and the number of district (*uezd*) doctors in St Petersburg gubernia between 1868–1903 rose from 10 to 13.[74] St Petersburg relied more and more on secondary medical personnel, with the number of feldshers, midwives and other secondary medical personnel increasing from 45 in 1870 to 169 by 1904, and the number of independent feldsher outposts rising from 55 in 1880 to 75 by 1898.[75] In addition, the aim was to improve the quality of feldsher training, to encourage peasant entrants as they were more familiar with peasant culture and to encourage women to become feldshers or midwives after 1870.[76] However, physicians opposed both these strategies: the first on the grounds that it would blur the difference between modern and folk medicine and the second due to male prejudice towards women.[77] As a result, there were still recruitment problems, thus the number of midwifery points in St Petersburg declined by 50% from 14 in 1877 to seven by 1898.[78] Bater concludes that 'whatever the intentions of (the) municipal authorities, limited financial resources imposed severe restrictions on action'.[79] Despite the financial restrictions, health services did expand, albeit from a very low base. For instance, in 1890, there were 441 hospital beds in state facilities, 176 in city district hospitals and 265 in rural district hospitals. By 1898, these totals were higher at 562, 190 and 372 respectively.[80] Shortages of finance, placed restrictions on the development of medical education and research, but nevertheless food hygiene, tropical medicine, public hygiene and other research institutes and clinics did still flourish.

By the early twentieth century health still occupied first place in the city of St Petersburg's budget. Public health expenditure increased from 11.1 million roubles in 1912 to 13.9 million in 1914 or by 25.6%, higher than the increase in Petrograd's budget which rose by 22.2%.[81] Some idea of what the money was spent on is indicated in Table 1.9.

Table 1.9 Public health expenditure (by item) in Petrograd, 1911–1914 (in thousands of roubles)

Category	1911	1912	1913	1914
Medical and sanitary aid	6.851	7,470.7	7.753	9,524.9
Hospital commission	53.7	60.0	62.5	151
Sanitary commission	33.5	39.5	39.2	65.8
City pharmacies	92.2	98.4	113.5	237
School hygiene	210	217.7	237	302.8
Sanitary upkeep of doss houses	193	226.8	218.4	175.2

(*continued*)

Table 1.9 Public health expenditure (by item) in Petrograd, 1911–1914 (in thousands of roubles) (*continued*)

Category	1911	1912	1913	1914
City water supply system	576	200.3	2,113.6	2,296.9
Cleaning and watering the streets	274.8	270.6	273.5	315.7
Maintenance of sewage pipes	203.5	200	318.8	278
Total	9,994.4	11,113.7	11,726.6	13,921.4
City budget expenditure	40,561.5	43,509.3	47,210.7	53,162.7
As percent of city budget	24.6%	25.5%	24.8%	26.1%

Source: Z. I. Frenkel', 'Sanitarnoe blagoustroistvo i vrachebno-sanitarnoe delo' in *Petrogradskaia gorodskaia duma v 1913-1915gg* (Petrograd 1915), 168

The category 'medical and sanitary aid' includes funds spent on the city's hospitals, including maintenance. The latter appear to have been in poor condition as the amount of money spent on repairs rose from 6.25 million roubles in 1912 to 8 million roubles by 1915.[82] Also included is hospital expenditure in order to maintain outpatient units, maternity and premature birth clinics, laboratories, medical equipment or money needed to combat epidemics. For instance, expenditure on anti-epidemic measures increased from 94,800r in 1912 to 103,400r by 1915; whilst the funds allocated to sanitary surveillance work or city laboratories rose from 170,800r to 202,700r over the same period.[83] The allocation of hospital commission funds enabled the number of beds in city hospitals to increase from 12,181 in 1912 to 15,620 in 1915 or by 21%.[84]

Prior to the start of the First World War, the St. Petersburg municipal authorities were prioritising improving the water supply network, keeping the streets as clean as possible and trying to provide the local population with better medical facilities by increasing the number of beds available and providing pharmacies with more funds. In addition, the municipal government hired more doctors, increasing the number to 72 by 1916. Forty of these doctors had particular responsibility for handling the fight against infectious diseases as the capital had nearly 30,000 registered cases in 1916.[85] It is important to recognise that at a time when Russia was at war, with money required for military purposes, 14.8 million roubles was still being spent on public health, a recognition of how much the body Russian was considered to be in danger.[86] In Bater's view 'the challenges facing municipal government were great, and although the response usually fell short of what was required, the possibility at least ought to be borne in mind that under the circumstances not much better might have been expected'.[87]

But even if adequate finances had been available there are other more compelling reasons, not always explicitly acknowledged as important by Bater, why the authorities would not have been able to maintain adequate standards of public health in St Petersburg. From the perspective of the later Soviet concept of the collective, the above situation reflects its lack of commitment to protecting the public, especially poor peasants and the new industrial working class. For instance, when the typhus epidemic hit the city in 1908 and cholera followed in 1909–10, the death rate soared, but the authorities failed to take necessary action. It took until 29 May 1911 for a law on the building of a sewage system and water supply network in St Petersburg to be passed. In 1912, a special city commission (*Spetsial'nogo gorodskogo kommissiei po ustroistvu i perestroitstvu vodosnabzheniia*) was set up to carry out this work under A. I. Guchkov as Chairman. Its preparatory work was finished in April 1913 and the Home Office (MVD) reviewed the scheme proposals between February-April 1914 and allocated 47.6 million roubles to construct a Ladoga water supply system and a further 2.8 million roubles was allocated to acquire the necessary land.[88] This was not the only case of inadequate city responses. Another example was the failure to take the necessary initiative after the cholera and typhus epidemics of 1908–10 regarding the problem of water pollution. In this instance, the city council did not act until 1912, when it decided to set up a filter-ozone system, equipped with a filter pump and ozonised water. In October 1913, another water supply station was set up in an attempt to reduce the fluoride in the water but using old English filters. Although the Petrograd Duma allocated nearly half a million roubles for water supply and sewage work in the Spring 1914,[89] the lack of a well thought out and coordinated strategy hampered efforts. We shall now turn to discuss how the medical profession responded to this situation.

The St. Petersburg medical establishment – radical and professional

The difficulty before 1917 was that each area of local government had its own medical facilities and all Ministries within the tsarist government had its own medical establishments, and this split jurisdiction across numerous local governments and Ministries, created a lack of clear direction and coordination. This situation, together with the local government inaction, industrialist indifference and divisions within the medical profession itself led to the failure to combat medical epidemics, improve life expectancy and reduce mortality rates.

According to John F. Hutchinson, the St Petersburg medical establishment consisted of various layers, the medical elite who served the Tsar, high society and the court and then a number of research and teaching institutions. One of the most senior posts was the chief of the military medical inspectorate and he commissioned greater than 12,000 Army officers, pharmacists and inspectors in all military hospitals. Other important roles included the Inspector of the Court medical branch and then below this was the Imperial institute of Experimental Medicine (dealing with bacteriology and infectious diseases), the Women's Medical Institute (offering general medical education and training those to deal with women and children's diseases), the Clinical Institute of Grand Duchess Elena Pavlova; the Heads of the most important hospitals such as the Obukhov, Marinskii and the Imperial Founding and the Imperial Military Medical Academy. These heads of department were said to be loyal to the tsarist regime and unlikely to upset the status quo.[90] Russian doctors had no corporate organisations, like the BMA or AMA, with legally recognised control over the licensing of medical practitioners. All Russian doctors were servants of the state, the worst off were those in the Army and Navy (who were required to serve for two years); zemstvo private doctors needed 'permission to practice' and although private practice was tolerated, it was not encouraged by the tsarist government. Zemstvo and private doctors could be conscripted during times of epidemics and to perform prison, police or forensic medicine, if other doctors were not available.[91] This section examines the emergence of medical organisations, such as the Society of Russian Doctors in St Petersburg (*Sanktpeterburgskogo obshchestva russkikh vrachei*), its goals, the background of the capital's physicians and the role which the tsarist government played in promoting the growth of zemstvo medicine, and the medical profession.

The Society of Russian Doctors in St Petersburg set up in 1833.[92] The *Trudy* and *Protokoly* of the Society reveal the leadership's objective was to formulate medical policies capable of resolving these health problems. Thus society members discussed the plagues of 1828–1829 and 1850[93] and the threat posed by typhus and cholera[94] and showed a keen interest in social medicine, the organisation of outpatient care in the city, industrial hygiene, the development of medical statistics and combating epidemics affecting the capital.[95]

Prior to the zemstvo reform of 1864, Russian social welfare institutions relied mainly on donations and charities. Thus the committees of public assistance (*Prikazy*) attempted to provide voluntary aid to children, the mentally ill, veterans and beggars.[96] In 1864, zemstvo institutions, self-governing bodies, were now given responsibility for serving local needs.[97] Through the imposition of taxes, the zemstvo built roads, set up schools and provided health care, all deemed necessary in the light of Russia's defeat in the Crimean War (1854–56) and the problems highlighted earlier.[98]

Members of the St Petersburg medical profession pushed for the creation of an adequate system of health care delivery, for more doctors and other medical personnel and for the extension of medical aid to all groups of the population. These questions were hotly debated in the Society of Russian Doctors in St Petersburg journal Medical Herald (*Meditsinskii Vestnik*) between 1861–65 and in the Society's proceedings, minutes and reports (*Protokoly zasedenii obshchestva russiskikh vrachei Peterburge*) from the 1850s onwards.[99]

Given the shortages of facilities and qualified medical personnel in the capital, differences of opinion existed on the pros and cons of the circuit (*raz"ednaia systema*) and the stationery (*statsionaia sistema*) systems of medical provision. The former involved the physician travelling throughout the city and its surroundings, visiting rural areas on designated days, with a circuit carried out every 30–40 days. If the physician was absent, the population was treated by a doctor's assistant (*feldsher*). The circuit was opposed because first, it reduced the level of actual medical care available by preventing easy follow ups if required; second, it did not provide a convenient place to treat patients; third, it did not allow privacy; and, finally, it did not allow for hospitalisation in cases of serious illness or injury. By contrast, the stationary system involved the physician being based at a city medical unit with patients needing care visiting the doctor from all areas of the capital. This system was also criticised because it denied peasants in remote areas of St Petersburg equal access to a doctor's care and also prevented doctors from meeting the specific needs of these and other patients.[100] Although from the 1880s, most zemstvos adopted the stationary system of health care delivery, in St Petersburg in 1880, no districts used the stationary system only, two used the circuit and six used both. It was not until 1900 that St Petersburg finally saw the merit of the stationary system of health care.[101]

Those who did manage to graduate from the Medical-Surgical Academy or were attending the Pirogov Society, later went into private practice or government employment. Thus between 1885–1893, of participants from St Petersburg, who went to the Pirogov Society Congresses, 735 went into private practice, 446 worked for the zemstvo, 624 served in hospitals, research and charitable organisations, 429 in universities, 207 in the civilian bureaucracy, 445 in the military, 109 in factories or railroads and 402 in other establishments.[102] Some work locations were clearly highly sort after and others potentially less popular, creating shortages in some areas of the St. Petersburg province. Of those in government service, it was the doctor in each medical sub-district (*uchastok*) who was responsible for ensuring that health care ran smoothly and effectively. This was a difficult task as doctors could not cope with the increasing number of patients demanding treatment, so doctors relied upon the use of feldshers, and many uchastok were in fact split into feldsher districts. St Petersburg was no exception.

Nancy Frieden's seminal work, *Russian physicians in an era of Reform and Revolution, 1856–1905* (1981) shows that during the nineteenth century most physicians served in the public sector – government institutions or the zemstvo. In terms of background, the majority of doctors, who entered the prestigious Medical-Surgical Academy, for instance, were from humble origins, with most coming from the clergy, tradesman and personal nobles in the period 1857–65 (see Table 1.10).

Frieden demonstrates how the Russian state played a dominant role in the training and organisation of the medical profession. The large majority of medical personnel served in the public sector. It was this 'state service ethic' which precluded the type of professional autonomy gained by the medical professions in Europe. Although some studies analysing the development of

Table 1.10 Social origins of students at medical surgical academy in St Petersburg, 1857–65

Children of:	1857 N=978 (%)	1859 N=867 (%)	1861 N=722 (%)	1863 N=663 (%)	1865 N=770 (%)
Nobles	23.0	25.7	25.6	19.3	16.1
Army officer (rank v-vii)	3.6	3.8	4.3	4.9	5.0
Army officer (rank vii-xi)	9.9	13.2	15.1	17.1	15.8
Clergy	26.0	24.3	19.6	19.3	15.3
Honoured citizens	1.4	1.2	1.2	1.5	1.8
Members of merchant guilds	3.7	2.6	2.3	11.3	9.8
Petty tradesmen, craftsmen and members of merchant guilds	18.0	14.1	13.4	9.9	12.2
Non-nobles	5.9	5.9	6.2	10.1	14.6
Foreigners	3.6	3.3	2.2	3.3	3.1
Jews	4.7	5.6	9.9	3.9	5.9

Source: N. M. Frieden, *Russian physicians in an era of reform and revolution, 1856–1905* (Princeton University Press 1981), 42

the intelligentsia from the 1860s have argued that physicians had radical leanings,[103] Frieden argues that

> this interpretation is misleading. The radical medical student, if he managed to avoid being expelled, learned to moderate his stance in order to complete his training and many physicians who openly criticised conditions and agitated for reform, focused on attainable goals.... Turning to social and political issues, physicians often referred to the 'body politic', diagnosed its enormous defects, and in keeping with their treatment of patients, recommended means to remedy, not bury the political system. Only a small segment of the medical profession allied itself with the radical intelligentsia.... If they did get involved in politics this was to achieve their 'professional goals.[104]

This book disagrees for reasons set out earlier with Bater who attributes public health problems primarily to financial difficulties and with Frieden who disassociates the medical profession with active politics. Instead it advances the argument that members of the medical profession became more politicised over time and started to link up with the Russian revolutionary movement. They did this for many reasons. The Populist ethos of serving the people (*narod*) and a desire for political change not just for professionalisation reasons but to eradicate the issues highlighted earlier.

From the early 1860s, medical students in St Petersburg embarked upon revolutionary activity. In 1861, for instance, students at the Medical-Surgical Academy took part in unrest and some were placed under police surveillance and student meetings were banned.[105] Despite government harassment, medical disorder continued. In 1867–69 unrest flared up again, with some within the Medical-Surgical Academy, such as Z. A. Ralli, associated with the Nechaev and Tkachev circles. This action resulted in the closure of the Medical-Surgical Academy on 15 March 1869 and the arrest of many of those involved.[106] This trend continued into the 1870s as 366 students from the Medical-Surgical Academy – trainee doctors as well as pharmacists, feldshers and midwives – were accused of being 'radicals' for participating in protests. This led official circles to distrust the Director of the Medical-Surgical Academy, Ia. A. Chistovich with the result that strict surveillance was put in place at the Academy by 1874.[107] In 1872 students on women's medical courses at the Medical-Surgical Academy began spreading propaganda among Petersburg workers.[108] Barbara Engel notes that female students in St Petersburg also showed a great interest in the trial of the '50' held in 1877–78, especially the case of Vera Zasulich.[109]

Although some medical students served at the Front in the Turkish wars in the 1870s[110], others continued their radical activity. Engel argues that of the 691 graduates of women's medical courses at the Medical-Surgical Academy between 1872–82, 10% were involved with the police,[111] whereas Johanson believes that 46 out of 648 women on these courses were arrested for revolutionary activity.[112] By the 1890s, disorder was reaching a peak. There was widespread unrest and growing opposition to the Tsar and the Russian working class was becoming more militant and an increasing number of strikes were held. Students demonstrated and distributed anti-tsarist propaganda whilst terrorists attacked government Ministers. Medical students and doctors in St Petersburg also got involved in these events. A total of 380 medical figures were involved in the Petersburg League for the Emancipation of the working class between 1895–98. Most of those associated with the League were arrested and sent into exile.[113] One participant, E, N. Federova, who knew Lenin and his wife Krupskaia, became interested in the 'workers' question' in 1892, distributed literature to workers in 1897 and later on in 1903 became a secretary of the St Petersburg branch of the Bolshevik wing of the RSDLP and subsequently played a key role in the 1905 Russian revolution.[114] Some medical students, such as N. A. Alekseev, Ia. M. Liakhovskii and V. P. Krasnuka started linking up with factory workers in the capital, and V. N. Katkin-Iartseva was involved in the strikes in the St Petersburg textile industry in 1895–96.[115]

Between the mid-1890s and 1905, many medical students had become politicised. At the end of February 1901, 700 students at the Women's Medical Institute joined the Petersburg League for the Emancipation of the working class demonstration on Nevskii Prospect in the centre of the city and others gathered at St Petersburg University or at the Technological Institute between 1903–04, setting up Bolshevik committees and discussing and distributing revolutionary literature.[116] On 24–25 February 1904, O. M. Genkin and E. D. Stasov, who ran a Bolshevik committee at the Women's Medical Institute got arrested but despite this, organisational and propaganda work (anti Russo-Japanese war messages and anti-government meetings), attended by 516 people were held at the Women's Medical Institute in Autumn 1904. Calls were made for an end to the war and more demonstrations until this objective was achieved.[117]

This political, as opposed to purely professionalisation angle, was typified by medical student and staff roles in the 1905 Revolution.[118] The Pirogov Society for its part greeted 1905 with enthusiasm calling it a 'historical moment' which 'ushered in the dawn of a new life'.[119] In support of 1905, strikes took place at the Women's Medical Institute and at the St Petersburg Military-Medical Academy.[120] Petersburg pharmacists were the first to protest against the 1905 'Bloody Sunday' by striking between 9–15 January 1905 and later on in April they formed an illegal Union of Pharmacists.[121] By September 1905, some 70 pharmacists were on strike and a resolution led to the closure of 87 pharmacies, only three for non-strike reasons.[122] Four hundred and thirty-nine Military Medical Academy (MMA) students by a two-thirds majority voted to strike in support of workers.[123] Workers from the Vyborg district of St Petersburg held meetings at the MMA to discuss if the Tsars October Manifesto was sufficient to meet demands.[124]

The above discussion confirms that medical students and other medical personnel were more than willing to get involved in political action. The Ninth Congress of the Pirogov Society was held at the end of 1904 and it passed resolutions which involved public denunciations of the Russian autocracy, calling for political and social reforms, including the abolition of capital punishment, greater access for women to higher education and criticism of restrictions of Jewish entry to university. This shows that doctors were not out of touch with broader debates on civil and human rights occurring at this time.[125] Pirogov Society doctors also called for welfare changes such as projects on hygiene education, better sanitary conditions in prisons and schools, as well as pushing for the provision of free medical care for the urban and rural poor.[126] Frieden maintains that their goals were primarily professional, but it is clear that some Pirogov Society doctors at this point were equating public health problems with the general malaise and lack of freedom in Russia in the early twentieth century. Thus when the Pirogov Society 'Cholera Congress' was held in March 1905, leaders and members demanded basic civil rights and freedoms, an end to the war with Japan and an amnesty for political prisoners, especially their medical colleagues.[127] Community physicians were becoming frustrated by the lack of political reform, excessive bureaucracy and by centralisation, which they perceived as being the main obstacles to addressing the health care issues highlighted earlier. As Hutchinson notes, there was a gradual awareness that 'the tsarist regime was the principal obstacle to the improvement of public health' and the Pirogov Society 'Cholera Congress' accused the 'government of administrative abuse, financial mismanagement and military adventurism'.[128] This motivated some St Petersburg physicians to participate in the 1905 Revolution, despite the harassment and arrest.[129]

The previous analysis shows that the medical profession in St Petersburg attempted to fulfil not just its professional but also its political aspirations. Frieden argues that doctors prioritised the former whereas this book argues that in the case of the capital, some parts of the medical profession gradually came to realise, like Lenin and the Bolsheviks that only political change would guarantee what they wanted – professionalisation and the transformation of the system of health care – and this necessitated a more radical approach.

This of course pitted doctor against doctor (conservatives versus radicals; young against old) as well as put radical doctors in conflict with the state. Hutchinson points out how the St Petersburg Mutual Assistance society, an offshoot of the 1899 Pirogov Society, made no mention of the Pirogov Society Congress's strongly worded resolutions in its proceedings. Similarly, when the next regular Pirogov Society convened in 1907, it was noticeable that many Petersburg luminaries, such as Professor S. N. Sirotinin of the Military-Medical Academy, Professor S. M. Lukianov of the Imperial Institute of Experimental Medicine and Professor G. E. Rein, who was soon to be named by Stolypin, as the President of the Tsarist Medical Council, were absent as they believed that the traditional ideals of Zemstvo medicine had been betrayed in March 1905 when some Pirogov Society members showed disloyalty to the Tsar.[130] Thus rifts were beginning to emerge in the Pirogov Society and its offshoots, with doctors taking different political sides.

After 1905, some medical students in St Petersburg continued to pursue this radical path in the ensuing period of reaction and reform (1906–14), partly via the new Union of All-Russian Medical personnel, which was seemingly more radical than certain parts of the Pirogov Society, and shared many of its radical aims and ideals. According to Mitsevich its first meeting in 1905 adjourned amid cries of 'Down with the monarchy' accompanied by the singing of revolutionary songs. The main aim of the Union was to provide a rallying point for all medical staff (physicians, pharmacists, midwives, dentists, even feldshers) and to give material and moral support to those harassed or dismissed from their posts due to their role in the 1905 Revolution. In August 1905, the Union approved the formation of an employment bureau to assist the former in finding jobs. In this regard the Union urged a boycott of all positions that had become vacant because of politically motivated dismissals and some members of the Union advocated strike action to get their members reinstated. Conservatives within the Union disapproved of this proposal and resigned.[131] No such line of action was eventually taken because of the concessions outlined in the Tsar's October Manifesto which promised reform, an end to the police state and the creation of a Duma with legislative powers. These hopes were soon dashed, and the Union of All-Russian Medical personnel only lasted a few more months.

The first and second Dumas of 1906–07 were somewhat liberal and opposed the Tsar, but when Stolypin came to the fore in the Russian government he dissolved both and there was a wave of reaction against liberalism.[132] Throughout 1906 and early 1907 many physicians suffered too. Those who had openly supported the revolutionary cause were dismissed, demoted or arrested as a tide of reaction swept through the Zemstvos.[133] More specifically, Stolypin's policies crushed radical physicians hopes of the establishment of democratically elected, all-class volost Zemstvo organisations which would give medical personnel the opportunity to renovate Russian society and its medical policy.[134] Although the Left and Right responded to Stolypin's policies by carrying out riots, naval uprisings (in Kronstadt, Svenborg and Reval), assassinations and strikes, the medical profession was in disarray at this point. The leadership at the April 1907 Pirogov Society Congress wanted to restore unity, and opted for a 'no political agitation policy'.[135] Traditionalists, such as S. N. Igumov and D. N. Zhdanov, feared a challenge to zemstvo health services or sweeping reforms. Hutchinson sees the Stolypin coup as a turning point that neutralised some sections of the Pirogov Society and points out that '[f]or the 6 months after the coup, the medical press was virtually silent, then began the laments, the recriminations, the soul searching which dominated the press for the next 6 years'.[136] It was not just Stolypin who might challenge community medicine, factory doctors had no desire to transfer their expertise to the zemstvo. Furthermore, bacteriologists, such as P. N. Diatroptov, L. A. Tarasevich and D. K. Zabolotnyi questioned the effectiveness of the public health work of zemstvos arguing that they had failed to take the necessary measures to combat epidemics using the latest developments in bacteriological research (following Pasteur's breakthroughs in the 1880s). All in all, between 1905–09, a zemstvo versus autocracy mentality prevailed, which assumed 'central government is bad, local government is good, private practice is wicked, public practice is noble (and that) zemstvo medicine is the envy of civilised work and must be kept from the profaning hands of St Petersburg bureaucrats'.[137]

Although the 1910 Pirogov Society Congress has been depicted as 'a spiritless and indecisive affair which made few decisions and avoided politically dangerous topics'[138] not everyone agreed with the Pirogov Society Congress's seemingly weak stance. Radical medical students in St Petersburg opposed it, set up a Bolshevik faction and circulated propaganda at the Women's Medical Institute in the capital.[139] Also in 1910, Rein, a member of the St Petersburg medical establishment, called for the creation of a Ministry of Public Health. This was supported by N. F. Gamaleia, D. K. Zabolotnyi and others, who had reviewed other centralised health systems in Europe and Britain and saw them in a positive way.[140] Certain sections within the Pirogov Society, however, opposed it and pushed for greater subsidies for the zemstvos and the municipalities instead. For instance, Ia. Iu. Kats argued that the new Ministry was not the solution. To deal with poverty (a cause of ill health) economic and social reform was needed; land reform and enforcement of housing standards was required for better housing and better policing and resolving the 'appalling physical and moral environment of the urban working class' as highlighted by the Alcoholism commission recommendations, via the abolition of prostitution, poverty, unemployment and encouraging temperance.[141]

This Rein proposal and the furious opposition to it, was nothing new. In the 1890s, the Botkin Commission advocated setting up a 'powerful central administrative agency to direct public health affairs' at a time of the 1892–93 cholera epidemics, but the 'Tsar's Ministers were less than lukewarm about establishing a Ministry of Public Health'.[142] Community doctors also objected because they believed zemstvo medicine was improving and it would be incompatible with the proposed new Ministry. Other Pirogov Society members, such as Dr. Erisman, were in favour, arguing the Ministry was needed in view of the vastness of the Russian Empire, adding that both state and society would benefit and doctors' lives would be easier as they could treat patients locally.[143] In the end, this move didn't go ahead as it was seen as a 'threat to zemstvo medicine' and there were worries about its field of jurisdiction, structure and that the new central organ might not be headed by a physician.[144] In relation to the 1910 proposal whilst some Pirogov Society members were progressive, putting them closer to the Bolshevik position, others, who were more ideologically dogmatic, seemed reluctant to experiment and innovate. From a different viewpoint, the 1910 proposal shows the Tsarist government's concern about deteriorating health conditions both in their own right and in relation to political instability and civil order issues as Russia headed towards war.

It is clear that the public health issues in St Petersburg/Petrograd outlined earlier had not been addressed for several reasons: ineffective local government, industrialists' failure to provide for the medical needs of their workforce, the failures of zemstvo medicine (not always doctors fault) and now we can add that certain members of the medical profession were also a major obstacle to change as some wanted to protect the status quo by retaining community medicine whilst other conservatives in the Pirogov society disliked political participation and engagement. Finally, there were other elements within the Pirogov Society who were in favour of implementing a Ministry of Public Health to coordinate medical responses and who were more politicised. Soviet historians tend to depict the medical profession as on the side of the Tsarist government and in opposition to the Bolsheviks. This chapter shows that this is view was too simplistic, the medical profession was divided, held different views and some were closer to the Bolshevik position than is normally acknowledged. This made cooperation after 1917 possible, another point overlooked in Soviet historiography.

The Bolsheviks and public health: putting workers first

As the working-class movement gained momentum during the late nineteenth century, meeting the needs of workers rose up the political agenda. In Russia, the Social Democratic parties, local and central government, and the medical profession, as we saw during the previous discussion of factory medicine, were all acutely aware of this challenge. We shall focus on Bolshevik responses here, using social insurance as our lens and means of assessing their thinking on health and welfare.

Lenin, in *The Development of Capitalism in Russia* (1899), highlighted arduous working conditions, the absence of labour protection and basic social insurance, the high level of industrial injuries and the general lack of medical care for the toiling masses, as indicators of the flaws in tsarist medical provision.[145] Although in 1895–96 the RSDLP pushed for a law making manufacturers accountable for injuries sustained during production and for them being responsible for the provision of aid for their employees,[146] its policy position on health and welfare was not fully outlined until the Second RSDLP Congress in July 1903. At this Congress emphasis was placed upon the following: an eight-hour working day; a weekly rest period; a ban on overtime work; prohibition of night work (9pm to 6am) unless essential and agreed with workers' organisations; forbidding the use of child labour of school age (6–16 years) and the imposition of six-hour limits on adolescent (16–18 years) employment; the prohibition of female employment in harmful industries; the granting of maternity leave four weeks before and six weeks after childbirth with full pay; the building of crèches for infants and young children and providing 30 minute feeding times for new mothers every three hours; social insurance against old age and incapacity financed through a tax on industrialists; the provision of adequate numbers of factory inspectors; the employment of female inspectors to cover branches of industry with high levels of female employment; the election of workers' representatives (paid by the state) to enforce factory legislation; health inspections in all factories; free medical aid for workers at employers expense; and a law making violation of labour protection provisions by employers a criminal offence.[147] Such measures were seen as crucial to protect the Body Russian, in particular the industrial working class and peasants.

In relation to these points, only piecemeal action was taken by the tsarist government, such as the introduction of the Workers Compensation Act of 2 June 1903, which provided owners insurance against liability for accidents, but only on a voluntary basis. This law covered cases of injury or death among factory, mining and metallurgical workers (about half a million in total), but its scope and coverage were deemed inadequate.[148] Although some, such as Litvinov-Falinskii, called upon the government to ensure owners complied with the new law,[149] it lacked the resources and sufficient central coordination to do this. Ewing concludes that 'this law demonstrated the government's unwillingness to impose obligatory insurance on the reluctant owners'.[150]

Such a view is only partly correct. This chapter argues that Ewing fails to fully acknowledge the forces compelling these groups to make concessions or to introduce new principles and labour policies to deal with the rising industrial working class and labour movement. It was the 1905 Revolution, which if anything, brought such matters to the forefront. Following unrest and a concern about the lack of civil rights, there was renewed interest in the 'social' or 'workers' question'. The Russian government realised that action was needed and set up the Kokovtsov commission, headed by the then Minister of Finance, who was charged with addressing 'workers' dissatisfaction' and containing working class militancy.[151] The goal of any legislation stemming from its work was to 'tie workers to the state while promoting stability in the factories and economic growth for the country as a whole'.[152] However, other variables, such as welfare issues being broadly defined as part of the state's role; public poor relief being obsolete[153] and the fact that Russia was failing behind other nations, such as Germany, and its welfare state, all became important in late nineteenth – early twentieth century and added pressure on the Tsarist regime. In the end, the scope of coverage and type of social insurance measures introduced in Russia in 1912, which were heavily influenced by Bismarck's model,[154] was based on self-administration by the insured party rather than the state and so each person made contributions to the fund in direct proportion to their representation.

The social insurance question was debated in the period 1906–12. The Minister of Trade and Industry, M. M. Fedorov, in a meeting 15–21 April 1906 urged the government to appease the workers, who were 'associating with political elements' by first, implementing coverage for illness, birth, death and industrial injuries; second, by establishing 'self-managed' medical funds in enterprises with 50 or more workers; and finally, by running arbitration courts to adjudicate in cases between insurance agencies and victims.[155] The debates continued with the idea of welfare funds (*kassa obezpecheniia*) rejected as they were used by strikers; but Ministry of Trade and Industry officials were in favour of full insurance for hired labour, self-managed funds, guaranteed minimum payments in event of illness and a 6–13 day recovery period and medical aid for workers.[156]

In 1908 at the Fifth RSDLP Congress, a resolution was passed calling for increased agitation and propaganda activity on the aforementioned 1903 Congress programme and in the Third Duma (1907–12) Bolshevik representatives demanded more action and less talk calling for legislation on labour protection and medical aid in the light of the catastrophes in the Donets Basin and Petersburg construction industry.[157] However in the period 1908–12, although social insurance and medical provision for workers was constantly debated, not much progress was made. Tim McDaniel explains why:

> Added to the government's conservatism was the lack of impetus from within the Duma, which was dominated by a moderate right-wing majority with little commitment to fundamental changes.[158]

As a result, the 'body Russian' in St. Petersburg continued to be adversely affected. For instance, the number of industrial injuries doubled from 15.7 to 32.3 per 1,000 workers between 1902–11 and consequently insurance companies paid out nearly 18,000r in accident benefits between 1904–10.[159]

During these debates about the need for social insurance legislation, two clear sides emerged: on the one hand, the Tsarist state and industrialists wished to introduce piecemeal legislation to reduce the threat from the working class and labour movement whilst on the other, the RSDLP, had no such desire to dampen down working class discontent or to see workers move closer to the State, so they pointed out that existing legislation was woefully inadequate and emphasised through the *Rabochii vopros* (workers' question), the social divisions within society and lack of civil rights. It was against this background that the 1912 insurance law was introduced.

The insurance law passed on 23 June 1912 consisted of three elements: first, sickness and accident coverage in factories with no less than 20 workers (in mechanised industries) or 30 workers (in non-mechanised industries); second, accident insurance was to be paid for by employers based upon occupational membership and categories of risk; and, finally, the law provided for benefits in cases of sickness and injury, but not for invalidity or unemployment. Regarding contributions, employers made them in all cases, apart from sickness, which was based on workers contributions. Two percent of the wage fund was put aside for this.[160]

According to the new law, which covered about a fifth of all industrial workers in Russia,[161] medical funds (*kassy*) were given the right to distribute financial aid to members and their families during illness, childbirth or in the event of death. These funds could be based in factories if they had more than 300 workers, and if not unified funds in key industries, operated the funds.[162]

Table 1.11 shows that sickness payments were highest in the metal-working industry. First came the Putilov, located on the outskirts of the Peterhof district, then the Metal Works followed by the Franco-Russian engineering works which was located in the heart of the Kolomna district. Vyborg's Lessner machine construction factory was next. Although both the Semenov engineering works and the Spasskii paper factory paid out negligible amounts, a total of nearly 123,500r was paid out in the first quarter of 1914.

After the implementation of the 1912 law, Vigdorchik calculates that the average industrial accident payment for insured workers was 10r for youths; 18r for teenagers and 30r a month for adults, as well as a one-off payment of 36r once the accident has been verified.[163] In this context, Strumilin estimates that in 1913 the average factory worker earned 295r a year including

Table 1.11 Expenditure by medical funds during the first 13 weeks of illness in various Petrograd factors in 1914

Factory	Expenditure by medical funds
Franco-Russian	11,898r 11k
Putilov	79,371r 17k
Lessner	10,405r 41k
Metal works	11,723r 42k
Semenov	957r 14k
Treugol'nik	8, 303r 14k
Spasskii	820r 17k

Source: G Baturskii, 'O 13 nedeliakh', *Strakovanie rabochik*, no. 11–12, November–December 1915, 11–12

allowances for welfare provision and housing,[164] so payments were pitiful, but the Act was still a breakthrough.

Medical provision was supposed to be rendered in these cases. This included first aid in cases of industrial injury on factory premises; treatment in out-patient departments; maternity care and/or treatment by office staff. Health care was free to fund members. Assistance was rendered for a period up to four months by a doctor or feldsher.[165] Article 52 of the 1912 Act set a minimum of one doctor per 1,000 workers and one bed per hundred workers. Workers' memoirs reveal that doctor's inspections of medical examinations of workers were rather basic and could hardly be deemed 'examinations' at all.[166] Moreover, even if problems were identified all doctors or factory inspectors could do was warn the employer, they were powerless to get them to act.[167] Industrialists accepted a worker's right to minimal medical aid, financed by employers, but wanted the illness funds to manage the day to day running of them, assisted by other institutions were necessary.[168] Finance was the greatest concern and so employers sought to keep their liability at a minimum.[169] An analysis of the journal Trade and Industry (*Promyshlennost' i Torgovlia*) for the period 1908–12 reveals that industrialists in general in St Petersburg favoured the new 1912 law,[170] but certain groups, such as the St Petersburg Society of Mill and Factory owners (*Peterburgskoe oshchestvo zavodchikov i fabrikantov*) and the Association of Trade and Industry (*Sovet s"ezdov prestavitel promyshlennosti i Torgovli*), both objected to the medical provision aspects of the new law.[171] In the end, although the industrialists were pleased that they only had to look after accident victims for 13 weeks (which benefited companies) they lost in two other ways: first, the insurance scheme was now extended to government-owned and non-industrial enterprises and second, the state bureaucracy and police had oversight of insurance institutions.[172] Nevertheless, the government and some industrialists saw the 1912 law as a move in the right direction to reduce worker discontent via relatively minimal changes.

The Bolsheviks, as shown by their coverage of social insurance issue in the journal, Questions of Insurance (*Voprosy Strakhovaniia*), criticised the new law because it made no provisions for large sections of the population, paid out inadequate benefits and compensation, gave the state and industrialists too great a role in determining its provisions and only permitted low levels of worker participation in managing the insurance funds.

This subject is important in its own right but more so as it indicates how the Bolsheviks saw health and welfare in relation to the educated and conscious parts of the industrial working class (a source of support and political change). By focusing in this final section on the Bolshevik social insurance campaign and its key elements – the creation of medical funds, a workers' section on the insurance council and the use of publications (insurance journals) to get their message and policy across – we will be in a position to analyse how the Bolsheviks framed health issues and the needs of key sections of the population, and most importantly when the Bolsheviks started to begin formulating their socialist principles and to develop a system that sought to protect the members of the collective, issues taken up later in the book.

When the Fourth Duma opened on 15 November 1912, in the midst of a strike by 23,362 workers from 59 St. Petersburg factories, one of the things on their mind was the new social insurance legislation. Russian workers demanded more self-managed funds; greater coverage for invalidity, maternity and unemployment; improvements in financial provisions, reduced dependency on bosses and a unified medical fund.[173] The Bolsheviks started agitating on these issues and for workers' representatives on the Insurance Council in December 1912. At the start nearly 14,000 workers from 13 Petersburg factories supported the campaign and a week later another 60,000 strikers joined them.[174] The Bolsheviks also urged workers to participate in the work of the funds and if necessary boycott the new 1912 insurance law.

Lenin urged RSDLP members and factory workers to combine together and defeat the bosses by becoming fully acquainted with flaws in the 1912 law and by getting themselves elected onto the Insurance Council, so that the required changes were made.[175] The Mensheviks in their insurance journal entitled *Workers Insurance (Strakhovanie Rabochik)* thought that boycotts were tactically wrong and not in workers' interests as it was better to negotiate with factory administrations and government.[176] However, the Bolsheviks disagreed and intensified their campaign via the creation of *Voprosy Strakhovaniia*, seeking to gain control of the funds and getting workers appointed onto the Insurance Council and Insurance office.[177]

The first medical fund in St Petersburg was opened in the Nevskii stearin candle factory in March 1913 with Ivanov as President and Ill'in as Secretary. Membership fees were set at 1r per month with insurance payments as follows: in cases of industrial injury 1,500r for 12 weeks; 6,000r in event of illness; 1,500r for a birth and 350r in the case of death. The sick were treated in the fund hospital between the hours of 10am and 6pm.[178] From this moment on, the number of funds in Russia increased from 2,326 in May 1914 to 2,900 by January 1916, with members rising from 2,049,000 to 2,152,770 in the same period. The expansion of funds in St Petersburg by 1913 is shown in Table 1.12.

Table 1.12 The Expansion of the insurance campaign in St Petersburg, 1913

Year/month	Number of medical funds	Number of members
March 1913	8	8,300
April 1913	20	15,300
May 1913	31	42,900
June 1913	53	58,800
July 1913	133	112,800
August 1913	188	141,500
September 1913	220	182,000
October 1913	286	277,000
November 1913	315	288,000
December 1913	393	326,000

Source: *Voprosy Strakhovaniia* No. 2, 11 January 1914, 15

The government was attempting to discourage the establishment of medical funds in places like St Petersburg, were the labour movement was strong, so growth was slow at first in March 1913 but rapid after July 1913 reaching nearly 400 funds by the end of the year. It was not just government opposition to the funds that hampered their growth. Bolshevik boycotts also played a part. Thus a ballot of workers at the Lessner factory on 16 February 1913 showed that only 221 were in favour with nearly 10 times more (2,067) against setting up a fund. Similar opinions were held at the Feniks, Semenov, Erikson and Nobel factories.[179] Following an All-Russian Workers Congress on Insurance questions in August 1913, a series of metalworking and engineering factories – Siemens-Halske, Langenzippen, Robert Krug, Franco-Russian – as well as others, such as the Skorokhod shoe factory and the Maxwell cotton mill, all agreed to campaign against boycotts and in favour of city wide medical funds, so that the highest possible benefits could reach their workers.[180]

The second challenge to success which the Bolsheviks insurance campaign faced was that large groups of workers were unprepared for the kassy and insurance agency elections. Thus press and metal workers in the Semenov Metal works and the Old Lessner all failed to put candidates forward for election, although those in the second Nevskii spinning manufacturer, the Nevskii candle, the Tregul'nik and the Resin factory were better prepared and nominated candidates.[181] As a result, in one St Petersburg campaign held in early 1913, only two out of five representatives were workers, the rest were Ministry of Trade and Industry nominees and town/gubernia governors. Some activists, such as Volgar, blamed uncultured (*nekul'turnyi*) or illiterate workers.[182] This is unlikely as literacy was high among workers in the capital.[183] A more plausible explanation is the fact that the police were breaking up meetings which impacted on attendance so success varied.[184] Some indication of the results is shown in Table 1.13.

Table 1.13 Election results to St Petersburg insurance establishments, 2 March 1914

Workers elected to:	Political affiliation					
	Bolsheviks		Mensheviks		Left SRs	
	a	b	a	b	a	b
Insurance Council	33–35 (47)	- (82.4)	- (10)	- (17.6)	- -	- (1.2)
Insurance Office	31–33 (37)	- (84.1)	- (7)	- (15.9)	- (4)	- -

Notes: a Absolute numbers   b Percentages

Sources: V. Sh. 'Vybory v strakhovyia uchrezhdeniia v Peterburge i zadachi edinstva', *Bor'ba, rabochii zhurnal* No. 6 June 1914, 2. Figures in brackets are from R S Rotenburg, 'Bor'ba rabochego klassa za gosudarstvennoe strakhovanie', *Voprosy istorii* 1958, No. 11, 140

Despite the above difficulties and political competition, workers associated with the Bolsheviks won the majority of places on the Insurance Council (82.4%) and Insurance Office (84.1%) in March 1914. On the significance of this victory, Ewing states '[t]hese election victories gave the Bolsheviks a tremendous advantage by making them the official spokesmen for the Insurance campaign'.[185]

These gains were cut short by the outbreak of war. In August 1914 the Russian Empire along with France and Britain (the Entente powers) went to war against Germany, Austria-Hungary and Turkey. This situation changed things dramatically in the public health sphere in the capital – medical students and personnel were drafted; zemstvo hospitals and dispensary services were put on a war footing and the journal Questions of Insurance was banned and did not resume publication until 20 February 1915. The kassy had been decimated (as many members went off fighting and did not return) and the Workers' Group on the Council of Workers Insurance ceased to exist as all but two of its members had been arrested.[186] Despite political oppression and closure, the Bolsheviks managed by the end of 1916-early 1917 to have 80 medical funds in Petrograd with 176,000 members, that is 45% of the city's workforce, but they were in a hopelessly battered state and in 1917 as the road to revolution intensified, they never proved effective in mobilising the workers to the Bolshevik cause. With regards to health care, the number of out-patient clinics and feldsher points declined from 170 in 1912 to 125 by 1917 for Petrograd guberniia as a whole (excluding Petrograd). There was also a corresponding fall in the number of people treated in these clinics from 734,164 in 1912 to 561,502 in 1917.[187] The public health budget was under great strain as it now needed to deal with the demands for war on top of domestic health challenges.

Pirogov Society physicians feared that whilst away at the Front, medical care might, out of necessity, fall into the hands of secondary medical personnel, such as the feldshers.[188] The only upside for Pirogov Society leaders was the announcement in September 1914 that Rein's plan for a Ministry of Public health was now shelved until the end of the war.

The First World War revealed that medical services for the Army were not adequate in view of German firepower and so the troops suffered. Community doctors were used to treat 5.2 million soldiers evacuated from the Front in hospitals at the rear, of which 2.8 million had various war wounds and 2.3 million suffered from infectious diseases, frostbite etc. and 15,000 from mental illness due to the trauma of war by 1915. The medical profession did the best it could to launch vaccination programmes against typhoid, cholera and dysentery including building a plague fort at Kronstadt[215] but in the end with over 689,000 killed in action and a further 2.6 million wounded in action, just over 970,000 dying of their wounds, 2.4 million contracting various forms of disease, and nearly 156,000 dying of disease, this was a major uphill struggle.[189]

Government actions during the Great War were frequently called into question, the February Revolution followed and, eventually, the Tsar abdicated on 2 March 1917. The Provisional Government then shared dual power with the Bolsheviks in the Petrograd Soviet. At this time, Pirogov Society leaders occupied key posts dealing with military and civilian medical affairs. Between March–July 1917, the Provisional Government was itself viewed increasingly with contempt and disregard, and pro-Bolshevik members of the Pirogov Society such as Z. P. Solov'ev and I. V. Rusakov, gradually distanced themselves from the Provisional Government. A debate took place in this period over the future direction of medicine and public health and a Central Medial Sanitary Council was set up in mid-July 1917. The July Days followed but by the Autumn of 1917, the Provisional Government was losing what remained of is limited authority, and by October, the Bolsheviks were in power – this left one major question unanswered: Would community medicine continue or would it be replaced by centralised, socialist medicine?

Conclusion

We saw earlier that zemstvo medicine emerged in the 1860s. Doctors were faced by a major challenge – high levels of disease, illness, poor hygiene, overcrowded housing and poor health care facilities for the rising industrial working class. Although the municipal authorities and community doctors were committed to improving standards of sanitation, it was difficult to properly address the adverse impact of industrialisation and urbanisation, given the shortages of finance and the tsarist state's lack of a leading role. The city and national government in St Petersburg lacked the drive and initiative to move things forward. The medical profession itself was split between those who wanted professionalization and those who desired much more – fundamental political change. Thus conservatives with the Pirogov Society and other medical organisations in St Petersburg were also part of the problem. Health and welfare in general, and social insurance in particular, were viewed as very significant issues among workers in the capital. Workers were willing to allow the Bolsheviks to use the medical funds as a political weapon and to push for welfare changes, but most importantly the Bolsheviks retained their power base and kept the pressure on the Tsarist regime from 1903 onwards. In public health terms, the legacy left by zemstvo medicine, the Pirigov Society and the insurance campaign was that the Bolsheviks gained extensive knowledge of the health conditions and plight of the industrial working class, a key component of the collective. After 1917, health care for the masses and in particular medical provision for the insured became a prominent feature of the new Soviet welfare state. The new Soviet regime wanted to move away from an elite health care system in which community medicine was underfunded and to remedy health inequalities by creating a welfare state. This involved expanded state support and prioritising the health of workers and peasants and other key members of the new collective.

Notes

1 James H. Bater, *St. Petersburg: Industrialisation and Change* (Edward Arnold, London 1976), 1.
2 James H. Bater, 'Some dimensions of urbanisation and response of municipal government: Moscow and St. Petersburg', *Russian History/Histoire Russe* 1978, 5, Part I, 46.
3 Robert B. McKean, *St. Petersburg between the Revolutions: Workers and Revolutionaries, June 1907-February 1917* (Yale University Press 1990), 2–3.
4 *Petrogradu po perepisi 15 Dekabria 1910 godu* (Petrograd 1914), tom 2, 1–23.
5 Bater, 'Some dimensions', 1978, 48.
6 McKean, *St. Petersburg*, 18.
7 Ibid.
8 *Materialy po statistike Petrograda, Vyp. 1* (TsSU Petrogradskoe stolichnoe statisticheskoe biuro, Petrograd 1920), 18.
9 'Sankt Peterburg' in F. Brokgauz and I. A. Efron (ed.), *Entsiklopedicheskii slovar'* (St. Petersburg 1900), tom. XXVIIIa, 314.
10 R. Glickman, 'The Russian Factory women, 1880–1914' in D. Atkinson and G. Lapidus (eds), *Women in Russia* (Stanford University Press, 1977), 63–83; W. Berelowitch, "L' evolution de la fécondite légitimite a Saint-Petersbourg-Petrograd-Leningrad (1860 – 1926)', *Annales de Demographique historique* Paris 1982, 252–253 and L. Edmundson, *Feminism in Russia, 1900–17* (Heinemann 1984), 142–143.
11 J. H. Bater, 'The social geography of St. Petersburg on the eve of the Great war', paper presented to conference on *The Social history of St. Petersburg/Leningrad, 1880–1930*, University of Essex, 3–5 July 1981. I am grateful of Dr Chris Ward of the University of Cambridge for supplying this source.
12 McKean, St. Petersburg, 38.
13 Bater, *St. Petersburg: Industrialisation and Change*, 24; McKean, *St. Petersburg*, 38.
14 'Sankt Peterburg' in Brokgauz and Efron, *Entsiklopedicheskii slovar'*, 314.
15 Ibid., 316.
16 McKean, *St. Petersburg*, 40.
17 Cited in Reginald E. Zelnik, *Labor and Society in Tsarist Russia: The Factory workers of St. Petersburg, 1855–70* (Stanford University Press, 1971), 242–243.
18 McKean, *St. Petersburg*, 39–40.
19 Ibid., 35.
20 Ibid., 35.
21 Bater, 'Some dimensions', 49.
22 Bater, *St. Petersburg: Industrialisation and Change*, 327; S. A. Smith, *Red Petrograd: Revolution in the factories, 1917–18 (Cambridge University Press* 1985), 9.
23 McKean, *St. Petersburg*, 39.
24 M. M. Steinin, 'Kanalizatsiia' in *Gorodskoe khozyiastvo i ustroitel'stvo Leningrada za 50 let* (Leningrad 1967), 164.
25 'Sankt Peterburg' in Brokgauz and Efron, *Entsiklopedicheskii slovar'* 1900, 316–317.
26 P. V. Novikov, 'Vodosnabzhenie' in *Gorodskoe khozyiastvo i ustroitel'stvo Leningrada za 50 let* (Leningrad 1967), 150.
27 Bater, *St. Petersburg: Industrialisation and Change*, 183–184.
28 Novikov, 'Vodosnabzhenie', 150.
29 Steinin, 'Kanalizatsiia', 165.
30 A. G. Woodhouse, 'Report', *British Parliament Papers: Diplomatic and Consular reports* XCVII, 1909, 943 cited in Bater, *St. Petersburg: Industrialisation and Change*, 352.

31 P. P. Anisimov et al., 'Leningradskaia promyshlennost' i etapy ee razvitia' in *Leningradskaia promyshlennost' za 50 let* (Leningrad 1967), 5.
32 Bater, *St. Petersburg: Industrialisation and Change*, 308.
33 Zelnik, *Labor and Society*, 252.
34 Cited in N. F. Izmerov, *Control of air pollution in the USSR*, Public health papers, No. 54 (WHO, Geneva 1973), 13.
35 Zelnik, *Labor and Society*, 252.
36 Ibid., 242–252.
37 Ibid., 252–262.
38 Cited in Bater, *St. Petersburg: Industrialisation and Change*, 188.
39 Zelnik, *Labor and Society*, 269–270.
40 Quoted in Zelnik, *Labor and Society*, 252. This is partly true. In 1865 there were 623 doctors, 32 employed by the police.
41 Zelnik, *Labor and Society*, 253.
42 Ibid., 268.
43 See 'Po povedu dela o pishche i pomeshchenii rabochikh na fabrike kuptsa Egorova', *Arkhiv sudebnoi meditsiny i obshchestbennoi gigieny* 1871, No. 1, sec iii, 124–143.
44 Medical report in 'Po povedu dela', 1871, 124–126. This case is also discussed in Zelnik *Labor and Society* 1971, 276–279.
45 Zelnik, *Labor and Society*, 412.
46 Bater, *St. Petersburg: Industrialisation and Change*, 351.
47 A. P. Zhuk, *Razvitie obshchestvenno-meditsinskoi mysl' v Rossii v 60–70gg XIX veka* (Moscow 1963), 303.
48 A. G. Rashin, *Nasekenie Rossii za 100 let (1811–1913gg): Statisticheskii ocherki* (Moscow 1956), 235.
49 Bater, 'Some dimensions', 51.
50 *Materialy po statistike Petrograda, Vyp. 1* (TsSU Petrogradskoe stolichnoe statis-ticheskoe biuro, Petrograd 1920), 30 and *Statisticheskii sbornik po Petrogradu i Petrogradskoi gubernii* (RSFSR TsSU Petrogradskoi gubernskii otdel statistiki 1922), 15.
51 L. P. Alekseeva, 'Voprosy gigieny i profilaktiki v trudakh obshchstva russkikh vrachei v Peterburge', *Sovetskoe Zdravookhranenie* 1957, No.5. 39–40.
52 Zelnik, *Labor and Society*, 244.
53 Zhuk, *Razvitie obshchestvenno-meditsinskoi mysl'*, 317–318.
54 S. N. Semenov, 'Fabrichnaia meditsina i russkie rabochie (Po materialiam Peterburga nachala XX veka), *Sovetskoe Zdravookhranenie* 1965, No. 12, 35; V. G. Pavlov, 'Meditsinskaia pomosh' rabochim peterburga v 1882–1886gg (Po materialam fabrichno-zavodskoi komissii)', *Sovetskoe Zdravookhranenie* 1979, No. 7, 59; Zhuk *Razvitie obshchestvenno-meditsinskoi mysl'*, 320–321, 327–328.
55 Zhuk, *Razvitie obshchestvenno-meditsinskoi mysl'*, 320–327.
56 V. A. Bazanov, 'Gigienisti peterburga i zemskaia meditsina', *Sovetskoe Zdravookhranenie* 1973, No. 6, 66
57 Alekseeva, 'Voprosy gigieny', 38.
58 Bazanov, 'Gigienisti peterburga', 67.
59 Pavlov, 'Meditsinskaia pomosh', 59.
60 Ibid., 60.
61 Ibid., 61.
62 E. M. Dement'ev, *Vrachebnaia pomoshch' fabrichno-zavodskim rabochim v 1907g* (St. Petersburg 1909), 13, 140
63 Smith, *Red Petrograd*, 41.
64 S. N. Semenov, *Peterburgskie rabochie nakanune pervoi russkoi revoliutsii* (Moscow), 140–141.

65 Semenov, *Peterburgskie rabochie*, 136–137; Semenov, 'Fabrichnaia meditsina', 36.
66 A. N. Vinokurov, 'Sanitarnoe sostoiane i meditsinskaia pomoshch' na fabrikakh i zaodakh peterburgskoi gubernii (1885–1908gg)', in *Trudy XI Pirogov S"ezda* (St. Peterburg 1911), 318.
67 Semenov, 'Fabrichnaia meditsina', 35; Semenov, *Peterburgskie rabochie*, 137.
68 Vinokurov, 'Sanitarnoe sostoiane', 318.
69 Smith, *Red Petrograd*, 42.
70 Ibid., 42.
71 Cited in McKean, *St. Petersburg*, 33.
72 Bater, *St. Petersburg: Industrialisation and Change*, 408.
73 V. P. Karavaev, 'Zemskie smety i raskladki' in B. Veselovskii and Z. G. Frenkel', *Iubileinyi zemskii sbornik*, 1864–1914 (St. Petersburg 1914), 167, 180.
74 B. Veselovskii, *Istoriia zemstva za sorok let* (St. Petersburg 1909), t. 1, 354.
75 Veselovskii, *Istoriia zemstva*, 341–342.
76 S. C. Ramer, 'The zemstvo and public health', in T. Emmons and W. S. Vucinich (ed.), *The Zemstvo in Russia: An experiment in local government* (Cambridge University Press 1982), 293–394.
77 Ramer, 'The zemstvo and public health', 296–297.
78 Veselovskii, *Istoriia zemstva*, 386–387.
79 Bater, 'Some dimensions', 55.
80 Veselovskii, *Istoriia zemstva*, 386–387.
81 Z. I. Frenkel, 'Sanitarnoe blagoustroitstvo i varchebno-sanitarnoe delo', in *Petrogradskaia gorodskaia duma v 1913*–1915gg (Petrograd 1915), 167.
82 Frenkel, 'Sanitarnoe blagoustroitstvo', 171.
83 Ibid., 173.
84 Ibid., 203.
85 *Statisticheskii spravochnik po Petrogradu* (Petrograd 1919), 60–62.
86 Ibid., 66.
87 Bater, 'Some dimensions', 61.
88 Frenkel, 'Sanitarnoe blagoustroitstvo', 181–182.
89 Ibid., 183–189.
90 John F. Hutchinson, *Politics and public health in Revolutionary Russia, 1890–1918* (The John Hopkins University Press 1990), 18–20.
91 Hutchinson, *Politics and public health*, 24–26.
92 Zhuk, *Razvitie obshchestvenno-meditsinskoi mysl'*, 39–40.
93 *Trudy Sanktpeterburgskogo obshchestva russkikh vrachei* (SPb meditsinskogo departmenta MVD 1836), chast 1, 1–75.
94 *Trudy Sanktpeterburgskogo obshchestva russkikh vrachei* (SPb meditsinskogo departmenta MVD 1843), chast 3, 114–131.
95 *Trudy Sanktpeterburgskogo obshchestva russkikh vrachei* (SPb meditsinskogo departmenta MVD 1852) chast 5, 152–159.
96 Zhuk, *Razvitie obshchestvenno-meditsinskoi mysl'* 1963, 70–71.
97 J. W. Walkin, *The Rise of democracy in pre-revolutionary Russia* (Praeger, London 1963), 155.
98 Nancy Frieden, *Russian physicians in an era of Reform and Revolution, 1856–1905* (Princeton University Press 1981), 37.
99 Zhuk, *Razvitie obshchestvenno-meditsinskoi mysl'*, 72–75.
100 Ramer, 'The zemstvo and public health', 290–291.
101 Vasil'evskii, *Istoriia zemstva*, and L. O. Kanevskii et al, *Osnovye cherty razvitiia meditsiny v Rossii v period kapitalizma* (Moscow 1956), 129.
102 Frieden, *Russian physicians*, 121.
103 D. R. Brower, *Training the nihilists: education and radicalism in Tsarist Russia* (London 1975), 72–78; K. I. Gurevich, 'Uchastie meditsinskikh rabotnikov v

revoliutsionnom dvizhenii v Rossii XIX-nachala XX veka', *Voprosy Istorii* 1972, No. 4, 203–206 and I. A. Slonimskaia, 'Uchastie peredovykh meditsinskikh rabotnikov v revoliutsionnom dvizhenii 1905–1907gg', *Sovetskoe Zdravookhranenie* 1955, No. 5, 41–42.

104 Frieden, *Russian physicians*, 13, 18.

105 T. G. Polinskaia, 'Studecheskie volneniia v Peterburgskoi mediko-khiruricheskoi akademii', *Sovetskoe Zdravookhranenie* 1967, No. 4, 54.

106 K. I. Gurevich, 'Studenty – mediki – "prikosnovennye" k protsessu Nechaeva', *Sovetskoe Zdravookhranenie* 1970, No.2, 70–75 and Polinskaia 'Studecheskie volneniia' 1967, 56–57.

107 V. S. Antonov, 'K voprosu o sotsial'nom sostave i chistlennosti revoliutsionerov 70-kh godov' in *Obshchestvennoe dvizhenie v poreformennoi Rossii: Sbornik statei* (Moscow 1956), 240 and S. M. Bagdasar'ian, *Ocherki istorii vysshego meditsinskogo obrazovaniiia: K istorii Voenno-meditsinskoi akademii* (Moscow 1959), 59.

108 A. V. Pavluchkova, 'Slushate'nitsy peterburgskikh vrachebnik zhenskikh kursov – uchastnitsy russkogo revoliutsionnogo dvizheniia 70-kh godov', *Sovetskoe Zdravookhranenie* 1974, No.3, 67.

109 B. A. Engel, 'Women medical students in Russia, 1872–82: Reformers or radicals?', *Journal of Social History* Volume 12, No.3, Spring 1979, 403.

110 Engel, 'Women medical students in Russia', 403; C. Johanson, 'Autocratic politics, public opinion and women's medical education during the reign of Alexander II, 1855–1881', *Slavic Review* Volume 38, No. 3, December 1979, 435.

111 Engel, 'Women medical students in Russia', 405, 408–409.

112 Johanson, 'Autocratic politics', 441.

113 K. I. Gurevich, 'Vrachi i student mediki – chleny "peterburgskogo soiuza bor'by za osvobozhdenie rabochego klassa"', *Sovetskoe Zdravookhranenie* 1969, no. 3, 60, 66–67.

114 F. Shalaev, 'Ye. N. Fedorova – chlen peterburgskogo "soiuza bor'by za osvobzhenie rabochego klassa"', *Sovetskoe Zdravookhranenie* 1986, No. 8, 67–69.

115 Gurevich, Vrachi i student mediki', 67.

116 G. Voronov, 'Slushatel'nitsy sankt-peterburgskogo zhenskogo meditsinskogo institute v period 1899–1904gg', *Sovetskoe Zdravookhranenie* 1978, No. 10, 75–76.

117 Voronov, 'Slushatel'nitsy sankt-peterburgskogo', 77.

118 Slonimskaia, 'Uchastie peredovykh', 42; A. G. Ianovskii, 'Meditsinskoe rabotniki v sovetakh deputatov v period revoliutsii 1905–1907gg', *Sovetskoe Zdravookhranenie* 1975, No. 6, 69–73.

119 Frieden, *Russian physicians*, 283–284.

120 M. A. Tikotin, 'Slushate'nitsy peterburgskogo zhenskogo meditsinskogo institute v pervoi russkoi revoliutsii', *Sovetskoe Zdravookhranenie* 1975, No. 4, 69–71 and N. F. Shalaev, 'Uchastie studentov Voenno-meditsinskoi akademii v revoliutsii 1905–1907gg', *Sovetskoe Zdravookhranenie* 1980, No. 8, 53.

121 P. Ye. Liubarov, 'Uchastie farmatsevtov v revoliutsionnom dvizhenie 1905', *Sovetskoe Zdravookhranenie* 1985 No. 11, 64–66.

122 Liubarov, 'Uchastie farmatsevtov', 66.

123 Shalaev, 'Uchastie studentov Voenno-meditsinskoi akademii', 53.

124 Ibid., 54. For more on MMA's role in 1905 see E. F. Selivanov, 'Studenty Voenno-meditsinskoi akademii v gody pervoi russkoi revoliutsii' in *Trudy Voenno-meditsinskogo muzeia* (Leningrad 1968), 5–10 and A. V. Shabunin, 'Uchastie studentov voenno-meditsinskoi akademii v pervoi russkoi revoliutsii, 195–1907gg', *Sovetskoe Zdravookhranenie* 1985, No. 11, 62–64.

125 Frieden, *Russian physicians*, 231.

126 Ibid., 233.
127 Peter F. Krug, 'Russian physicians and revolution: The Pirigov Society, 1917–1920', PhD, University of Wisconsin-Madison 1979, 48.
128 Hutchinson, Politics and public health, 45.
129 Tikotin, Slushate'nitsy peterburgskogo', 70.
130 Hutchinson, Politics and public health, 6–7.
131 John F. Hutchinson, 'Society, corporation or unity? Russian physicians and the struggle for professional unity', Jahrbucher fur Geschichte Osteuropas 30 (1982), H 1, 45–46 and E. I. Rodiodova, Ocherki istorii professional'nogo dvizheniia meditsinskikh rabotnikov (Moscow 1962), 61–62.
132 See G. A. Hosking, The Russian Constitutional Experiment: Government and Duma, 1907–1914 (Cambridge University Press 1973); R. T. Manning, The Crisis of the Old Order in Russia: Gentry and Government (Princeton University Press, NJ 1982).
133 John F. Hutchinson, 'Russian physicians and medical politics in the Revolution of 1917', Canadian Bulletin of Medical History 3 (1986), 10–11.
134 Hutchinson, 'Society, corporation or unity?', 48–49.
135 Ibid., 49–50.
136 Hutchinson, Politics and public health, 73.
137 Hutchinson, 'Russian physicians and medical politics', 20–22, 25; Hutchinson, Politics and public health, 75
138 Hutchinson, 'Society, corporation or unity?', 1982, 50.
139 M. A. Tikotin, 'Peterburgskii zhenskii meditsinskii institute v revoliutsionnom dvizhenii', Sovetskoe Zdravookhranenie 1981, No. 7, 51.
140 Hutchinson, Politics and public health, 73.
141 Hutchinson, 'Society, corporation or unity?', 1982, 46–47 and John. F. Hutchinson, 'Medicine, mortality and social policy in Imperial Russia: Early years of the Alcoholism Commission', Histoire Sociale volume 7, no. 4, November 1974, 206–211.
142 Hutchinson, Politics and public health, 78.
143 Ibid., 79.
144 Ibid., 77.
145 K. E. Tarasov and O. Pavlovskii, 'Partiia v bor'be za okhranu zdorov'ia naroda (K 70-letiiu s"ezda RSDRP)', Sovetskoe Zdravookhranenie 1972, No. 2, 5.
146 Mark G. Field, Soviet socialised medicine: An introduction (Free Press, New York 1967), 35–36.
147 B. Pearce, 1903: Second Ordinary Congress of the RSDLP (original 1904; this edition New Park publications, London 1978), 7–8; A. I. Nesterenko, 'Voprosy okhrany zdorov'aia trudiashchkhsia v pervoi programme partii, priniatnoi II s"ezdom RSDLP v 1903g', Sovetskoe Zdravookhranenie 1973, No.8, 66; Tarasov and Pavlovskii, Partiia', 1972, 6.
148 B. G. Danskii, strakhovaia kompaniia: Rabochie, khozyiaeva chinovniki i vyredenie strakhovamiia (St. Petersburg 1913), 5–6 and N. A. Vigdorchik, strakhovanie ot neschatnykh sluchaev v Rossii (Petrograd 1916), 8–12
149 V. P. Litvinov-Falinskii, Organizatsiia i praktika strakhovaniia rabocikh v Germanii i usloviia pomoshchogo obespecheniia rabochikh v Rossii (St. Petersburg 1903), 221–222.
150 Sally E. Ewing, 'Social insurance in Russia and the Soviet Union, 1912–22: A study of legal form and administrative practice', unpublished PhD in Sociology, Princeton University, 1984, 66.
151 M. Kheisin, 'Gosudarstvennoe strakhovanie rabochikh v Rossii', Nasha Zaria 1911, No. 11, 28
152 Ewing, 'Social insurance in Russia and the Soviet Union', 6.
153 On this see A. Lindenmeyr, Poverty is not a vice: Charity, Society and the State in Imperial Russia (Princeton University Press, 1996).

154 D. Zoller, 'Germany' in P. A. Kohler and H. F. Zacher (eds), *The evolution of social insurance, 1881–1981* (St. Martin's Press 1982), 24–27; G. A. Ritter, *Social welfare in Germany and Britain: Origins and Development* (Berg, Leamington Spa 1986), Chapter 2, 176.

155 Cited in Kheisin, 'Gosudarstvennoe', 29.

156 Kheisin, 'Gosudarstvennoe', 31–32.

157 KPSS rezolutsiiakh i resheniiakh s"ezdov, konferentsii i plenomov TsK (7th ed. Moscow 1954), 199 and G. A. Beilikhis, 'Bolsheviki deputaty III i IV gosu-darstvennykh dum v bor'be za okhrany zdorov'iia rabochikh', *Sovetskoe Zdravookhranenie* 1968, No. 6, 48.

158 Tim McDaniel, *Autocracy, Capitalism and Revolution in Russia* (University of California Press 1988), 140

159 V. Ezhov, *Bol'nichnaia kassy i vrachebnaia pomosh' rabochim po zakony 23 iuniia 1912g* (St. Petersburg 1913), 3 and R. S. Rotenburg',Bor'ba rabochego klassa Rossii za gosudarstvennoe sotsial'noe strakhovanie (1900–1914), *Voprosy Istorii* 1958, No. 11, 131.

160 Kheisin, 'Gosudarstvennoe', 34–41.

161 McDaniel, *Autocracy*, 140.

162 N. N. Shchepkina, 'Sotsial'noe zakonodatel'stvo s tochki zreniia spravedlivnosti i gosudarstvennyi neobkhodimosti', in *Tret'iia Gosudarstvennaia Duma. Fraktsiia narodnoi svobody v period 15 Okt. 1910 goda – 15 Maia 1911 goda, Ch. II: Rech'i chlenov fraktsii v chetvertoi sessii tret'ii Dumy* (St. Peterburg 1911), 96–108

163 N. A. Vidgorchik, *Strakhovanie ot neschastnykh sluchaev v Rossii* (Petrograd 1916), 18.

164 S. G. Strumilin, *Problemy ekonomiki truda* (Moscow 1964), 453, 474.

165 Ezhov, *Bol'nichnaia kassy*, 29–30.

166 See P. Timofeev, 'What the Factory worker lives by' in Victoria E. Bonnell (ed.), *The Russian Worker* (University of California Press, London 1983), 91.

167 See F. P. Pavlov, 'Ten years of experiences (Excerpts from reminiscences, impressions and observations of factory life)', in Bonnell, *The Russian Worker* 1983, 148.

168 R. Amende Roosa, 'Workers' insurance legislation and the role of the indus-trialists in the period of the third State Duma', *Russian Review,* October 1975, 422.

169 Roosa, 'Workers' insurance legislation', 448.

170 See for instance, 'Zakonoproekty po strakhovaniiu rabochikh', *Promyshlennost' i Torgovlia* 1 July 1908, 14–15; 'K zakonoproektam o strakhovanii rabochikh', *Promyshlennost' i Torgovlia* 1 December 1908, 627–629; 'Strakovanie rabo-chikh ot neschastnykh sluchaev', *Promyshlennost' i Torgovlia* 15 March 1909, 339–341 and 'Po rabochemy voprosu', *Promyshlennost' i Torgovlia* 15 December 1910, 635.

171 P. A. Berlin, *Burzhvaziia v storoe i novoe vremiia* (Moscow 1922), 253.

172 Roosa, 'Workers' insurance legislation', 449.

173 B. G. Danskii, '"Pravda" i rabochaia strakhovaia kampaniia', *Proletarskia revo-liutsiia* 1930, No. 7–8, 172.

174 A. E. Badaev, *Bol'sheviki v gosudarstvennoi duma* (Leningrad 1929), 80–82 and *Rabochie dvizhenie v Petrograde v 1912–1917gg: Dokumenty i materialy* (Lenizdat, Leningrad 1958), 86.

175 Cited in S. M. Shvarts, *sotsial'noe strakhovanie v Rossii v 1917–1919 godakh* (Russian Institution, Columbia University, New York 1968), 26–28.

176 Danskii, '"Pravda"', 173–175.

177 S. Shvarts, 'Rabochaia strakhovaia kampaniia v Peterburge', *Nashe Zaria* 1913, No. 4–5, 26–34 and 1913, No. 7–8, 74–83.

178 I. M. Ivanov, 'Pervyi shagi zavod', *Stakhovanie rabochik* 1913, No. 9, 26–29.

179 N. Morozov, 'Strakhovanie kampaniia v Perterburge', *Stakhovanie Rabochik* 1913, No. 6, 26 and 'Vserossiiskoe rabochii s"ezd po voprosam strakhovaniia', *Stakhovanie Rabochik* August 1913, 3–7.

180 G. Baturskii, 'Strakhovaia kampaniia v Petersburg', *Stakhovanie Rabochik* No. 11–12, 1913, 22–24.

181 B. G. Danskii, 'Strakhovanie kampaniia', *Prosveshchenie* 1913, No. 4, April, 76–77.

182 This complaint was made by Volgar see 'Khoziaskii plan strakhovanii kanpanii (Petersburgskoe "Obchestvo zavodchikov in fabrikantov" o strakhovoi kampanii)', *Proveshchenie* No. 7–8, July-August 1913, 100.

183 T. Hasegawa, *The February Revolution: Petrograd, 1917* (University of Washington Press, Seattle 1981), 80–81 and Smith, *Red Petrograd*, 34–35.

184 G. Osipov, 'Pervye vybory rabochikh predstavitelei v strakhovoi sovet', *voprosy Strakhovaniia* 8 November 1923, 34.

185 Ewing, 'Social insurance in Russia', 111.

186 Hasegawa, *The February Revolution*, 86–88.

187 *Statisticheskii spravochnik po Petrogradu* (Petrograd 1919), 65 and *Statisticheskii sbornik po Petrogradu i Petrogradskoi gubernii* (Petrograd 1922), 318.

188 Hutchinson, 'Society, corporation or unity?', 52.

189 P. Gatrell, *Russia's First World War: A social and economic history* (Pearson/Longman 2005), 65.

2   The health of the Petrograd collective under War Communism, 1918–20

This chapter examines the impact of the revolution and civil war on health care in Petrograd. Using the local press, key public health journals, statistical handbooks and new material from the declassified Narkomzdrav (Ministry of Public Health) archives, we assess the main challenges to social transformation (trends in morbidity, mortality, health service development, the socio-economic and political context and its impact on health policy and decision-making, and above all relations between the medical profession and the state) and the degree of success or failure in redefining Russian welfare strategies between 1917–20. We will discuss the continuing notion of a 'collective health' and how the new Soviet regime wanted to modernise health and welfare in view of the health conditions highlighted in the previous chapter. We examine key indicators of reconfiguration, reform and modernisation in relation to health care, such as Lenin's aim to provide free health care to all, free access for all, and the role played by the state in relation to welfare provision and policy. It will argue that medical issues became a political issue for two reasons: the need to survive amidst foreign intervention and the reliance upon tsarist trained doctors and medical personnel. A final concluding section assesses how far Lenin got in creating a new socialist health service underpinned by collectivist values by the end of the civil war.

Life and death in Petrograd, 1917–20

The first part of this section analyses changes in demographic, health and sanitation patterns in Petrograd and how the Party, State and medical profession dealt with the challenges. The data furnished in Table 2.1 shows that in Petrograd the population fell in this very short period from 2.3 million in 1917 to only 740,000 by the end of the civil war in 1920. This was the product of the First World War losses, followed by revolution and the civil war. Workers and peasants were driven out of town by hunger. The birth rate initially fell from 18.8 in 1917 to 13.8 by 1919 but had recovered to 21.8 per 1,000 in 1920. The death rate doubled between 1917 and 1918 from 23.3 to 46.6 before increasing to 77.1 in 1919 and then falling to 50.6

Table 2.1 Population of Petrograd, 1918–20

Year	Size of population	Number of births	Births per 1,000	Number of deaths	Deaths per 1,000	Rate of natural increase/ decrease
1918	1,469,000	25,380	17.3	68,533	46.6	−29.5
1919	900,000	12,365	13.8	69,381	77.1	−63.3
1920	740,000	16,119	21.8	37,429	50.6	28.8

Sources: *Materialy po statistika Leningradu i Leningradskoi gubernii, Vyp.* 6 (Leningrad 1925), 202 and *XV let diktatory proletariata: Ekonomiko-statisticheskii sbornik po gor. Leningradu i Leningradskoi oblasti* (Leningrad 1932), 135

by 1920, which was still considerably higher than in 1917. The birth rate fluctuation was connected partly with an increased marriage rate from 8.9 in 1917 to 27.7 by 1920,[1] social disruption (men away fighting, families forced to migrate) and with illegal abortions, whilst deaths were mostly accounted for by infectious diseases.

Thus typhus, which was endemic throughout the civil war, increased from 0.63 cases per 10,000 in 1913 to 1.9 in 1917 climbing as high as 404 per 10,000 in 1919 before falling to 255.2 per 10,000 a year later. Similarly, relapsing fever rose from 0.48 to 12.7 cases per 10,000 between 1913–17, reaching 94.0 per 10,000 at the end of the civil war. Excluding dysentery, which rose from 32.4 in 1913 to 101.7 per 10,000 by 1920, all other diseases exhibited a decline. For example, typhoid morbidity fell from 65.8 per 10,000 in 1913 to 10.9 by 1920, as did measles (from 73.7 to 4.8), scarlet fever (39.8 to 11.3) and diphtheria (from 29.5 to 11.2). This was, of course, a truly extraordinary situation in which various infectious diseases were rampant, posing huge problems for the Petrograd health service.

Table 2.2 arranges the individual registered causes of morbidity and shows that morbidity from airborne diseases as a percentage of overall causes of ill-health declined from 59.3% in 1913 to 7.8% by 1920. Water and food borne diseases also fell from 40.2% to 30.6% over the same period. Data on morbidity from other vectors, indicates a dramatic increase from 0.45% in 1913 to 86.7% of overall causes of illness in 1920.

Particular epidemic diseases caused major problems for local public health administrators as they hit the city in short, sharp waves thereby putting a strain on medical and other resources. Infectious diseases in Petrograd in 1919–20 were more frequent in the winter rather than summer months. Morbidity as a whole was highest in March–April 1919 and in February–March 1920.[2] These were the months when food supplies were also at their worst, so malnutrition was a factor compounding illness in Petrograd during the civil war.

Epidemics of typhus and dysentery were the worst, hitting all age groups but especially the infirm, the weak and the very young.[3] Those living in working-class districts of the city, where sewage systems were non-operational, water supplies contaminated and housing stock in a state of

Table 2.2 Incidence of infectious diseases in Petrograd, 1914–20 (rates per 10,000 population)

Type of disease	1914	1915	1916	1917	1918	1919	1920
Typhoid	48.2	40.5	21.6	5.2	7.6	4.8	10.9
Typhus	0.94	2.1	1.0	1.9	74.7	404.0	255.2
Relapsing fever	0.26	0.7	8.4	12.7	5.6	17.9	94.0
Smallpox	10.6	15.4	5.5	4.4	8.6	62.9	15.1
Measles	97.7	70.9	18.3	n.a.	1.1	37.4	4.8
Scarlet fever	42.5	50.9	31.8	5.4	3.4	11.2	11.3
Diphtheria	30.1	28.5	18.4	4.5	7.9	14.5	11.2
Dysentery	22.3	29.0	12.8	n/a.	6.7	62.3	101.7
Total	252.6	238.0	117.8	34.1	115.6	615.0	504.2

Source: GARF f. A-482 op. 10. d. 292, lists 27–35

disrepair, suffered particularly badly. For instance, Aleksandr-Nevskii, Moscow and Vyborg districts had the highest morbidity from typhus and cholera in 1918, when compared to the Admiralty district.[4] Overcrowding accounts for disease in some cases. Thus, Aleksandr-Nevskii wards II and III were found to have the highest concentration of inhabitants per room (3.7 and 3.9 respectively) in 1918 while Admiralty wards I and II had one of the lowest density levels (1.1 and 1.2 respectively). In 1919–20, the situation remained largely unchanged, despite boundary differences, when infectious diseases were highest in Petrograd side, Narvskii-Peterhof and Smolnyi districts and lowest in Admiralty district.[5]

In overall terms, a year by year breakdown shows that in 1913–14, morbidity was greatest from measles and typhoid; in 1915–16 from measles, scarlet fever, typhoid and diphtheria and in 1917 from typhus, smallpox and measles. During the civil war, the highest morbidity levels were caused by typhus, smallpox and measles in 1918–19 and by typhus, relapsing fever and measles in 1920.

The changing causes of mortality are shown in Table 2.3 which indicates that certain diseases predominated in particular years: dysentery and all forms of typhus in 1917; dysentery, typhus, typhoid and diphtheria in 1918; typhus, dysentery, smallpox and measles in 1919 and in 1920, as the civil war drew to a close, most deaths resulted from typhus, dysentery and relapsing fever.

Breaking the causes of death down by vector during the period 1917–20, shows that airborne diseases, as a percentage of overall deaths, declined from 31.4% in 1917 to 23.0% by 1920 while water and food borne diseases rose slightly from 9.7% to 10.9% over the same period. It was morbidity from other vectors which increased most markedly from 0.6% to 19.5% of the total causes of death between 1917–20.

Mortality in Petrograd varied according to time of the year, sex, age-group and social class. Data collected by Petrograd statisticians shows that mortality was higher among males than females in all age-groups in

Table 2.3 Death rate from various diseases in Petrograd, 1917–20 (rates per 10,000 population)

Type of disease	1917	1918	1919	1920
Typhoid	5.2	7.6	4.8	10.9
Typhus	1.9	74.7	404.0	255.2
Relapsing fever	12.7	5.6	17.9	94.0
Smallpox	4.4	8.6	62.9	15.1
Measles	-	1.1	37.4	4.8
Scarlet fever	5.4	3.4	11.2	11.3
Diphtheria	4.5	7.9	14.5	11.2
Dysentery	-	6.7	62.3	101.7
Total	34.1	115.6	615.0	504.2

Source: GARF f. A-482 op. 10. d. 292, lists 27–35

this period. The gap in mortality between the sexes was initially rather wide standing at 13.3 per 1,000 for males and 9.5 per 1,000 for females in 1917, but as the civil war got underway, the gap narrowed: in 1918 to 25.3 and 21.4 respectively; in 1919 to 38.6 and 38.5 before increasing to 28.7 for males and 21.9 for females by 1920. Thus the death rate by gender was wider in 1920 than 1917, with more males than females dying.[6]

We saw in the previous chapter that in St Petersburg mortality was highest amongst the poor migrant peasant and working-class inhabitants of the city. After 1917, the situation is made more complicated by the rapid social changes that occurred. By 1917–18, the court, aristocracy, wealthy business and foreign community had gone, although in 1920, some members of the nobility, honoured citizens, merchants and the intelligentsia remained in Petrograd.[7]

As a result of the changes in housing policy documented below, residential mixing became more widespread during the civil war than before 1913, but despite this mortality was still greater in some Petrograd districts such as Vyborg, Aleksandr-Nevskii and Moscow.[8]

The decline in Petrograd's population was a consequence of revolution, civil war, foreign intervention, epidemics and hunger, all of which meant that migration from the city was high. The surplus of deaths over births was 130,993 meaning that only 8.4% of the net decline in population is attributable to this variable.

Petrograd faced major mortality crises as a consequence of severe hunger (*golod*)[9] between July 1918–August 1919 (deaths peaked at 90 per 1,000 population at Easter 1919) and then between November 1919–April 1920 (once again deaths peaked at 90 per 1,000 population, this time in February 1920). The hunger has been estimated to have accounted for 15% of the extra mortality registered at the peak of the famine period in 1918–21.[10] Medical facilities were most stretched in January–March 1917, May–August 1918, January–April 1919 and January–March 1919.

The prominent Petrograd statistician, Novosel'skii argued that in 1920 hunger exhaustion (*golodnogo istocheniia*) caused 2,737 deaths (or 37.7 per 10,000 population) which was far less than the level of mortality caused by infectious diseases such as typhus (4,752 or 64.2 per 10,000) or tuberculosis of the lungs (3,733 or 50.4 per 10,000).[11] In seeking to examine the reasons for birth and death variations in the city, we will analyse the food supply, fuel shortages and housing.

Shortage of food was one of the major factors weakening the population of Petrograd. In October 1917, the Bolsheviks faced a situation in which food stocks were said to be 'dangerously low', rationing was in place and bread and other foodstuff prices were rising quickly.[12] Although some people left the city, those who remained in McAuley's view were 'nearly starving to death'.[13] In the winter 1917, the food position was said to be 'extremely grave' and food procurement was placed under local government control.[14] The food supply continued to be grave in Winter-Spring 1918, then serious in late 1919 and acute in the summer of 1920. For example, the quantity of rye fell from 52.5 poods in 1917 to 42.9 poods in 1920; oats from 54.2 poods to 35.9 poods; barley from 44.9 poods to 29.6 poods and potatoes from 723.1 poods to 421.8 poods between 1917–20.[15]

Average daily consumption of food was low and the population of Petrograd was relying on low calorie diets for its survival. By December 1918, daily calorie intake fell to as low as 1,500 calories[16] when the recommended level was 2,300 calories.[17] The Petrograd local authorities focused on procuring grain, distributing bread and other foodstuffs and creating co-operatives. The new Soviet regime closed private restaurants (due to an anti-free trade stance) in October 1918 and replaced them with communal eating facilities, but despite these measures it was still necessary to introduce a ration system. There were four broad categories: category I – heavy physical labour; category II – white collar workers (including doctors working in state hospitals or medical staff teaching in universities); category III – members of the intelligentsia, home and stall owners; and category IV – the 'bourgeois'.[18]

Table 2.4 details the percentage of different population groups in Petrograd in each ration category. The large majority of the city's population were in the first 3 categories and in June 1919, there were 771,156 in category I; 136,604 in category II and 12,747 in category III. Figures for category IV were not specified.[19]

Doctors in state establishments were in the second food ration category as Table 2.4 shows. This table needs interpreting with caution as the categories may have been fixed but people changed occupations in order to try and shift ration categories, thus aristocrats took jobs as clerks and traders went to work in factories which had not yet closed.[20] The state also reclassified people as the pressure increased. Hence during the 1918 cholera epidemic, doctors and other medical personnel were moved from food category II to I in view of their importance in combating the public health crises.[21]

Table 2.4 Percentage of population in different food rationing categories in Petrograd, 1918–1920

Food ration category	October 1918	January 1919	January 1920	April 1920
I	52.3	61.1	63.0	63.0
Children	-	20.0	30.0	30.0
II	38.6	16.5	7.0	6.5
III	8.9	2.2	0.2	0.1
IV	0.2	--	-	-

Source: M. McAuley, *Bread and Justice: State and society in Petrograd 1917–1922* (Clarendon Press, Oxford 1991), 288

By January 1919, there were 33 different ration cards in operation for bread, potatoes, tobacco, cotton and flax, fabrics, boots, soap, milk, butter etc in Petrograd.[22] Cards were issued on a monthly basis and rations were low. Using Trudy TsSU data, Wheatcroft estimates that at no time during the civil war did calorie intake reach the recommended level. Among working class families in Petrograd, the situation was 1,578 calories per person in March, 2,415 calories in July and 2,976 calories in December 1919. By May 1920, levels fell to 2,690 calories.[23]

The staple diet, according to McAuley, consisted of bread (when available), thin soup, cabbage and salt fish, which was all the Petrograd government could provide. By mid-1919, sugar, cereals, fats and eggs had disappeared and potatoes became a luxury.[24] Workers were eating half as much bread, a third as much meat and about the same amount of potatoes as in 1908. A year later in 1920, workers were eating half as much food as they had just before the First World War in 1912–14.[25]

Due to food scarcity, money prices became increasingly meaningless and bartering now ruled. Smith suggests that prices rocketed in 1917 and into 1918 and Wheatcroft adds that throughout 1919, as hunger became more widespread, food prices steadily increased.[26] As a result, the cost of a loaf of bread increased from 25k in January 1919 to 2r 35k in November 1919; the cost of nearly half a kilo of potatoes rose from 9k to 82k; the price of nearly half a kilo of meat from 26k to 4r 25k; of nearly half a kilo of fish from 22k to 2r 20k and nearly half a kilo of butter from 82k to 15r 83k over the same period.[27] Grain prices in the free market reached their peak in the winter of 1919–20. By mid-February 1920, a loaf of bread cost 30r, nearly half a kilo of potatoes cost between 9r 50k to 14r, fish 50r and butter 200–260r.[28] To put these figures in perspective, a specialist could be earning 3,500r and a worker 500r, meaning that by late 1919, a director was earning 15 times more than an office cleaner.[29] These price increases show just how difficult it was for some groups to purchase food and survive.

In Petrograd, workers tended to consume more food than their white-collar counterparts in June and December 1919 and in May and November 1920 and only in April and September 1919 did office workers consume more. During the civil war, workers consumed more than the average for the city of Petrograd as a whole, with the exception of April 1919.[30] This reflected the fact that the city's food policy prioritised workers, especially industrial workers and the Red Army. Despite this, more and more of the population still had to engage in bartering, buying and selling in order to keep alive, as money wages declined in importance.[31]

In this situation, at first workers used their savings, which quickly became exhausted, then they borrowed money from friends and relatives, and the poorest among them sold their possessions or begged. Some left for the countryside to avoid hunger. Those workers who remained, tended to resent the estimated 1,000 members of the bourgeois living in Petrograd in October 1918. Those defined as 'bourgeois' included higher ranking tsarist civil servants, police chiefs, bankers, industrialists (with a workforce of 20 or more) or landowners (with less than 20 desiatina of land), who were all seen as class enemies.[32] Members of the bourgeoisie or 'former people', who were put in the lowest food ration category, naturally did not have things easy either. They too were also forced to use their servants to sell precious linen, and when this ran out, the wives of the former well-off tended to sell their other luxury goods on the open market. Of course, it was the traders (later nepmen) who benefitted most from this situation, as they overcharged for goods and services. Speculators also made money on goods sold to them by desperate people in Petrograd.

Either way, the poor diet and malnutrition made Petrograd citizens susceptible to illness and sometimes death. Lenin acknowledged the seriousness of the situation pointing out:

> Typhus in a population already weakened by hunger and sickness and without bread, soap and fuel, may become such a scourge, as not to give us an opportunity to undertake socialist construction. Its eradication must be our first step in our struggle for survival.[33]

The civil war not only caused food shortages, it generated fuel supply difficulties. After the particularly bad winter of 1917–18, factories were closed, the transport system was paralysed (trams failed to run and horse drawn taxis stopped, as the horses were dead) because fuel was dwindling fast. This was partly as a result of the signing of the Treaty of Brest-Litovsk in March 1918, which led to the loss of the Donbass and the ceasing of oil from Baku, followed by the outbreak of the civil war in Autumn of 1918.[34]

This caused a fuel crisis in Petrograd. According to Rudenkov's calculations, fuel consumption by Petrograd industry in 1917–18 declined as follows: coal from 56,449 thousand poods to 12,150 poods; oil from 39,989 to 8,650 poods; and firewood from 44,654 poods to 34,110 poods.

Only peat fuel consumption increased from 593 poods to 8,000 thousand poods in this period.[35]

One estimate suggests that by 1919, the fuel available for consumption (other than domestic) was 40% of its 1916 level.[36] Petrograd now required fuel from elsewhere to survive. In 1917, 185.6 thousand poods of fuel arrived; in 1918, 61.7 thousand poods; 1919, 39.3 thousand poods; and finally, only 57,000 poods of fuel in 1920.[37] Even with this help and sacrifice elsewhere, the fuel supply situation reached crisis level in late 1918 and throughout 1919 before becoming catastrophic by winter 1919.[38]

Fierce cold, caused by lack of fuel and severe winter weather, coupled with a poor diet as detailed above, made the population more likely to get ill or die. It is no coincidence that this was also a period of epidemics of infectious disease. Victor Serge reflects on the situation in his memoirs:

> The Winter of 1917–18 was frightful. In the larger cities that were ravaged by famine and typhus, people were deprived of fuel water and illumination. The water and sewage pipes froze up inside the buildings. Families would crowd together around little stoves (and) old books, furniture, doors and floor boards were used in lieu of firewood. In Petrograd and Moscow ... water closets no longer worked, piles of excrement accumulated in the courtyards, shielded by constant snowfalls, but storing up epidemics for the Spring.[39]

A related issue was housing which was not in short supply given the huge fall in the population, meaning the population-apartment ratio was reduced from 5 persons per apartment in 1918 to 2.8 persons by 1920.[40] By June 1918, there were 8,000 empty apartments in Vasilevskii island and Petrograd side of the city and this number increased to 53,822, for example, in Spasskii and Novoderevenskii districts and in Vasilevskii Island by the time of the 1920 census.[41] The number of apartments fell by 15% during the civil war as buildings were used to provide firewood.[42] The Petrograd Bolsheviks confiscated property and moved poor and needy families from unsanitary working-class districts to bourgeois apartments in the city. This housing policy and process was approved in November 1917 but did not start until somewhere between March-Summer 1918.[43] No reliable statistics are available on the number of people re-housed, but figures for April 1919 suggest that 12,848 workers' families were allocated new houses. Also 1,362 apartments were allocated to communists; 568 to Communist clubs and 1,424 to Commissariats. The process then slowed down between March–September 1919, when 2,000 workers' families received housing and a further 4,000 were allocated to Red Army and Red Sailors personnel.[44] Sosnovy argues that in overall terms 550,000 people were re-housed in Petrograd during the civil war.[45] In this context, McAuley notes: 'Despite their efforts, the new authority's could not halt the deterioration in the physical environment and services; all they could do was to distribute what (housing) was available rather more equally (than under Tsarism)'.[46]

Ideologically, a housing nationalisation programme and the removal of the bourgeoisie to make space for workers, wherever possible, was the policy pursued but doing this in practice proved problematic. By April 1918, only 200 houses had been nationalised on the Petrograd side of the city for instance. This figure slightly increased to 258 in February 1919, rising to 900 by April 1919, so that by the summer of 1920, 2,000 houses belonged to different Commissariats in that part of the city. In overall terms, according to McAuley, 6,400 houses belonged to the new regime but far more (9,400) were still in private hands at this point.[47]

The shortages of good quality housing meant that when the 1920 census was carried out, 721,296 people were occupying 17,657 houses in Petrograd. There were 273 houses with less than five people in them; 3,162 with 6–10 people; 3,624 with 11–25 people; 2,684 with 26–50 people; 2,667 with 51–100 people; 1,456 with 101–200 people; 379 with 201–500 people and 43 houses with 500 people or more.[48] So ill health in Petrograd might have been partly caused by communal living under War Communism in some districts (Vyborg, Aleksandr-Nevskii, Narva and Lesnoi), but it was the failure to supply habitable and decent housing which was one of the biggest challenges facing the population and the local authorities.

One of the ways the Petrograd council tried to improve the housing stock was through the collection of rents. Mary McAuley argues that housing rent collection was good in the central Liteinyi district but bad in Peterhof and Nevskii districts. This situation meant that revenues did not always cover the cost of repairs of housing, sewage and sanitation. In Peterhof in 1918, for instance, 185,000r was collected in rents but repairs cost 41,000r; water supply maintenance 33,000r; garbage collection 84,000r; yardsman's pay 98,000r; and housing department staff pay 127,000r. So the housing department was living beyond their means.[49]

To try and ease the strain, if people's income in Petrograd was under 400r then they were exempt from rent payments, but the wealthy were still charged a property tax in order to raise much needed revenues. Because those who owned houses faced property tax charges, many owners simply abandoned their houses, leaving them to the housing committees, so this was nationalisation by default, but some of these dwellings were in such a bad condition that they were more of a burden than an asset.

Unfortunately, re-housing and low or no rents for workers failed to solve the housing crisis, as any revenues raised did not cover costs, so the city council and council districts were unable to maintain housing quality. The lack of maintenance meant that many houses were in a dilapidated condition. Thus in 1920, according to Binshtok, 6.8% of city centre housing, 4.4% in Petrograd side, 2.8% in Smolnyi, 1.3% in Vasilevskii Island, 2.4% in Vyborg and 2.1% in Nevskii district were in a very poor state.[50]

So high rents were no longer an issue and workers did not have to live in cellar apartments that were flooded or corners of rooms as in pre-revolutionary times, which was a significant improvement. However other problems still remained. Lots of houses in the city of Petrograd lacked basic amenities. In April 1919, of the 3,350 houses owned by the municipality, according to the newspaper *Krasnaia Gazeta,* 1,800 needed their water supply repaired and 1,000 needed sewer system repairs.[51] The situation got worse a year later. Of the 48,132 buildings surveyed as part of the 1920 census, 16,578 houses (or 34.4%) had a functioning water supply; 2,164 houses (4.5%) had a water supply in place but it did not work and 10,698 houses (22.2%) had no water system at all. Similarly, 13,801 houses (28.6%) had a functioning sewer system; 2,742 houses (5.7%) had a sewer system that was not operational and 2,199 houses (4.6%) had no such facilities.[52] The water supply fell from 10.2 million vedro in 1917 to 8.17 million vedro by 1920, which was lower than its 1913 level of 8.57 million vedro. The average daily per-capita use of water in Petrograd rose from 11.6 vedro in 1917 to 31.8 vedro by 1920.[53] The problem was the impurity of the water supply which was associated with the epidemics of infectious diseases such as cholera and typhoid discussed earlier.

As we saw in Chapter 1, before 1917 the city cellars were closely located to accumulated excrement and refuse and tons of filth was piled up in courtyards. After 1917, the city of Petrograd was still full of rubbish, and sewage was either dumped in the street or the canals. In McAuley's words, Petrograd was by the end of the civil war 'a city of empty apartments, broken sewers and water pipes, rats and piles of garbage'.[54]

The Petrograd Council's shortage of staff meant that although it was concerned about this situation, its hands were tied.[55] This unhygienic situation led to complaints about the mismanagement of housing policy and its impact on health and sanitation. For example, at one meeting held in the Putilov factory on 14 December 1920, the chairman of the district council was informed that there were 150 houses with no doors or windows; dripping water was a frequent problem and rats were everywhere. The audience complained that there were insufficient ponies (14) to clear away garbage from the streets.[56]

The Petrograd city Duma spent nearly 1.1 million roubles on the purification and repair of the sewage system in 1919 and in the first 6 months of 1920, it succeeded in repairing 56,409 sections of the old system and in setting up 16,056 new ones.[57] Purification of the city's canals began in the winter of 1917–18 and throughout the civil war period, the population was mobilised to clean the streets, factories, homes and the local water supply.[58] Chlorination programmes were also devised and filter stations were set up on the river Neva.[59] Unfortunately none of these efforts prevented the *vibrio cholera* contaminating local supplies.[60]

Poster 1 shows the dangers that unclean food, which cannot be washed, caused to key parts of the collective in this case – a soldier. This soldier

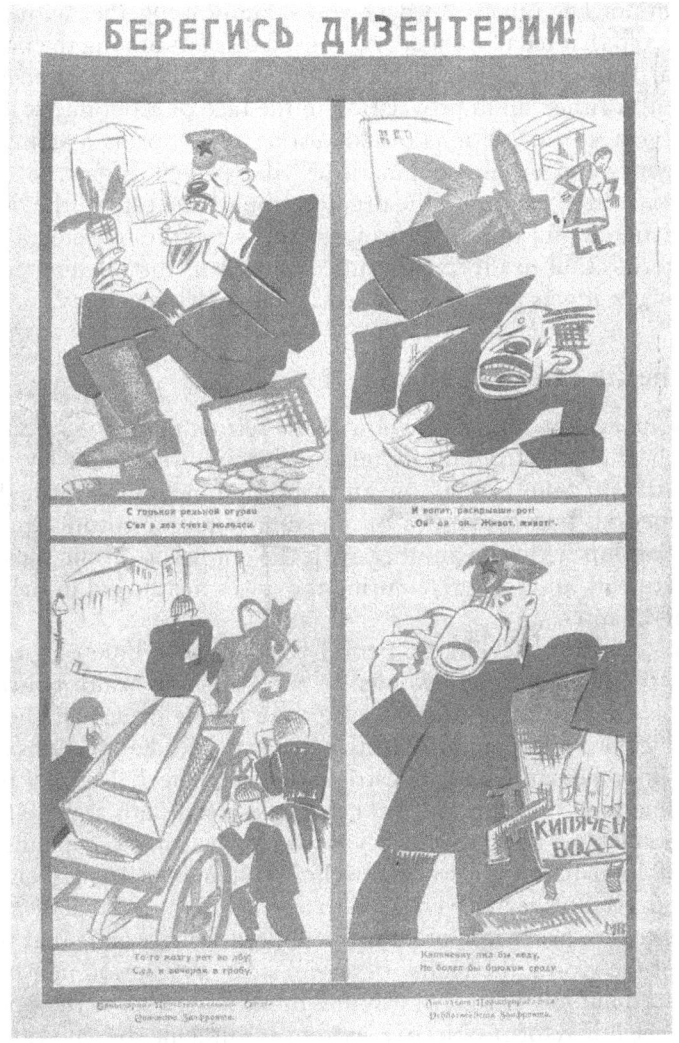

Poster 1 Dysentery caused by unclean food and water

Source: 'A Soviet soldier dies of dysentery as a result of eating unwashed vegetables'. Colour lithograph by M.V., c. 1920, for the Sanitarno-Prosvetitel'no Otdel Sanchasta Zapfronta. Credit: Wellcome Collection, Wellcome Library, London (CC BY 4.0)

depicted in red, to symbolise the Red Army, eats unclean vegetables in panel one, this leads to dysentery and severe health problems (panel 2) and eventually causes his death (depicted by the coffin in panel 3). The final panel, number 4 in bottom right, depicts a healthier soldier apparently drinking clean water from the tap with the words 'boiled water' written in red.

Thus in stark contrast to the pre-war period, it was not overcrowding, but a decline in housing quality, hygiene and sanitation together with poor diet and fierce cold that led to hunger and caused diseases among the population in civil war Petrograd. The policies of War Communism themselves, which can be seen as either 'an improvisation in the face of economic scarcity and military urgency in conditions of exhausting war'[61] or as a 'compound of war emergency and socialist dogmatism'[62] also played its part.

The next section examines the organisational structure of the health service in Petrograd and the extent to what this structure reflected a response to the deteriorating health conditions explored in the opening section or whether or not it was primarily shaped by Bolshevik ideology.

Socialist health care in Petrograd

This section begins with a discussion of the setting up of the Commissariat of Public health in Petrograd, its relationship with the Ministry of Public health (*Narkomzdrav*) in Moscow and with its functioning throughout the civil war period. It concentrates on the subordinate institutions and their inter-relationship with one another, with the emphasis on the most important departments and their role during the crises mentioned in the first section of this chapter.

The post-October Revolution period was clearly a time of great uncertainty, but the Bolsheviks still wanted to reverse tsarist health policies. They inherited, as we saw in the previous chapter, a totally inadequate health care system, which provided minimal health care for the neediest sections of Russia society – poor peasants and industrial workers. The Bolsheviks possessed no clear blueprint, but they did want to modernise health and welfare. This involved eradicating the tsarist legacy (so there was an anti-capitalist dimension) and a desire to move towards a welfare system built along socialist lines.

Although the Bolsheviks were keen to transform the old, backward tsarist system of welfare provision into a truly modern welfare state that would be the envy of the world, the reality of Soviet rule – revolution in a backward country faced initially with civil war and hunger, together with opposition – made this health reform objective extremely difficult to achieve from the outset. As a result, the modernisation of Russian welfare did not proceed smoothly and debates occurred about what were the most appropriate methods for bringing about change and also about the speed of change necessary.

Over time, as we shall see in this book, the objectives of welfare modernisation changed from the simple eradication of the tsarist legacy to the desire to create a Soviet welfare state that was far superior to its Western counterparts. Moreover, as Stalinism developed apace the goal was to use welfare as a tool to ensure that the Soviet Union was able to catch up and overtake the West in economic and technological terms. However, as this book demonstrates, the failure to prioritise welfare initially under NEP, then Stalin, and thereby ensure that it kept pace with Soviet modernisation drives elsewhere, especially in the economy, had adverse knock on effects, which put severe constraints on the ability of the Soviet state to cater for the needs of the collective. In the long-term, as the later chapters show, Soviet welfare never truly recovered from this lack of priority, economies and its Stalinist legacy, as the Nazi's invaded in 1941 and Leningrad was faced with a siege lasting 900 days until 1944.

According to C. A. E. Winslow, Professor of the Yale Medical School 'In spite of advances made in the great cities, the rural population of Russia lived and died practically without medical care'[63] and in Nikolai Semashko, Soviet Russia's First Health Minister, view:

> The tsarist government left Soviet power a terrible heritage of unsanitary conditions. The exceptionally bad material conditions of the working masses of town and country, the police oppression which stifled all public activity, the merciless exploitation of the workers and poorer peasants, the low cultural level of the population and the consequent low sanitary culture, all combined to create a favourable soil for epidemic diseases among the population.[64]

These verdicts show the extent of the difficulty facing the Bolsheviks when they took power in October 1917. From the outset, Soviet leaders and Marxist theoreticians saw pre-1917 welfare provision as backward and exploitative. Thus Maistrakh noted how 'tsarist health care lacks uniformity of plan or method of operation'.[65] The reasons why this occurred, according to Russian Marxists, were first, a lack of a centralised medical service because each tsarist Ministry had its own medical divisions which competed with various religious, philanthropic and public organisations; second, the fact that health and welfare provision was unevenly distributed across the Russian Empire and among social classes; and, finally, although welfare was provided by dedicated zemstvo and other staff, they were over-stretched and poorly funded by the Tsarist government. Above all, following Marx and Lenin the new Soviet government believed that the environment and Capitalism in particular, created ill health. Lenin and the Bolsheviks were fully aware that Russia's pre-revolutionary health and welfare system lacked the infrastructure and resources to combat epidemics, hunger, a high death and infant mortality rate, and it was not in a position to reverse the falling birth rate.[66]

It was against this background that Lenin embarked upon his modernisation of Russian welfare policy. In Semashko's words, this was to be based on 'a radical revolution in order to bring about order out of the chaos'.[67] The strategy put in place involved a reorganisation 'of the entire public health system both in the principles on which it was based, in its organisation and its practical aspects, along entirely new lines'.[68] The new Leninist principles of health and welfare included: state responsibility for public health – hence greater state interventionism, the development of public health within the framework of a single plan (not really discussed until the 1920s and put in place until after 1928), centralisation of health care, provision of free and comprehensive medical aid, an emphasis on preventive medicine (with a belief in the impact of 'environment') and unity of theory and practice.

On 26 October 1917, the first step in this direction was taken and the medico-sanitary department of the Military-Revolutionary committee of the Petrograd Soviet was set up. It was run by M. I. Barsukov and B. N. Bonch-Bruevich, assisted by A. N. Vinokursov, S. I. Mitskevich and others.[69] The aim was to reorganise the medical service in Petrograd.[70] As a result of the economic collapse and the chaos, this department was unable to function properly. In November 1917, calls were made for local medico-sanitary departments to be attached to local Soviets (Councils) of Workers, Peasants and Soldiers deputies.[71]

The Bolshevik leadership had its own notions and ideas of developing and implementing a health policy that sought to protect the collective, but in the absence of sufficient resources, distribution and supply problems in relation to food, fuel and problems providing hygienic and sanitary housing, this idea of a socialist health service, which was captured in the term 'Communism' was more of a theory and rhetoric from 1917–20, due to the circumstances of the civil war.

Under Tsarism, responsibility for public health was divided between the zemstvo and various Ministries of the Interior, Education, Finance, Justice, Trade and Industry, Navy and Army, and other government departments and committees. This dispersal of medical facilities across a wide range of state, social, private and philanthropic organisations, led to shortages of funds but most importantly to uncoordinated medical services and provision. This did little to protect the health of the non-wealthy sections of society, or what the Soviets called the 'collective'. Lenin favoured a central single unified health care organisation would could administer public health affairs throughout Soviet Russia but he acknowledged that conditions immediately after the October 1917 Revolution made such a move impractical. Lenin, therefore advocated, in early 1918, the creation of local public health sections. This approach culminated in the formation of a Council of Medical Boards (*Sovet vrachebnykh kollegii*) which was responsible for monitoring progress towards this goal.[72]

The first local medical section to come into being was the Petrograd health service (*Kommissariata zdravookhraneniia Petrogradskoi trudovoi kommuny*) on 24 March 1918.[73] According to Sigal and Bazanov, the aim of this medical organisation was to create a comprehensive health service network in the city to meet the population's needs.[77] A former member of the Council of Medical Boards, Evgenii Porif'evich Pervykhin, was made head of the Petrograd health service, following a Sovnarkhom meeting, held on 24 March 1918.[74]

Regarding the first principle of the new Soviet health care system, Semashko declares 'the organisation of prophylactic and medical aid for the population of the USSR is regarded as one of the basic duties of the state.

Medical care is not to be left, as it was before the Revolution, to private charitable institutions or to private enterprise'.[75] As a result, the State was given sole responsibility for public health and welfare in order to overcome past Tsarist deficiencies. This new health system was based upon two guiding principles: *nationalisation*, whereby private ownership was to be abolished and state control implemented, and *municipalisation*, which meant increased local government control over health and welfare.

At a meeting on 6 April 1918, Pervykhin called for the introduction of a state-controlled health service in Petrograd containing seven departments: hospitals, sanitation, pharmaceutical, veterinary, statistics, administration and military (Red Guards and Army).[76] His plans were given the official go ahead at a Council of Medical Boards session of 16 May 1918.[77]

This was a time of constant reorganisations and so the Petrograd health service became the Commissariat of Public Health for the Northern Region (*Soiuza Severnoi Oblast'*). Now the Petrograd health service was responsible for meeting the needs of residents from Petrograd, Pskov, Olonets, Vologda, Archangel, Novgorod and Cherepovets provinces.[78] This was an extremely large area which undoubtedly put a great strain on resources. The Petrograd health service retained this form until July 1919 when it became the city of Petrograd public health department (*Petrogradskoi gorodskoi otdel zdravookhraneniia*). Subsequently in October 1920, it was reorganised once more into the Petrograd provincial public health department (*Petrogradskii gubzdravotdel*).[79] These changes were a product of the civil war and Bolshevik ideology.

The Petrograd health service attempted to introduce a socialist health policy which pledged itself to disease prevention via mass programmes in hygiene and prophylaxis. Thus one article on 'The socialisation of medicine' published in *Petrogradskaia Pravda* on 12 October 1918 declared:

> Our aim is to encourage the population to get involved in public health matters; to provide free health care and to carry out fundamental reform in all medical areas. These reforms seek to eliminate the problems facing urban and rural medicine; to provide more doctors and to nationalise all medico-sanitary establishments, such as hospitals, sanatoria, bacteriological units, pharmacies, laboratories and so forth.[80]

These are very close to overall principles of Soviet medicine on which Narkomzdrav (the Ministry of Public Health) was later founded on 11 July 1918.[81] The Petrograd Health service came into being 3 months before Narkomzdrav and Bazanov maintains that the creation of the Petrograd Health Service played a significant role in the eventual establishment of Narkomzdrav. He states 'the organisation of the Soviet health service in Petrograd was utilised when the People's Commissariat of Public Health, RSFSR, was founded'.[82] From early 1918, Pervykhin, the head of the Petrograd Health service, as a member of the Council of Medical Boards, had been privy to early discussions regarding the foundation of Narkomzdrav, and eventually on 14 June 1918, Pervykhin alongside Z. P. Solov'ev put forward proposals regarding Narkomzdrav. These were discussed in depth at the First All-Russian Congress on Medico-Sanitary departments on 15 June 1918.[83] The discussions indicate the extent to which Narkomzdrav was willing to follow Petrograd's example.[84] Solov'ev was in favour of a central public health administration as this organ would be able to coordinate all medical affairs by setting tasks for all departments and commissions to attain. This would also facilitate the coordination of medical and scientific research, with the assistance of the Scientific Medical Council[85] and by exercising strict financial control. Pervykhin wanted a leading organ of Soviet medicine in order to achieve greater unity. To achieve this objective, Narkomzdrav needed to be based on collective and corporate principles, which involved the service being run at managerial level by specialists from all fields of medical inquiry, with each representing the interests of their department and staff. The retention of individuality (*individual'nost'*) was in Pervykhin's opinion, vital to Narkomzdrav's success.[86] It was this clear qualification of the principle of centralisation which distinguished the two approaches. In the end Solov'ev's proposal was accepted rather than Pervykhin's (probably out of fear of too much autonomy)[87] and on 14 July 1918, a Sovnarkhom decree approved the setting up of Narkomzdrav.[88]

Thereafter the ties between Narkomzdrav and the Petrograd health service grew stronger. Two indications of this are Pervykhin's election onto the Narkomzdrav Board on 21 July 1918 and D. K. Zabolotnyi's nomination onto Narkomzdrav's Scientific Medical Council.[89] These appointments led Leonov and Bazanov to assert that under Pervykhin's leadership the Petrograd health service played a key role in realising Narkomzdrav's objectives during the War Communism period.[90] In this context, Semashko, speaking at the First Congress of Medico-Sanitary departments of the Northern Region in November, commended the Petrograd health service for its excellent work in defending the city and in assigning the Red Army priority in medical services. Later, at a Narkomzdrav Board meeting on 18 February 1919, Semashko declared: 'We recognise the necessity not only of maintaining this organisation, but also of expanding its activities in view of Petrograd's importance as a scientific and medical centre'.[91]

Narkomdrav officials retained their interest in the Petrograd Health service after the civil war. In fact, a symbiotic relationship seems to have existed between the two organisations throughout the 1920s, as shown by Pervykhin's appointment as Head of the Administrative department at Narkomzdrav in 1923.[92]

For the Petrograd Health service to be a dependable institution which was capable of contributing to health provision and disease prevention, each sub-section and/or department had to evolve and develop in such a way that it became an integral part of the entire Petrograd health service. Roles had to be assigned and staff training offered. But most of all, Petrograd health service activities had to be well coordinated by the relevant local and central bodies, in order to operate as efficiently and effectively as possible in the midst of a civil war, good communication channels were therefore essential, together with the necessary finance and resources. The main problem during the civil war was that no well-developed philosophy of medicine had been devised by the Petrograd Bolsheviks, only broad operational principles. In line with the transfer of responsibility for public health to the state, for example, private practice or the operation of charities, in theory, was not permitted. The introduction of a city wide centralised medical system was aimed at organising medical care more efficiently by distributing both medical personnel and resources to the neediest areas and parts of the collective.[93] However, economic and political constraints, prevented these goals from being fully achieved in the period up to 1920 and also prevented the state from having total control over all medical resources. Hence, private practice still existed into the 1920s.

The second guiding principle, the development of all public health services in accordance with a plan, was not implemented under War Communism, but discussed during the New Economic policy period and then put in place from the very late 1920s onwards. This will be dealt with in Chapter 4. Both the aforementioned two principles were inter-connected and involved turning private health establishments into publicly owned ones that were run at a local level.

The possibility of legalising pharmacies had been debated when the 1912 social insurance legislation was enacted, but the reform was never implemented due to the outbreak of the First World War. This transfer never got underway until the municipalisation of all private pharmacies was approved by the City Duma (*Petrogradskaia gorodskaia duma*) in January 1918[94], with management responsibility passing onto the Pharmaceutical Commission (*Aptechnoi komissii*) in March 1918.[95] In the same month, the Pharmaceutical Department was formed. Its main tasks, together with the Commission, were to oversee the nationalisation of pharmacies, train cadres, set drugs prices (providing them free wherever possible) and regulate their supply to different social groups and areas of Petrograd, as well as eliminate the black market in drugs and to prevent strikes.[96] Given the prevailing circumstances, many of these objectives were not attained.

The third modernisation principle – open and free access to health care – was geared towards making access to health care based not on class or ability to pay but on need. For a whole range of reasons from War Communism, throughout NEP and into the Stalinist era, this principle was never strictly adhered to. 'Class' was an important determinant of access, at least until the mid-1930s, but fees of one sort or another always applied. For instance, drugs were only available free to pupils and teachers, the insured and industrial workers.[97]

A drugs shortage[98] existed partly because of the civil war blockade. In October 1919, for example, the Pharmaceutical Society was producing two million tablets and 300,000 pills daily, but this was insufficient to meet demand.[99] Unfortunately production was slow and supply quotas remained unfulfilled. According to some estimates, the Petrograd pharmaceutical department only fulfilled 40% of its orders in 1919.[100] Furthermore, although by 1920, Petrograd was receiving 10% of the Soviet government's drug supplies, the widespread epidemics discussed above, drained drug resources quickly.[101]

Further problems included the fact that training was of poor quality;[102] staff were also in short supply and drugs were marketed before the necessary quality control had been carried. As a consequence, diseases continued to spread because poor control measures rendered some drugs ineffective.[103] Finally, any attempts to eradicate privately owned (*chasnovadel'skii*) chemists, only met with limited success. Thus one delegate speaking at a Congress of Medico-sanitary departments, Northern Region in November 1918, declared that 'the process of eliminating the extremely large number of private pharmacies and transferring them from private hands to the State was too slow'.[104]

In the end, a sustained nationalisation programme and rationalisation reduced the number of pharmacies in Petrograd from 600 in June 1918 to only 174 by 1920.[105] This process began in earnest in early 1919, when the Russian Society for Trading in Pharmaceutical goods and other private pharmacies (such as Stol' and Shmidt, Shaskol'skii, Gofman and Buller) were all nationalised.[106] Mary Schaeffer Conroy argues in relation to pharmacies, for instance, that this new policy led to conflicts between staff and the new management of the municipalised pharmacies over how these new establishments would be run and also over pay and work hours. Shortages of staff in some areas such as Petrograd further hampered things. In the end, calls were made in the case of pharmacies for a transfer of ownership not from private to local but to central authorities, a move resisted in Petrograd.[107]

The Pharmacy Employees Union (*Soiuza sluzhaschikh v aptekakh*) was asked to play a key role by unifying all pharmacy workers (private and State employees) together. A meeting was held on 16 February 1920 to discuss the merger with the Union of Medical Workers (*Soiuz medrabotnikov*).[108] However, conflicts broke out. Members of the communist faction within the Union of Pharmaceutical Workers (*Soiuz aptechnykh rabotnikov*), for example, argued that unification was in everyone's interests but Mensheviks disagreed arguing this was not feasible as both unions represented different groups and did not share common goals or policies. When a vote was taken, only three were against and proposal was approved. Menshevik members were criticised for opposing the new regime.[109]

It is interesting to note, that in fact many members of the Petrograd branch of the Union of Medical workers were non-Party affiliated. This applied to 102 out of 230 (44.4%) members in February 1920 and to a larger proportion of members by October 1920 – 173 out of 234 (74%). Newspaper reports at the time, nevertheless, pointed out that a limited number of medical workers retained Menshevik opinions which created disagreements on health policy. On top of the problems highlighted earlier, this difference of political opinion hampered the Petrograd health service from introducing socialist principles in the early years of Soviet power. Nevertheless, despite these challenges, the Petrograd Medical workers Union was now in a position to set up a Pharmacy section.[110]

The hospital department of the Petrograd health service was a site at which peasants, workers and other key members of the new collective experienced Soviet health care directly. At the time of the 1917 October Revolution, hospitals in war torn Petrograd were in a general state of disrepair. By 1918, there were fewer hospitals than in 1913 (down from 352 to 75) but the number of hospital beds was slightly higher (701 more). More importantly the ratio of beds per 10,000 population (due to the population decline discussed above) witnessed a three-fold increase (see Table 2.5).

It was conditions within the hospitals themselves that was the major issue during the civil war. Thus Dr Shamov of the Military-Medical Academy pointed out that by 1920:

> the stock of surgical instruments which had not been renewed since 1917, got so outworn that many could no longer be used. Often one had to work for many months in the operating room with one curved needle and one pair of forceps. There was also a lack of gloves, silk sutures and surgical dressings.... Silk sutures were replaced by common thread, and even this was difficult to get. In order to economise surgical dressings were washed over and over again, but this could not be done systematically, owing to the irregularity of laundry pick-ups.[111]

Such a situation meant that it was difficult to perform surgery, stitch up injuries and to ensure that those undergoing surgery had their wounds dressed in a hygienic way. Additional challenges included the fact that X-ray machines could not be used because no tubes or plates were available which might have hindered effective diagnosis. Given the pharmaceutical issues detailed above, drugs were not always available to hospital patients in civil

Table 2.5 Number of hospitals and beds in St Petersburg and Petrograd, 1913–20

Year	Number of hospitals	Hospitals per 10,000 population	Number of Hospital beds	Hospital beds per 10,000 population
1913	352	1.66	19,984	93.6
1914	113	0.51	20,838	94.0
1915	74	0.32	20,022	86.5
1918	88	0.60	29,618	201.6
1919	101	1.13	27,723	308.0
1920	75	1.02	20,685	279.5

Source: *Statisticheskii materialy po sostoianiiu narodnogo zdraviia i organizatsii meditsinskoi pomoshchi v SSSR za 1913–1923gg* (Moscow "Narkomzdrav" 1926), 82–83, 86–87

war Petrograd. Other problems facing hospital doctors were far more basic, as simple but essential things like hot water or soup were lacking.[112]

Prior to 1917, many hospitals were either run by the church, attached to factories (though only 7 by 1917) or under the jurisdiction of the medical funds (*kassy*) as we saw in the previous chapter. These Tsarist charity, church and kassy hospitals were nationalised in March 1918. Hospital doctors and other medical personnel opposed this and went on strike. A Hospital Council (*Bol'nichnyi Sovet*) was formed to deal with staff problems, food norms and strikes.[113] Furthermore, a hospital commission (*Bol'nichnaia komissiia*) investigated food supplies, fuel, the provision of medical equipment etc to ensure that supply, wherever possible, met demand.[114] Both the Hospital Council and commission were under the jurisdiction of the Petrograd health service hospital department[115] which in turn carried out repairs, distributed medical supplies, linen, beds etc and monitored the living and working conditions of hospital medical staff.[116] Given the general disruption and turmoil, it was not always easy to fulfil these goals. Dr Shamov of the Military-Medical Academy notes:

> At the time of the fuel crisis nearly all the hospital heating was discontinued ... the immense windows, even though double, were covered by ice ... which when thawing, overflowed into the operating room; the wet putty, and the stucco on the walls cracked and fell off in bits. During the winter of 1918–19, when the population had not yet adapted itself to the struggle with the cold, the temperature went to 6° or 8° below zero.[117]

The fuel shortages outlined above led to hospital closures putting increased pressure on existing facilities. Even though beds were reserved for infectious disease patients,[118] unfortunately people were treated in hospitals that lacked food and basic medical supplies. Unhygienic conditions also helped to spread disease. Dr Grekov of the Obukh hospital in Petrograd states:

> A physician who worked here in 1913, visiting the same place in 1917 would hardly recognise it, so changed were the surroundings and patients. The corridors were dirty, the floors falling in, the ceilings and walls damp, black and mouldy; the air so saturated with the exhalations of patients and the odour of purulent wounds. The patients were extremely emaciated or oedematous and very pale and yellow, and in the throws of agony; and then nurses and physicians stalked like ghosts.[119]

Following the abolition of the hospital council due to a 'great number of mistakes'[120] the hospital sector was reorganised in mid-1919 to facilitate expansion and to enable a more even distribution of hospitals throughout Petrograd.[121] In addition, in early 1920 new accounting methods were introduced to increase efficiency and improve the quality of hospital administration which was now under Party and trade union control.[122] In this context, in late January 1919, hospital staff were elected committee members of the Union of Medical Workers in Petrograd.[123] This was all part of a strategy geared towards incorporating the old bourgeois medical profession into the new social order. Political commissars were frequently appointed to hospital posts during the civil war. For instance, they held posts at the Forel central psychiatric hospital, the Smol'nyi hospital for the chronically ill and the Novoznamenskii psychiatric hospital. Party cells, under the auspice of communist workers, were also opened at this time. The Erismann hospital had one such cell with 13 members and the Obukhov also had one with 16 members. These Party figures were largely junior medical and administrative staff.[124] The low-ranking nature of Party cell medical personnel is important suggesting that they were relatively recent recruits to the socialist cause rather than well-established former Tsarist officials who were viewed as politically suspect.[125]

Pervykhin himself advocated the setting up of the Petrograd health service maternity department (*Otdel okhrany materinstva i mladenchestva*) in November 1918 and this was followed by a Council for the Protection of Women and Infants (*Sovet okrany materinstva i mladenchestva*) on 3 December 1918.[126] The maternity department was made up largely of midwives, gynaecologists and paediatricians and their role was to monitor women's health before and after pregnancy, to combat infant mortality, combat prostitution, reduce illness and death among women and children from tuberculosis, venereal diseases etc and to set up a series of maternity departments and to monitor school sanitation and hygiene.[127] According to Alexandra Kollontai, the aim of this department was to move 'the burden of motherhood' from the shoulders of women onto the collective'.[128] The setting up of the maternity department was not just there to assist women it was also geared towards reducing the infant mortality rate (IMR) shown in Table 2.6.

The number of infant deaths rose from 9,421 in 1897 to 13,141 in 1916 then, after the October Revolution, the number of infant deaths fell from 10,459 in 1917 to 3,002 in 1920. Using the adjusted infant mortality rate per 100 births, the level rose slightly from 27.0 to 28.9 between 1897–1916, falling thereafter from 24.1 in 1917 to 20.9 in 1920. Population undernourishment and maternal illness during pregnancy were undoubtedly

Table 2.6 Infant mortality rate in St. Petersburg and Petrograd, 1897–1920

Year	Number of deaths in age group 0–1 year	Official infant mortality rate per 100 live births	Adjusted* infant mortality rate per 100 live births
1897	9,421	26.5	27.0
1913	12,972	23.1	23.6
1914	13,704	24.7	25.2
1915	13,165	25.3	25.8
1916	13,144	28.4	28.9

(continued)

Table 2.6 Infant mortality rate in St. Petersburg and Petrograd,
1897–1920 (continued)

Year	Number of deaths in age group 0–1 year	Official infant mortality rate per 100 live births	Adjusted* infant mortality rate per 100 live births
1917	10,459	23.6	24.1
1918	6,780	26.4	27.1
1919	4,980	31.4	31.9
1920	3,002	20.4	20.9

Note: *Allowances have been made for differences in definition as Soviet scholars exclude infants of less than 28 weeks gestation, 1000g in weight, 35cm in length and those who die within 7 days (UN Population and Vital Statistics Report, Statistical Report Series A, Volume 21, No. 3, 1969, footnote 22, 7). An adjustment was made in this column by multiplying the official figure by a factor of 1.00617 and adding 4.8 infant deaths per 1,000 live births. This formula is taken from P. D. Mazur, 'Expectancy of live at birth in 36 nationalities in the Soviet Union, 1958-60', Population Studies, Volume 23, No. 2, July 1969, footnote 24, 230
Sources: Statisticheskii sbornik po Petrogradu i Petrogradskoi gubernii (Petrograd 1922), 15; Z. I. Frenkel', Petrograd perioda voiny i revoliutsii: Sanitarnoe usloviia i kommunal'noe blagoustroistvo (Petrograd 1923), 21 and Statisticheskii spravochnik po gor. Leningradu 1930 (Izd. Leningradskogo oblispolkoma 1930), 29

contributory factors. The adjusted infant mortality rate was highest in 1919, also a year of food rationing, which is no coincidence. Abortions may have also damaged the female reproductive system and poor housing – impure drinking water, low levels of hygiene and a lack of basic amenities – could also have affected the IMR.

The notion of 'preventive medicine' (the fourth aspect of Lenin's welfare modernisation strategy) occupied a central place at the start, with Semashko remarking that '[p]rophylactic measures are the basis of the entire health service'.[129] The aim was to prevent disease rather than cure it. In line with this philosophy, a comprehensive series of measures were gradually introduced to prevent the spread of disease. Using the discipline of social hygiene (sotsial'naia gigiena)[130] which was defined by Semashko as 'the study of the harmful influence of social factors on the health status of the population and their eradication'[131], the prevention of disease, in this case with regard to women and children, was achieved by eliminating factors at work, at home or in relation to the individual themselves. As Semashko explained in 1927, 'preventive medicine involves not simply the treatment of disease, but more important it involves rendering the population healthy by eradicating the causes of disease at source'.[132]

For Russian medical experts and Marxists – poor housing, sanitation, environmental pollution, diet and difficult working conditions (poor ventilation, light and the absence of safety measures) – all caused ill-health. In this case, Dr Antonova believed that the lifestyles of mothers (high alcohol consumption, heavy smoking, a past history of venereal disease, a record of mental illness), mother and midwives lack of knowledge of a young baby's diet, physiology and need for correct feeding, are all major factors creating a high infant mortality rate.[133]

Health propaganda advised women that it was a mother's role to care for the baby, to feed it at the right times[134] but also as we shall see in later chapters, mothers were also expected to bathe, keep their children warm and above all free of any negative environmental factors. In this way women and children as key members of society, protected the collective and the future of the state and nation as they guaranteed the healthy upbringing of Soviet children. This was also part of the construction of motherhood[135] and the medical profession played a key role in generating Soviet models of childrearing thereby shaping the collective identities of women and this visual material became part of the literature used by Lenin and Stalin to give advice and, in the process, redefine the 'body Soviet'.

To support women, the Maternity Council introduced a number of policies. Midwifery schools were reorganised and courses restructured;[136] obstetrical and midwifery points and maternity homes were also reorganised in April 1919 with the express intention of preventing infant deaths and closely monitoring mothers in pre and post-natal phases.[137] Closer cooperation also took place between maternity and children's homes, women's consultation clinics (*konsul'tatsiia dlia veremennykh*) and pregnant women's refugees (*ubezhishcha dlia veremennykh normal'nykh i patologicheskikh*).[138] Advice was also given on habits harmful to women or children's health, such as heavy alcohol consumption or smoking.[139] Some efforts in these areas, however, was hampered by a shortage of trained staff and facilities. Thus the number of maternity hospitals fell from 31 with 1,161 beds in 1913 to 21 with 838 beds by 1918. Fewer patients were admitted with the number declining from 37,510 in 1913 to 15,027 in 1918 before falling further to 2,404 in 1921.[140] To try and rectify these difficulties, children's prophylactic units (*detskikh profilakticheskikh ambulatorii*) were created. The first one emerged in 1917 and by 1920, Petrograd possessed seven children's prophylactic units.[141] In addition, kindergartens and women and children's health points were set up. The maternity network was therefore, firmly established by the end of 1920. The Petrograd health service maternity department had 26 units across the city, six baby homes, eight baby units, two mothers and infants homes, 23 crèches and 23 maternity homes staffed by 345 children's doctors and 215 medical personnel.[142] It was clear that women's and children's health was a priority and that as a result the volume of child deaths and the infant mortality rate was lower in 1920 than in 1913, and as we shall see in the next chapter, this decline continued on into the 1920s.

The military medicine department was founded in September 1918 to ensure that the Red Army and Baltic Fleet received the necessary medical services and supplies after the civil war began.[143] Its staff tended to be military personnel or political commissars and its work covered the entire Northern Region offering the sick and wounded, medical assistance and combating counter-revolutionary activity to defend Petrograd between 1918–20.[144]

Other departments included health statistics which was set up in January 1919 with the aim of collecting and developing a classification system to rank and identify illnesses and deaths from specific diseases.[145] The School Hygiene department, with the help of the Commissariat of Education (*Narkompros*) monitored health conditions in schools and the health status of the pupils.[146] The legal section which gave advice on medical issues, liaised with the medical expertise section (*otdel meditsinskoi ekspertizy*) and trained various medical experts including judicial doctors (*sudebnoi vrachei*).[147]

The health education department, existed to boost people's awareness of basic hygiene and sanitation (via health education lectures and materials), to educate them about the nature and availability of health services and to offer advice on following government guidelines.[148] We will use some of the posters produced by Narkomzdrav throughout this book. In this context, David Hoffman points out that 'The October Revolution had seemingly wiped away everything from the past, including all pre-existing morals and values'.[149] What this book shows is that whilst the new Soviet government hoped this was the case and hence they could enthusiastically set about creating a New Soviet Person, in reality it was far from easy for the government under either Lenin or Stalin to instil socialist values in all members of society.

In relation to the themes explored, the goal was the establishment of health 'norms' that governed hygienic attitudes, drinking, sexual behaviour and child raising to name but a few areas, with collective values promoted through official speeches, in the press, medical journals and above all in health propaganda posters. The aim was to inculcate the values of cleanliness, sobriety and motherhood, for example, and to use the above principles to overcome the backwardness left by the tsarist regime, not just in terms of provision but in health values. Hoffman argues that the goal was 'to civilise the lower classes and create a more perfect society'.[150] Victoria Bonnell believes that the key attributes of these posters were that the messages were clear and positive and they offered advice in relation to health related matters in the context of combating certain diseases whilst trying to build socialism.[151] We must remember however that there were changes over time in terms of the images used but the goal remained the same, namely to create, in Christopher Read's words, the 'correct consciousness' and sanitary 'enlightenment'.[152] Read concludes that the goal of Soviet health policy was 'to win over the ordinary population not just to its policies but equally important to its values'.[153] This required the use of Party members and health propaganda to spread the 'party's slogans and decisions to the masses' and to ensure that the so-called 'consciousness gap' was plugged by Soviet institutions and organisations.[154]

In the context of this book, the emphasis in the Petrograd/Leningrad health education department's work was on the dangers of different types of behaviour and its consequences for the individual and more importantly, the collective as a whole, society and the Soviet system. This centred around the development of a greater consciousness and a more cultured approach (*kul'turnost'*) to public health matters by ensuring that members of the collective protected their own bodies, and that of the nation, by following the new Soviet regime's advised 'correct' hygienic habits at home and at work as projected in Soviet health education posters and propaganda.

Health norms where set by the government through official discourses regarding what was or was not acceptable behaviour. Lenin and Stalin's policies used this approach to devise a new civilised health culture to achieve the desired social transformation through the establishment of health models for the masses to follow. The aim of Soviet leaders was to change people's health habits, attitudes, desires and above all their way of life (*byt*) and to do this, as this book shows, hygiene and health education campaigns were launched throughout the Soviet period covered in this book.

There were many attempts to enlighten Petrograd and Leningrad workers and peasant migrants and some members of society conformed to this health code of conduct, either partially or superficially, at least in public, whilst other members of society rejected these official health norms and were seen and portrayed as a threat to nation, society and communist values. In the latter case, offenders' behaviour was sometimes defined as 'bourgeois', 'decadent' or deemed to be influenced by 'class enemies' because the population of the city failed to adhere to the new socialist health values and thinking and instead of following the spirit of collectivism fostered by the Soviet state and facilitating the creation of a new, healthy Soviet Person, one with collectivist consciousness, some people's health behaviour threatened the 'body Soviet'.

It was not just the Soviet state who had responsibly for people's health, the citizens of Petrograd and Leningrad were expected to transform themselves, to eradicate any backward attitudes to hygiene, sex, drinking, feeding and upbringing children and to reorganise their lives using the new communal housing, dining halls and nurseries provided by the state. Communist Party members, as the vanguard who led the country, were expected to be role models for other members of society to follow. They were not supposed to get drunk, be careerists, focus on their own personal enrichment and Party members were supposed to speak, dress and behave with decorum. If the Party activists were a 'bad' example, then how could they credibly police themselves and above all carry out sanitary surveillance amongst society.

This raises important questions about what is 'proper' conduct, or health behaviour, and what is not. It will become clear throughout the following chapters that citizens in the Soviet state who are defined as 'unhygienic' or 'corrupt' tended to be those who are viewed as 'backward' and it was argued that these people had not as yet eradicated their 'traditional' 'bourgeois' or 'Capitalist' tendencies, the remnants of Capitalism from the pre-1917 period. These individuals were nevertheless breaking the new health norms by excessive drinking, engaging in what was deemed to be 'immoral' sexual behaviour and conducting lifestyles that were seen by the state, and some health officials, as a deviation, which in turn created medical disorder, 'moral degeneration' and the actions of these individuals was said to corrupt others over time. As we shall see, in Chapter 4, by the 1930s, such patterns of health behaviour were increasing equated with political unreliability, brought into question people's loyalty to the collective and these dangerous individuals were said to endanger the state itself, as the unhealthy had started to associate with or be influenced by class enemies whose lifestyles and behaviour were deemed unacceptable and inappropriate.

In addition to the health education department of the Petrograd health service, there was also a dentistry department which provided dental care to adults and children in state establishments.[155] Various medical supply units distributed fuel, food and boiled water, supplied hospitals and other establishments with medical instruments and equipment, combated theft and misappropriation and generally sort to cut down wastage and loss, wherever possible.[156] The scientific section of the Petrograd health service examined the need for ordinary and capital repairs, construction projects etc and then allocated funds and monitored their use to ensure they were utilised in the correct way and for the right purpose.[157] Repair disinfection brigades carried out purification work on at railway stations and on boats[158] and the sanitary transport division provided basic and emergency medical facilities to transfer the seriously ill or wounded to hospitals. However, because of the fuel difficulties outlined above, staff relied not only on motorised vehicles but on horses wherever possible.[159] The general kontrol' section checked, inspected and monitored the work of all departments in the Petrograd health service and with the help of the control-inspection commission (*kontrol'no-inspektsionnaia komissiia*), staff tried to ensure via spot checks and audits (*revizii*) that each and every department was running as efficiently and effectively as possible under the adverse conditions prevailing.[160]

At this point, we will discuss the role of the medical funds in Petrograd's public health system during War Communism in view of the importance of factory (*zavodskaia*) and insurance medicine (*strakhovaia meditsina*) in the 1920s and beyond.

Factory medicine

On 12 December 1917, new regulations were drawn up regarding the Council of Workers Insurance (*Sovet po delam strakhovaniia rabochikh*) and workers' representatives made up 32 out of the 48 members.[161] A decree of 22 December 1917 transferred responsibility for medical care for the insured to the medical funds (*kassy*) which were funded from worker contributions.[162] Nine days later, another decree was issued which placed the management of the kassy in workers' hands enabling them to elect their own representatives and set up their governing body.[163] This was clearly in line with the drive for workers' control in industry in Petrograd.[164] When the elections were actually held on 24 January 1918, 25 workers' representatives were elected out of the 48; 19 came from the insured, one each from the Central TUC, Central Council on Factory Committees and the Society of Mill and Factory Owners and three from the Ministry of Labour (*Narkomtrud* of NKT for short). No representatives were put forward from the agricultural committees, the People's Commissariat of Justice, city administrations, doctors or lawyers. In the end, Osipov was elected President, Podzrin and Gogelev his assistants and Fedorov, the Secretary of this Insurance council.[165] However, factory owners still refused to provide the necessary funds to set up the city kassy, despite a January 1918 Ministry of Labour ruling to this effect. Despite this resistance, sickness funds were merged into general city kassy in January 1918 and henceforth they handled a heavier workload – sickness, accident and unemployment insurance – following the introduction of these forms of social insurance in late 1917–early 1918.[166] At the Third Petrograd Insurance Conference on 2–3 January 1918, contributions from the wage bill were set as follows: 10% of wage to cover illness; 4% for old age; 3% for invalidity and unemployment and 2% for maiming.[167]

Petrograd's network of medical facilities for the insured expanded rapidly. In the first six months of Soviet rule, 49 medical establishments and 100 medical points were opened by workers' kassy. These included a therapeutic-pediatric institution, a summer sanatorium for TB sufferers, a clinic for VD patients, maternity homes, 20 pharmacies and a central pharmaceutical warehouse.[168] By the end of 1918, Petrograd's insurance medicine network was staffed by 500 doctors, 150 feldshers, 400 nurses and orderlies and 100 pharmacists. High standards regarding facilities were set. These included one bed per 100 kassy members; one doctor per 25 kassy patients; the location of out-patient clinics no more than 21km away; a minimum of six visits per doctor and a minimum of 6–10 patients per hour.[169]

Following a debate on whether or not the kassy were working-class or state organs, the sickness kassy were abolished in October 1918 and their functions put under the jurisdiction of the People's Commissariat of Social Security (NKSO). This measure, which was largely a response to civil war conditions, caused great friction between NKSO and Narkomzdrav because the latter had created its own medical department to deal with the insured earlier on in July 1918.[170] Subsequently, a February 1919 decree eliminated insurance medicine in favour of a more unified Soviet medicine.[171] The frequent reorganisations of social insurance and insurance medicine during the period 1917–19 shows that things did not go smoothly and also helps explain why the kassy were phased out.[172] This was, however, only a temporary setback because under NEP insurance medicine flourished again as we shall see in Chapter 3.

Finally, we shall deal with the role of the various commissions and councils in combating officially designated social diseases (tuberculosis, alcoholism and venereal diseases) in the civil war.

Social diseases

Before 1917, the fight against tuberculosis (TB) was only in an infant state, with the entire Russian Empire only having 43 TB clinics and 18 TB sanatoria with 307 beds. Anti-TB work was undertaken by the Pan-Russian League for the fight against TB, which was funded by collections and private donations. During the First World War, however, its activities were severely curtailed, so by 1917 the League largely existed on paper.[173] After October 1917, the fight against TB was renewed on a new basis. Responsibility for dealing with TB was transferred from private charities to the Soviet state. The TB department of the Petrograd health service was opened in December 1918, and it was of immense importance because TB was a major killer at this moment in time (see Table 2.7).

The number of deaths from TB increased from 7,129 cases in 1913 to 8,470 cases in 1917, falling in each year of the civil war until there were only 4,127 deaths from TB by 1920. However, the TB death rate per 10,000 population rose from 33.6 in 1913 to 36.8 by 1917 and from then on it went on increasing, reaching a peak of 55.7 per 10,000 by 1920, namely 22.1 per 10,000 higher than in 1913.

The Soviet anti-TB campaign centred around the use of health education campaigns, the organisation of dispensaries and the placement of TB patients in rest homes and health resorts located in areas with an excellent climate.[174] Treatment was guaranteed by law and available free for all insured wage earners and their families.[175] After staff (either health visitors or district nurses) had made a study of the living and working conditions of TB patients, a plan of action was devised. In the large majority of cases, this involved isolating sufferers, drawing up a special diet and giving advice on how to avoid contracting the disease. TB was said to be related to overcrowding, poor health or diet and linked to lifestyle (drug[176] or alcohol abuse) or homelessness.[177] Apart from overcrowding, which was not an issue in civil war Petrograd, all the other variables prevailed as members of the city's population potentially lived with or had contact with someone who was infected with TB. The food supply issues highlighted above meant that 'special diets' could not be guaranteed.

TB patients were often referred to sanatoria for treatment. In cases of partial work incapacity, they were treated at night sanatoria. The routine was as follows. TB patients changed clothes and went there after work. After showering they had one to two hours' rest and spent between 8–10pm relaxing

Table 2.7 Mortality rate from Tuberculosis (TB) in St. Petersburg and Petrograd, 1913–1920

Year	Number of TB cases	TB rates per 10,000 population
1913	7,129	33.6
1914	7,422	33.6
1915	8,470	35.6
1916	8,675	39.5
1917	8,470	36.5
1918	5,675	38.6
1919	4,322	48.0
1920	4,127	55.7

Sources: *XV let diktatory proletariata: Ekonomiko-statisticheskii sbornik po gor. Leningradu i Leningradskoi oblasti* (Leningrad 1932), 144 and Gert Meyer, 'Gesundheitsstatiken der stadt Leningrad (1909–1929)' in W. Beck et al, *Pax Medica: Stationen arztlichen Friedensengagements und Verirrungen arzlichten Militarismus* (VSA-Verlag, Hamburg 1986), 129

in the sanatoria club. This was the time that medication was administered. Patients then slept until 6am and after breakfast and exercise, they returned to work. Using this method, a patient's progress could be regularly monitored and treatment took an average of two to three months.[178] Separate TB facilities were also created for children who were either treated in their own sanatoria on the same basis, as for adults, between 9am–7pm or referred to doctors for a period of treatment and rest in health resorts located in Southern Russia.[179] By 1920, a special commission to combat children's TB (*Spetsial'naia komissiia po bor'be s detskim tuberkulezom*) had been set up under the able leadership of Professor V. O. Mochan.[180] Despite these efforts, TB remained a health challenge in the civil war period.

The Alcohol and Spirits Collegium played an important role, but in order to fully comprehend it we need to examine the extent of alcoholism in Petrograd and the policies used to combat it in the period from the October Revolution until the end of the civil war.

The hard life, difficult living conditions and harsh treatment at the hands of their bosses may have encouraged the local population to drink, as one observer noted:

> Vodka was the cure for poverty, cold and all human unhappiness. Half a litre of the state brand red-label cost sixpence, and the addict, as soon as he came out of the state monopoly shop, had the knack of loosening the cork by banging the bottle just above his knee, emptying the contents in one gulp and then falling with arms outspread in the snow.[181]

One survey conducted in 1910 found that 92% of male workers in St Petersburg regularly drank alcohol.[182] The Tsarist state had an alcohol monopoly and in 1913 taxes on spirits raised 93 million roubles or 5.4% of Russia's national income.[183] For both these reasons and Russia's drinking culture, Patricia Herlichy refers to Russia as an 'Alcoholic Empire'.[184] A Temperance movement and an Alcoholism Commission attached to the Russian Society for the protection of Public health emerged consisting of a wide range of groups – clergy, medical profession, members of the Duma, military etc. – and they blamed alcoholism on poverty, lack of civil rights and the absence of recreation for workers. Different professionals disagreed with one another over the cause and solution of alcoholism with some, advocating prohibition laws, rigorous policing and moral persuasion of so-called 'uncultured workers' (*nekul'turnye rabochie*); and others calling for the eradication of the bad economic and social environment detailed in Chapter 1, as it was the nature of pre-revolutionary Russia which created this social disease.[185] Many of these approaches re-emerged in the Soviet era.

Although Nicholas II banned alcohol on the eve of the First World War, this did not stop, as demonstrated in Table 2.8, the death rate from alcohol poisoning reaching 30.2 per 100,000 in 1914. The rate declined thereafter to 20.6 by 1916, so perhaps the ban and the adoption of dry areas started to have an impact. However lost revenues[186] the tendency to find and use substitutes

Table 2.8 Mortality rate from alcoholic poisoning per 100,000 population in Petrograd, 1913–1920

Year	Deaths for alcoholic poisoning
1914	30.2
1915	24.6
1916	20.6
1917	12.6
1918	6.9
1919	6.6
1920	8.6

Source: *Statisticheskii spravochnik po Leningradu 1930g* (Leningrad 1930), 36

such as moonshine (*samogon*), which also produced grain shortages, created issues not just from a health perspective but also from an economic viewpoint. Thus in September 1917, the Provisional government passed a law making it illegal to use grain for distilling.[187] Drink did not just undermine the social fabric of Russia, it also helped pushed Russia towards Revolution.

Alcohol riots took place in Petrograd in November-December 1917 as workers celebrated their victory over their former oppressors. The Bolsheviks responded by destroying alcohol stocks and closing wine outlets.[188] On 1 December 1917, the Military-Revolutionary Committee created an Alcohol and Spirits Collegium headed by G. Blagonravov, which later became part of the Petrograd Health Service, and a Committee for combating Pogroms, was also established under the leadership of V. D. Bonch-Bruevich.[189] These steps were not only taken because alcoholism was associated with the city's crime wave,[190] but because of doctors genuine concern regarding deaths from alcoholic poisoning due to excessive consumption on a low quality diet or drinking alcohol containing a high level of toxic impurities. Alcoholism was said to be so widespread because vodka was cheap and readily available in private stores.[191] To reduce production and consumption, stocks were ceased;[192] the production of moonshine was banned as of May 1918; home brewing was made a criminal offence (punishable by up to 10 years imprisonment) and distilleries were nationalised.[193] In 1918 alone, the police (*militsia*) uncovered 1,521 hidden stills.[194]

Representatives from the Ministries of Internal affairs, Justice, Labour and Finance introduced a 'Dry law' (*sukhoi zakon*) via a Sovnarkom decree on 19 December 1919 which led to the confiscation of distilling apparatus, distillers' property, to five-year sentences for those convicted and to one year's jail for intoxication in public.[195] Russian and Western scholars concur that alcohol consumption fell not so much as a result of the new law, but for practical reasons. As Neil Weissman points out, the reduction in alcohol consumption 'was the natural result of the foreign blockade and a pressing shortage of grain for distilling'.[196] In fact the 1919 legislation was largely ineffective. At best, it was sporadic and poorly enforced.[197] In all fairness, the approach was more administrative than medical. Nikolai Semashko, the Minister of Public Health, emphasised that drinking (which was deemed a 'social evil') caused ill health, divorce and falling productivity. Thus alcohol was a threat to the collective in the broadest sense. In the short term, calls were made to improve the cultural level of the masses in Petrograd via the provision of more leisure facilities,[198] with the hope in the longer term that alcoholism would be 'eliminated by the further development of socialist construction'.[199] This optimism proved unfounded because under NEP in the 1920s and Stalinism in the 1930s, anti-alcoholism campaigns were stepped up in Petrograd/Leningrad.

The last commission was that addressing the issue of venereal disease (*Komissiia po bor'be s rasprostraneniem venericheskikh zabolevanii*). The VD commission was set up in the winter of 1918 and it was attached to the Women's Medical Institute.[200] VD was not a new problem, as Semashko acknowledged when he wrote 'The tsarist regime left to the Soviet state a sordid heritage of widespread venereal disease'.[201] In this context, by 1913, the number of syphilis cases in St Petersburg stood at 49,606 and gonorrhoea cases at 39,136.[202] The overall number of venereal diseases was 33.6 per 10,000 population in 1913 rising to 36.2 in 1916, falling slightly to 35.8 in 1917 before reaching 51.0 per 10,000 by 1920.[203]

This Petrograd health service VD commission was responsible for monitoring the work of VD departments in hospitals, out-patient facilities and VD dispensaries. With the help of health education personnel, an anti-VD campaign was launched. It involved new regulations governing the registration of VD cases, a health advice programme[204] and a sustained campaign against prostitution, as prostitution was said to contribute to the growing number of cases of VD in Petrograd.[205] To reduce VD by eradicating prostitution, the goal was to draw women into the labour force, emancipate them and provide more social support and other social services.[206] Only the first of these aims was partly achieved, the second existed primarily on paper and the third fell short, as few meaningful social reforms were implemented during the War Communism period.[207]

Having previously shown how the civil war and the health problems prevailing largely shaped the structure of the Petrograd health service and the organisational changes made, it must also be acknowledged that Bolshevik ideology determined the social and collectivist principles of it. The health system was primarily shaped by the Tsarist legacy and civil war conditions.

The Petrograd medical profession: co-operation not conflict

As we saw earlier, after October 1917 the Bolsheviks wanted to implement a radical public health programme and in the midst of civil war, widespread epidemics and hunger in the period 1918–20, they needed members of the former tsarist medical profession and organisations to work with the new socialist regime. I have shown elsewhere that a range of medical professionals participated in strike activity from January 1918 to February 1919, but most of these disputes were of an economic rather than political nature centring around wages, length of working time or dismissals.[208] It was also the case, according to one estimate, that 25% of the medical profession emigrated after 1917.[209]

Soviet historians (Barsukov[210] and Zhuk[211]) and some Western experts, such as Field,[212] have interpreted this situation as evidence of bitter and irreconcilable differences between the medical profession (especially the Pirogov Society) and the new Soviet state. This view still prevails. Thus Musaev argued in 2000 that '[m]any doctors did not support the Revolution'.[213]

This book argues that such a view is exaggerated at least in Petrograd's case.[214] The argument will be advanced that the epidemics of the civil war period brought health crises to the forefront of public, state and medical profession concern. As Lenin declared at the Seventh Congress of Soviets in December 1919: 'Either the lice defeats Socialism or Socialism the lice'.[215] The seriousness of the situation is captured in Poster 2.

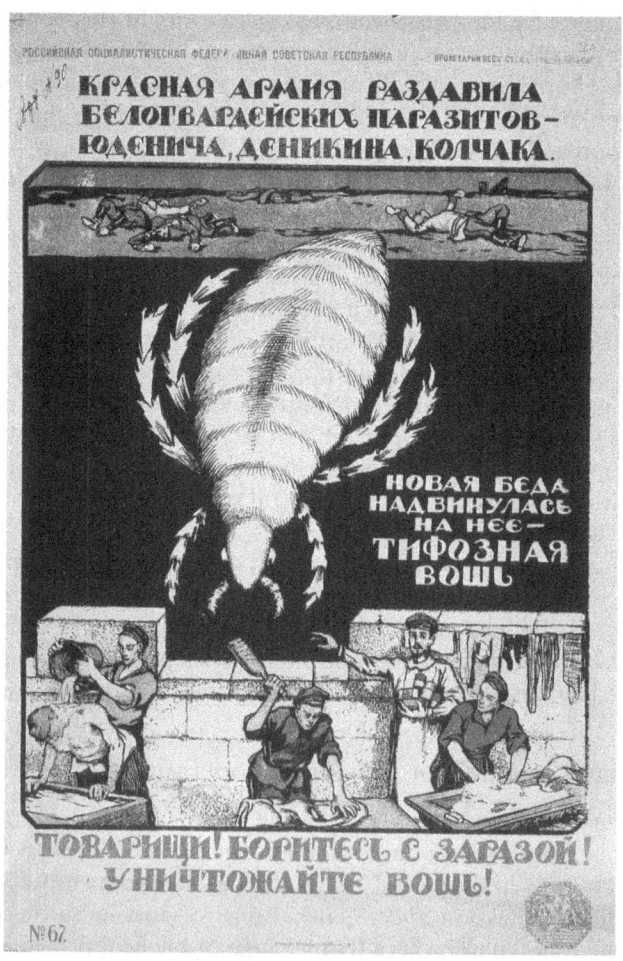

Poster 2 Anti-typhus poster, civil war period Russia

Source: 'After the defeat of the White Army, a new white peril threatens in the form of the typhus louse, against which the Red soldiers fight by washing themselves and their clothes vigorously'. Colour lithograph, c. 1921. Credit: Wellcome Collection, Wellcome Library, London (CC BY 4.0)

Poster 2 states that after the Soviet regime has successfully defeated the Whites in the civil war, a new peril, in the form of typhus, now threatens the Soviet state, and it urges the Red Army soldiers depicted to combat the louse by washing themselves and their clothes thoroughly in order to prevent the disease from spreading.

The epidemics meant that both sides – old tsarist zemstvo medical personnel and the new Soviet state – needed to cooperate and compromise. As Lenin pointed out:

> Of course, there are still doctors who regard the working-class government with prejudice and distrust and prefer to receive fees from the rich rather than throw themselves into the hard struggle against typhus, but they are in the minority, their number is growing less and less. The majority are of the kind who are willing to struggle to solve the fundamental problem of the salvation of our culture, and these doctors are devoting themselves to this hard and difficult task with as much self-sacrifice as a military specialist. They are prepared to give their strength to the promotion of the common cause.[216]

Despite political differences, former zemstvo doctors in this situation proved indispensable to the new state and were required to deal with such public health crises despite suspicions about their political reliability. As Sheila Fitzpatrick points out: 'The physicians with a strong political health orientation often had a positive attitude to state intervention and found it relatively easy to adjust to the new order'.[217]

The old medical profession and the new Soviet state both wanted some sense of stability and normality but they could not just utilize the old tsarist Ministerial structures in revised form in the case of public health as no such structure or organisation existed. The Bolsheviks and members of the old medical profession had to build a new welfare state together. In the confused civil war context, the system was not yet very centralized at least at the start and some self-governing of health and welfare was therefore still possible. It was only later in the second half of 1918–early 1919 that greater centralization started to occur, as the Bolshevik party and its medical profession allies sought to eliminate major public health crises. This situation enabled bourgeois specialists to actually participate in the revolutionary, state building process. Whilst some members of the medical profession did this for pragmatic reasons, others who had opposed the tsarist regime and its health policies did it for political reasons. But the situation is more complicated than this overall scenario suggests.

Members of the old medical profession believed in community medicine (now termed protecting the health of the collective) and so they cooperated with the new government to combat this problem. The social responsibility ethic, that had characterised the tsarist medical community, was retained when they carried on working in the Soviet period. It is also important to remember that Russian zemstvo physicians took great pride in their position as servants of the people. As S.N. Igumnov, a Pirogov Society doctor put it, the zemstvo physician

> is a community physician who satisfies the needs of broad strata of the population and who studies its sanitary condition, and not a clinician who shuts himself away in his chamber or operating room; he is a physician – sociologist who has the broad masses of population for the object of his study and activity, and not a physician-individualist who is interested in a particular sick organism.[218]

As the previous chapter showed, zemstvo doctors saw their mission as one of gradually winning the trust of peasants and workers and changing their lives (especially health and welfare) for the better. In providing medical services to the peasantry, zemstvo doctors sought to act as a link between the growing urban population and the illiterate Russian village, especially as migrant peasants arrived in relatively large numbers from the last quarter of the nineteenth century onwards in St Petersburg. The new Soviet workers' state also sought to serve the peasants and workers. So both groups had some views in common.

Furthermore, zemstvo and Soviet doctors had also witnessed poverty, illiteracy, housing problems, undernourishment (due to poor diet), a lack of hygiene, environmental pollution, widespread alcoholism, and social diseases, such as VD, tuberculosis and prostitution before 1917. Both bourgeois and Soviet doctors, though the product of different political contexts and beliefs, strongly believed that diseases were caused by the environment, so they sought to prevent disease at a group (collective) level rather than just cure the individual, as the benefits could be maximised through the use of preventive medicine.

Some sections of the Pirogov Society, like Lenin and the Bolsheviks also wanted change, as Nancy Frieden acknowledges:

> Working primarily in the public sector, they [physicians] argued that they could not prevent or control disease if the population continued to be economically and culturally deprived.... Their reputation as social reformers had become integral to the physicians' self-image as humanitarians, responsible citizens and scientific experts.... Portraying themselves as honorable citizens and advocates of the nation's welfare, the physicians began to question the ethical foundations of the tsarist state.... In effect, they questioned the regime's right to rule.[219]

The zemstvo doctors and the Soviet regime had the above and other things in common. Sanitary education and health advice literature was a feature of numerous pre-revolutionary campaigns, such as those against infant mortality[220] or alcoholism[221] and this tradition was continued in the Soviet period. This propaganda targeted what was termed the 'lower-class' before

1917 or the 'uncultured' after 1917, and this literature sought to transform so-called 'backward' groups in society and to win them over using the new Soviet propaganda state.[222] The perception of certain groups in society as 'backward' and 'ignorant' (usually but not exclusively peasants or those with 'traditional' values), prompted medical physicians and experts (former tsarist staff now working for the Soviet regime) to deploy hygiene and health propaganda that would be used as a means of overcoming the remnants of capitalism and their values after 1917. This shared progressive or civilizing framework was what also partly facilitated cooperation between the 'old' medical profession and the new regime in the early Soviet period, a point previously overlooked in Soviet historiography.

The negative view of medical profession-Soviet state relations has led historians to perhaps forget that doctors who were trained or qualified in the tsarist era wanted to fight disease and the serious cholera and typhus epidemics that prevailed in the Russian civil war. This cost many of them their lives. Thus a report of 15 June 1920 pointed out that during the Petrograd typhus epidemic the mortality rate amongst doctors (former tsarist and Soviet) was at 45–50% as against 8–9% for the general population.[223]

The 'old' and the 'new' members of the medical profession all suffered the chronic shortages of food, fuel and unhygienic housing depicted earlier, but nevertheless the Bolsheviks tried to build cooperation with the 'old' and ensure loyalty of the 'new' medical profession by putting them in a high ration categories, giving them higher pay[224] and most importantly allowing both bourgeois and pro-Soviet staff to play a leading role in shaping and reshaping early Soviet health policy and research.[225] This strategy was highly successful.

Whilst some members of the Petrograd medical profession disliked Soviet policies on wages,[226] private practice[227] or any moves to replace allegedly 'rich' members of the tsarist medical profession with new proletarian cadres,[228] this did not stop the old and new members of the Petrograd medical profession cooperating to defeat the common enemy – disease. Thus many former Pirogov doctors including Zabolotnyi, Gamaleia, Gran, Mol'Kov and Sysin either worked in local public health organisations or for Narkomzdrav.[229] One newspaper article declared in August 1918 that 'Pirogovtsy and Bolshevik members of the Petrograd Union of Doctors have put their 'class demagogy' behind them to fight the common enemy cholera'.[230]

By 1920, when a census was carried out of nearly 75,000 medical personnel throughout Russia, it was discovered that the large majority (93%) of these medical practitioners had in fact graduated from medical institutes or university medical faculties in the period before 1917.[231] Archival sources provide a more detailed analysis of a sample of 102 Narkomzdrav staff in 1921 indicating that some staff had 25–30 years medical service, the large majority were born between the 1860s–90s, had qualified on the eve of the First world war, and 90% were trained before the October Revolution and only 10% afterwards.[232]

The Soviet state was heavily indebted to these bourgeois medical specialists who assisted the Bolsheviks in putting a new health service in place. Lenin may have wanted central control but cooperation on medical issues was more important in the civil war period. Both sides got what they wanted. The health crises gradually subsided and the medical profession survived and defended its interests and throughout the 1920s influenced policy and enjoyed a considerable degree of autonomy that lasted until at least the end of the NEP period. This was because former zemstvo doctors and other medical personnel possessed the skills and knowledge that the Soviet government required and were active in government public health roles locally in Petrograd/Leningrad and nationally in Moscow.

Some members of the bourgeois medical profession had therefore started to define their place in civil war Petrograd society as an individual and collectively. They had thus become a part of the revolution in socialist health care and no longer remained on the outside. Some may have done this out of idealism (the pre-1917 pro-Soviet figures), pragmatism or out of cynicism. This suggests that the traditional interpretations of hostility as a reason for any failures in health strategy in the early Soviet era is flawed, as the Petrograd health service was run by and composed of former doctors and other medical personnel who were trained and practiced under the Tsarist regime. Although their situation and lives were difficult, it was the financial constraints that existed after 1917 and during the civil war that created the largest challenge. Thus although public health expenditure rose from 11.7 million in 1913 to 46.4 million by 1 October 1918 before rising to 1,656.9 million in 1919 and to 2,261.8 million in 1920,[233] these allocations were eroded by inflation, and so the health service was running a deficit.[234] Despite the constraints – economic and political – Petrograd's health leaders and staff of all political persuasions used a series of emergency measures to deal with infectious disease epidemics. A discussion of cholera will illustrate the point.

The sanitary epidemiological department, Council and Bureau came into being between March–May 1918 and they had responsibility for fighting cholera, Spanish influenza and typhus.[235] In July 1918, an inter-departmental extraordinary commission on cholera was set up. The first cases of cholera occurred in June 1918 – followed by 628 cases in July, with 14 deaths in the first five days.[236] Of all the 1919 cases: the age pattern was one case among those under one year old; seven among 1–5-year-olds; 16 among those 6–10 years; 45 among 11–15-year-olds; 101 in 16–20 age group; 116 among 21–30-year-olds; 101 cases for those 31–40 years old; 150 cases those aged 41–60 years old, 21 cases among 61–70 and six cases amongst those above 71 years.[237] Cases hit all districts of the city of Petrograd in 1919, with the lowest number of cases in Kazan district (six) and the highest number of cases at 141 in Petrograd side of the city.[238]

The Petrograd health service and local Council (*Sovet*)[239] acted quickly when the first cases of cholera were diagnosed in July 1918, allocating 12 million roubles to combat it and 10,000 staff were involved in this campaign.[240]

A cleaning and purification programme was launched in the city. Trains and boats were cleaned, anti-pollution measures were taken regarding the river Neva and boiled water was produced and distribution points were set up to provide cleaner water.[241]

The population of the city was warned of the dangers of cholera. Health Education Poster 3 consists of a panel of four images, mainly showing that

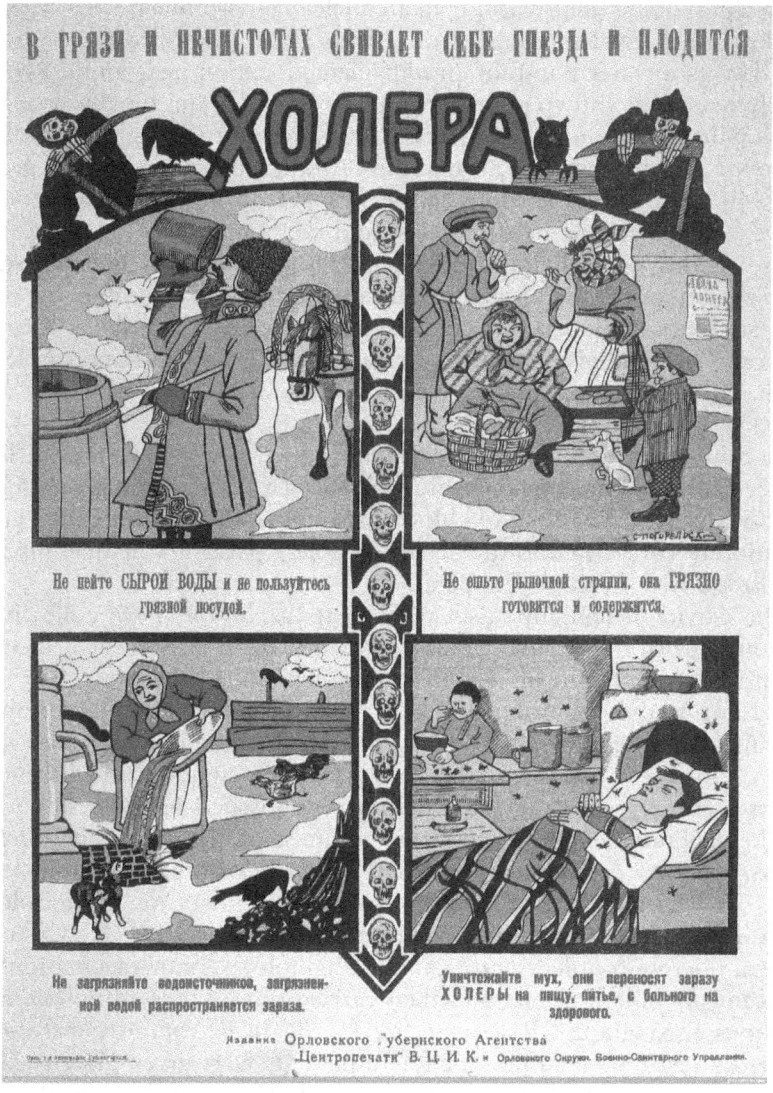

Poster 3 Causes of cholera in civil war Russia

Source: 'Unhygienic practices which lead to death from cholera'. Colour lithograph by S. Pogorelskii, c. 1920. Credit: Wellcome Collection, Wellcome Library, London (CC BY 4.0)

cholera was caused by drinking contaminated water or food contaminated with the bacteria *vibrio cholerae*. The grim reaper representing death is reproduced twice at the top of this poster and lots of skulls split the four panels, each showing different sections of the population drinking water in an unhygienic setting. In panel one (top left), a person is drinking water from a barrel with a horse in the background, implying it might be water only fit for horses. The second panel (top right), shows a group of four (three adults and a child) doing their washing in an unclean environment with an animal nearby and the washing basket on a dirty floor. The third panel (bottom left) depicts a water pump in an unhygienic location near animals and an elderly woman is shown pouring water down the drain. Finally, a sick person is lying down on the bed in the last panel (bottom right) with flies, a source of diseases, buzzing around him. Another person in the foreground, eats a meal in the same room as the sick person, implying to the viewer that cholera is spread by filth (flies) and contaminated food. This poster focuses upon people living in filthy conditions and how their unhygienic practices, in relation to water contamination, can cause cholera. It also suggests that victims are not looked after properly. Such 'backward' and 'ignorant' behaviour regarding water helps cholera spread and can lead to death. The Soviet civilising dimension and modernisation of health values is clearly evident in Poster 3.

In connection with improving water supply purity, a Petrograd health service Collegium meeting of 9 July introduced a chlorination programme of the Neva using 409,500kg of chlorine substances. It also called for greater attention to be devoted to the needs of cholera patients (the one in panel 4 of Poster 3 was possibly neglected).[242]

The Soviet leadership also wanted to serve the new collective by unifying health theory and practice which was an important principle in Lenin's modernisation of welfare policy. This fifth strategy refers to the Soviet notion that scientific and medical research findings must be applied to clinical settings. In Lenin's time, this meant immunization and inoculation. On the 9 July 1918 the network of vaccination and inoculation points were expanded and instructions were issued to those administering the programme. A vaccine serum commission (*vaktsino-syvorotchnaia komissiia*) was created in April 1918 under Zabolotnyi's able leadership. The Commission, Petrograd vaccination institute, bacteriological and other research institutes pooled resources and staff.[243] Newly trained cholera doctors (*kholery vrach*) and epidemiologists ran vaccination units and central cholera points and then carried out 34,000 anti-cholera vaccinations throughout 1918 rising to 45,786 in Petrograd gubernia as a whole by 1920.[244] In addition, cholera patients were given priority in hospital bed allocations. Sigal argues that in 1918, 3,000 beds in Petrograd hospitals were set aside for this purpose with the number increasing to 8,000 by 1919. Other patients were treated at cholera points or by medical brigades.[245]

Poster 4 suggests that the population of Petrograd needs to put its faith in the medical profession in the fight against infectious diseases, in this case via the use of cholera inoculations, so a doctor is depicted injecting a member of the collective. This view seems justified as this activity reduced the level of cholera cases from 628 in July 1919 to 247 in August 1919. Figures fell to 28 in September 1919 and levels were down to only 1 case in October 1919,

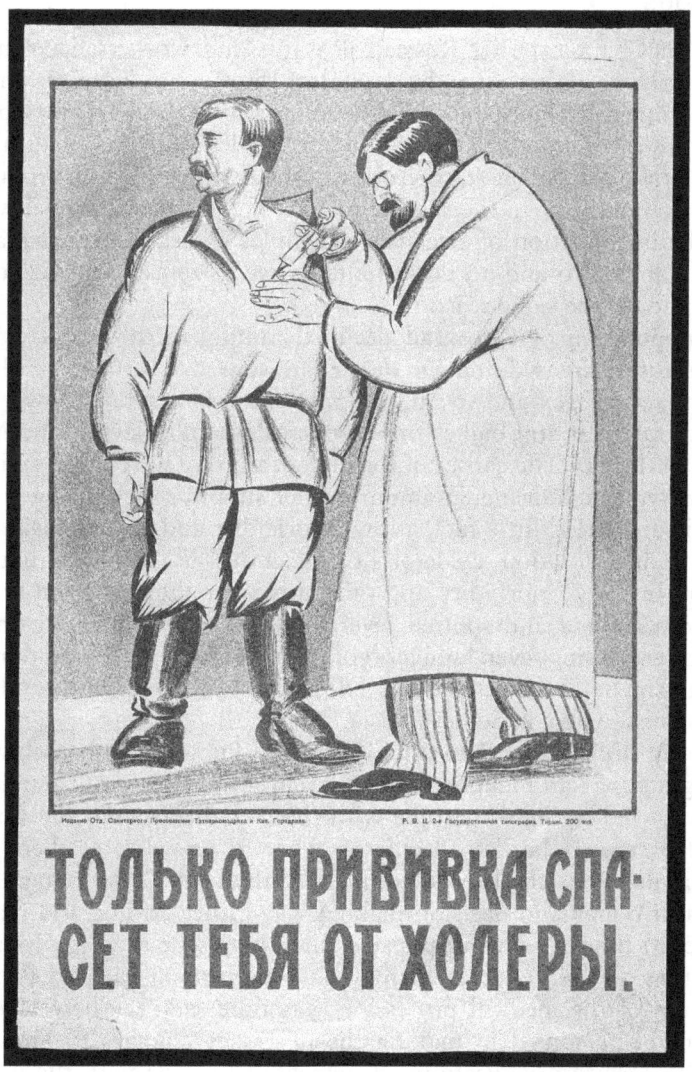

Poster 4 Doctors and inoculation programme to combat infectious diseases

with no further cases in that year.[246] There were only 22 cholera cases in 1920.[247] The number of preventive inoculations for all infectious diseases increased from 11,741 in 1913 to 698,738 in 1920 for the city of Petrograd, meaning that three quarters of the population had been vaccinated by the end of the civil war.[248] Such state and medical profession cooperation was highly effective in dealing with cholera.

Conclusion

We saw in Chapter 1 that Russian peasants and workers lived in misery in late tsarist St. Petersburg, the capital of the Russian Empire. This has a decisive impact on Bolshevik health policies after 1917. They wanted to reverse pre-revolutionary policies and a reorientation of medical policy started to take place. This restructuring of the Petrograd health service under Pervukhin took place in the specific historical context of the civil war. As a result, the introduction of 'socialist' principles of health care management was not adhered to and no radical alternative to zemstvo medicine was as yet possible for the same reasons.

The population of Petrograd declined rapidly in the period 1918–20, the birth rate increased and the death rate soared. Mortality levels varied according to age, sex and social group. Despite the levelling down process, the death rate was still highest in Vyborg, Aleksandr-Nevskii and Moscow districts of the city. The causes of the high death rate were a low standard of living, unhygienic housing, an impure water supply, a lack of sewer systems and basic amenities, little fuel, a low-calorie diet and environmental pollution. In such a situation, epidemics of infectious diseases and hunger were common. In 1917, morbidity and mortality were greatest from typhus; in 1918 from cholera and spotted fever; in 1919 from typhus again and in 1920 from relapsing fever. Hunger (*golod*) did exist in Petrograd during War Communism, but it did not have as a decisive impact on health conditions in the city, as elsewhere in Soviet Russia.

Recently declassified Russian Ministry of Public Health archive material suggests that an inexperienced Russian government and public health officials started trying to grapple with these challenges but the Bolsheviks found it extremely hard to decide on what to prioritise as there were so many simultaneous challenges, not just health crises. These materials reveal that health policy and decision-making was rather ad hoc and reactive in character at times.[249] This response cannot simply be attributed just to the circumstances. The government may have been inexperienced but a large proportion of the medical profession was time served. These tsarist staff aided Soviet personnel in making the necessary changes to and running the health service organisations in Petrograd to cope with the worsening health conditions. The Petrograd health service was frequently reorganised after May 1918, with new departments or staff added, as staff left or died or as circumstances changed. With time, however leaders gathered more ability and confidence and this gave some order to the chaos. Naturally such changes were justified in ideological terms as were the target groups.

Contrary to the conventional historical interpretation, this chapter shows that the Petrograd health service was not really hampered by a hostile medical profession, in fact in Petrograd the opposite was true. This was not just because the new Soviet regime took the necessary steps (offering preferential food supplies, good salaries, the opportunity to play a key role in public health policy and decision making, union representation), it was primarily because of a shared belief in a number of things – serving the community (now referred to as the 'collective'), the importance of medical science, preventive medicine and a belief in the environment as a cause of disease and death. Sections of the old, bourgeois medical profession were not simply coerced or co-opted into serving the communist regime, they willingly co-operated with the new Soviet order in the hope of gaining autonomy, professional recognition and being able to retain some of the principles of zemstvo medicine, in a new context, modified perhaps, but in some form after 1917.

The outcome of continuity of staff and certain values in the civil war meant that both the Petrograd health service and local authorities (both made up of some former tsarist officials) were able to respond quickly to epidemics of infectious disease, show their commitment to the needs of the 'community', to highlight areas of shared concern and above all to show their professional willingness, despite the political divide, to take the necessary initiative in order to avert a serious public health crisis. Thus the victory of Bolshevik ideology over the professional autonomy of the medical profession was not predetermined in civil war Petrograd and former zemstvo doctors served the regime, its collective and took a great step towards achieving its professionalization and in defending its interests. The longer-term challenge, explored in future chapters, was whether or not the Soviet state would subordinate the medical profession to state interests during NEP, the so-called face to industry and agriculture policies and during industrialisation and collectivisation or alternatively if the medical profession would retain some of its autonomy gained in the civil war period.

Given the social and economic conditions, and the meagre resources and finance available, remarkable successes were achieved, as our discussion of the common desire to combat cholera showed. Despite a deterioration in health conditions, the medical profession and the state and government in Petrograd coped relatively well. Of course, many structural problems prevailed – shortages of medical personnel, facilities, supplies – and the lack of finance prevented the Petrograd health service from resolving all the issues confronting them. The responses detailed in this chapter were mostly influenced by civil war expediency rather than ideology per se. As a result of economic constraints, and the desire for political survival, many of the Bolshevik's socialist principles – provision of free and comprehensive medical aid; the development of public health within the framework of a single plan; centralisation of health care – were not implemented fully.

However, a sense of state responsibility for public health; an emphasis on preventive medicine (with a belief on the impact of the 'environment') and the unity of theory and practice – were all evident between 1918–20.

The masses no longer lived in cellars, hovels or shacks and some, perhaps due to unfortunate circumstances, saw the inside of a hospital and clinic for the first time in their lives. This was evidence of the new regime's 'collective' policies in action. Although, for reasons beyond their control, there was a clear gap between health theory and practice, some of the bare foundations of a socialist health service had been laid in civil war Petrograd. What happened in the 1920s is the subject of Chapter 3.

Acknowledgments

Earlier versions of parts of this chapter have been published in 'War, medicine and revolution: Petrograd doctors, 1917–20', *Revolutionary Russia*, 4 (2), December 1991, 259–288.

Notes

1 *XV let diktatory proletariata: Ekonomiko-statisticheskii sbornik po gor. Leningradu i Leningradskoi oblasti* (Leningrad 1932), 142.
2 *Materialy po statistike Petrograda, Vyp. I* (Petrograd 1920), 108–109 and *Materialy po statistike Petrograda, Vyp.IV* (Petrograd 1921), 118–119.
3 *Materialy po statistike Petrograda, Vyp. I* (Petrograd 1920), 104–105 and *Materialy po statistike Petrograda, Vyp.IV* (Petrograd 1921), 116.
4 I. G. Fedorova, 'Epidemia sypnogo tifa v Petrograde, 1917–1918gg', *Izvestiia komissariata zdravookhraneniia Souiza kommun severnoi oblasti* No. 3–4 January–February 1919, 36.
5 *Materialy po statistike Petrograda, Vyp.IV* (Petrograd 1921), 106–107, 117.
6 S. G. Wheatcroft, 'Famine and factors affecting mortality in the USSR: The demographic crises of 1914–22 and 1930–33: Appendices', University of Birmingham SIPS Discussion paper No. 21, 1982, 17.
7 M. McAuley, 'Bureaucracy and Revolution: The Lesson from Leningrad, 1917–1927', *University of Essex, Russian and Soviet Studies Centre Discussion paper* No.4, October 1984a, 1.
8 M. McAuley, 'Party and Society during the civil war', *Sbornik: Journal of the Study Group on the Russian Revolution*, 45.
9 The Russian term golod can be translated as hunger or famine. The term hunger is more appropriate in Petrograd's case in my view.
10 S. G. Wheatcroft, 'Famine and factors: Appendices', 6, 17.
11 S. Novosel'skii, 'Estvestvennoe dvizhenie naseleniia v Petrograde v 1920g', *Materialy po statistike Petrograda, Vyp.V* (Petrograd 1921), 40.
12 S. G. Strumulin, *Problemy ekonomika truda* (Moscow 1964), 350; S. A, Smith, *Red Petrograd: Revolution in the Factories, 1917–18* (Cambridge, CUP 1983), 88 and M. McAuley, *Bread and Justice: State and society in Petrograd 1917–1922* (Clarendon Press, Oxford 1991), 280.
13 McAuley, *Bread and Justice*, 280.
14 V. Gogolevskii, *Petrogradskii sovet v gody grazhdanskoi voiny* (Leningrad 1982), 121; A. N. Chistikov, 'Deiatel'nost' Petrosoveta po reshcheniiu prodovol'stvennogo voprosa v 1917–1920gg', in *Leningradskii sovet v gody grazhdanskoi voiny v sotsialisticheskogo stroitel'stva 1917–1937gg* (Leningrad 1986), 87–88.

15 McAuley, *Bread and Justice*, 280.
16 McAuley, *Bread and Justice*, 280.
17 *Statisticheskii spravochnik 1922* (Petrograd 1922), 60. A pood is equivalent to approximately 16.38kg. The figure of 2,300 comes from *Ekonomicheskaia Zhizn'* 12 July 1919, 1. Western scholars concur see McAuley, *Bread and Justice*, 294.
18 McAuley, *Bread and Justice*, 286.
19 'Prodovol'stvennaia statistika', *Izvestiia Petrogradskogo Soveta*, 11 June 1919, No, 128, 2.
20 S. Malle, *The Economic organisation of War Communism, 1918–21* (Cambridge University Press, London 1985), 421.
21 McAuley, *Bread and Justice*, 287–288.
22 Ibid., 288.
23 S. G. Wheatcroft, 'Famine and factors: Appendices', 14.
24 McAuley, *Bread and Justice*, 293.
25 Ibid., 295.
26 Smith, *Red Petrograd*, 45 and S. G. Wheatcroft, 'Famine and factors: Appendices', 14.
27 G. K. 'Vol'nye tsifry v Petrograde', *Izvestiia Petrogradskogo Soveta*, 5 December 1919, 2. For an extensive discussion see A. M. 'Prodovol'stvennoe snabzhenie Petrograde', *Ekonomicheskoe vozrozhenie* 1922, No. 1, 73–76.
28 'Vol'nye tseny na prudukty', *Izvestiia Petrogradskogo Soveta*, 18 February 1920, 2.
29 McAuley, *Bread and Justice*, 200.
30 *Statisticheskii sbornik po Petrogradu i Petrogradskoi gubernii* (Petrograd 1922), 255–259.
31 McAuley, *Bread and Justice*, 300–301.
32 *Krasnaia Gazeta*, 6 October 1918, 4. This land measure is equivalent to 2.7 acres.
33 Quoted in M. G. Field, *Soviet socialised medicine: An introduction* (Free Press: New York 1956), 50.
34 *Materialy po statistike Petrograda, Vyp. 3* (Petrograd 1921), 3.
35 I. Rudenkov, 'Toplivnyi krizis i mery bor'by s nim', *Novyi Put'* No. 1–2, January 1919, 20.
36 M. Dobb, *Soviet economic development since 1917* (R.K.P. London 1966), 98.
37 *Kratkii statisticheskii spravochnik po Petrogradu i Petrogradskoi gubernii* (Petrograd 1922), 33.
38 See *Izvestiia Petrogradskogo Soveta*, 8 December and 22 December 1919 as well as *Petrogradskaia Pravda* 3, 5 and 7 December 1919.
39 V. Serge, *Year One of the Revolution* (translated and edited by P. Sedgwick) (Allen Lane, Penguin Press, London 1972), 363.
40 *Materialy po statistike Petrograda, Vyp. 3* (Petrograd 1921), 8.
41 McAuley, *Bread and Justice* 1991, 265 for 1918 figure and *Statisticheskii sbornik po Petrogradu i Petrogradskoi gubernii* (Petrograd 1922), 202–203 for 1920 figure.
42 *Materialy po statistike Petrograda, Vyp. 3* (Petrograd 1921), 8.
43 March 1918 is suggested by McAuley, *Bread and Justice* 1991, 272 whereas M. N. Potekhin, 'Pereselenie Petrogradskikh rabochikh v kvartiry buzhazii (Oktiabr' 1917–1919gg)', *Istoriia SSSR* 1977, No. 5, 142 gives a start date of Summer 1918.
44 McAuley, *Bread and Justice*, 267.
45 T. Sosnovy, *The Housing problem in the Soviet Union* (Research Program on the USSR, New York 1954), 54. This figure seems extremely high.
46 McAuley, *Bread and Justice*, 269.
47 Ibid., 270.
48 *Statisticheskii spravochnik 1922* (Petrograd 1922), 66.
49 McAuley, *Bread and Justice*, 270.
50 V. Binshtok, 'K zhilishchomu voprosu v Petrograde' in *Materialy po statistike Petrograda, Vyp. I* (Petrograd 1920), 64.

51 *Krasnaia Gazeta* 27 April 1919, 2.
52 *Statisticheskii spravochnik 1922* (Petrograd 1922), 76.
53 *Statisticheskii sbornik po Petrogradu i Petrogradskoi gubernii* (Petrograd 1922), 201. A vedro is the equivalent of 12 litres.
54 McAuley, 'Party and Society', 1984b, 45.
55 The Central Executive committee on housing matters had 310 staff in 1919 whilst the district housing committees had 608 personnel (Potekhin, 'Pereselenie Petrogradskikh rabochikh', 1977, 144 footnote 29).
56 *Krasnaia Gazeta* 15 December 1920, 3.
57 *Petrogradskaia Pravda* 16 February 1920.
58 *Izvestiia Petrogradskogo Soveta*, 16 November 1920.
59 *Izvestiia Petrogradskogo Soveta*, 31 December 1920.
60 V. A. Bazanov, 'Bor'ba za sanitarnoe blagopoluchie Petrograde v 1918g i stroitel'stvo pervykh sovetskikh organov sanitarnoe nadzora', *Gigiena i Sanitariia* 1969a, No.2, 63.
61 Dobb, *Soviet economic development*, 122.
62 W. H. Chamberlain, *The Russian Revolution, 1917–1921, Volume 2* (Universal library, New York 1965), 96
63 C. E. A. Winslow, 'Public health administration in Russia' in *Public Health Reports* 28 December 1917 (US Public Health Service, Washington Government Printing House, 1918), 3.
64 N. A. Semashko, *Health protection in the USSR*, London, Gollancz 1934, 11.
65 K. V. Maistrakh, *Organizatsiya zdravookhraneniya*, (4th ed., Moscow 1956), 8.
66 N. A. Semashko, *Des'yat let Oktiabria i sovetskaya meditsina*, Moscow, Izd. Narkomzdrava RSFSR, 1927, 3
67 Semashko, *Health protection*, 11.
68 Ibid., 15.
69 B. M. Khromov and A. V. Sheshnikov, *Zdravookhranenie Leningrada: Kratkii istoricheskii ocherk* (Leningrad 1969), 29.
70 B. S. Sigal, 'Pervye gody Sovetskogo zdravookhraneniiia v Leningrade', *Sovetskoe Zdravookhranenie* 1957, No. 7, 52.
71 Khromov and Sheshnikov, *Zdravookhranenie Leningrada*, 29.
72 N. A. Semashko, 'Osnovye Sovetskoi meditsiny', *Voprosy Zdravookhraneniia* 1928, No. 19, 7–8.
73 V. A. Bazanov, 'Organizatsiia zdravookhaneniia v Petrograde v pervye gody Sovetskoi vlasti', *Sovetskoe Zdravookhranenie* 1969b, No. 12, 51.
74 *Izvestiia komissariata zdravookhraneniia Souiza kommun severnoi oblasti* No. 1 November 1918, 14. For his biographical details see I. T. Leonov and V. A. Bazanov, 'Komissar zdravookhraneniia Petrogradskoi trudovoi kommuny E P Pervykhin', *Sovetskoe Zdravookhranenie* 1968, No. 2, 68–72; 'Evgenii Porif'evich Pervykhin, 1873–1941' in Ye. I. Lotova and B. D. Petrova (ed.), *Vrachi-bolsheviki-stroiteli Sovetskogo zdravookhraneniia* (Moscow 1970), 206–208 and V. A. Bazanov and A. I. Nesterenko, 'Novye straintsy biografii E. P. Pervykhin (K 100 letiiu so dnia rozhdeniia)', *Sovetskoe Zdravookhranenie* 1973, No. 12, 69–73.
75 Semashko, *Health protection*, 17.
76 Sigal, 'Pervye gody', 1957, 55 and Bazanov, 'Organizatsiia zdravookhaneniia', 52–53.
77 Bazanov and Nesterenko, 'Novye straintsy', 71.
78 Sigal, 'Pervye gody', 55.
79 *Zdravookhranie v g. Leningrade gubernii: K dokladu zavediaiushchego Leningradskom gubzdravotdelom na plenume Leningradskogo Soveta 29 iiulia 1927g* (Leningrad 1927), 3–4.

80 *Petrogradskaia Pravda* 12 October 1918. These principles were reiterated in a 1927 document which states that the aim of the Petrograd health service was 'to create a comprehensive, universal, health care service which would be provided by the State, seek to render preventive medical care to the local population and aim to ensure that full workers' participation in health service activities took place' (*Zdravookhranie v g. Leningrade gubernii: K dokladu zavediaiushchego Leningradskom gubzdravotdelom na plenume Leningradskogo Soveta 29 iiulia 1927g* (Leningrad 1927), 4).

81 H. E. Sigerist, *Socialised Medicine in the Soviet Union* (Gollancz, London 1937), 84; G. Hyde, *The Soviet health Service: A historical and comparative study* (Lawrence and Wishart, London 1974), 38–39; M. Kaster, *Health care in the Soviet Union and Eastern Europe* (Croom Helm, London 1976), 38–39; C. Davis, 'Economic problems of the RSFSR Health System, 1921–30', CREES University of Birmingham SIPS Discussion paper No. 19, 1978, 2 and V. George and N. Manning, *Socialism, social policy and the Soviet Union* (R.K.P, London 1987), 105. The reasons for the establishment of Narkomzdrav and its evolution in these early months of Soviet rule are traced in M. I. Barsukov, *Velikaia oktiabr'skaia sotsialisticheskia revoliutsiia i organizatsiia Sovetskogo zdravookhranenia (Oktiabr' 1917g-iiul' 1918g)* (Moscow 1951), Chapter 11 and A. I. Nesterenko, *Kak byl' obrazan Narodnyi komissariat zdravookhraneniia RSFSR: Iz istorii* Sovetskogo *zdravookhraneniia (Oktiabr' 1917g-iiul' 1918g)* (Moscow 1965), 3–4.

82 Bazanov, 'Organizatsiia zdravookhaneniia', 58.

83 Barsukov, *Velikaia oktiabr'skaia*, 46, 251–252 and E. D. Gribanov, *Vserossiskie S"ezdy zdravotedelov i ikh znachenie dlia praktiki Sovetskogo zdravookhraneniia* (Moscow 1966), 15, 18.

84 The following account is based on 'Postanovleniia 1-go vserossiiskogo s"eda medico-sanitarnykh otdelov sovetov', *Izvestiia Sovetskoi meditsiny* No. 5–6, 25 July 1918, 15–16. On its work see M. P. Mul'tanovskii, 'Dela i liudi uchebnogo meditsinskogo soveta na pervom etape ego deiatel'nosti (1919–1928)', *Sovetskoe Zdravookhranenie 1959*, No. 4, 18–25 and V. A. Bazanov, 'Organizatsiia uchebnogo meditsinskogo soveta narodnogo komissariata zdravookhraneniia RSFSR i ego sostav v 1918–1929 godakh', *Sovetskoe Zdravookhranenie 1974*, No. 6, 78–81.

85 Gribanov, *Vserossiskie S"ezdy*, 18–19.

86 Ibid., 31.

87 Barsukov, *Velikaia oktiabr'skaia*, 279 and Gribanov, *Vserossiskie S"ezdy*, 31.

88 Gribanov, *Vserossiskie S"ezdy*, 33; Leonov and Bazanov, 'Komissar zdravookhraneniia', 69 and Bazanov and Nesterenko, 'Novye straintsy', 71.

89 Bazanov and Nesterenko, 'Novye straintsy', 71.

90 'S"ezd medico-sanitarnykh otdelov Soiuza kommun Severnoi oblasti 2–7 noiabria 1918g v Petrograde', *Izvestiia komissariata zdravookhraneniia Souiza kommun severnoi oblasti* No. 2 December 1918, 76–77. According to this source, 30,000 military personnel were assisted with doctors working up to 12 hours a day to help the wounded.

91 Bazanov and Nesterenko, 'Novye straintsy', 71–73.

92 Ye. I. Lotova and B. D. Petrova (ed.), *Vrachi-bolsheviki-stroiteli Sovetskogo zdravookhraneniia* (Moscow 1970), 207.

93 Semashko, *Health protection*, 17.

94 Ia. Iaroslav, 'K voprosu o natsionalizatsii aptechnogo dela', *Izvestiia komissariata zdravookhraneniia Souiza kommun severnoi oblasti* No. 1 November 1918, 53. On the pre-revolutionary legacy see Mary Schaeffer Conroy, 'Pharmacy in Pre-Soviet Russia' *Pharmacy in History*, Vol. 27, No. 3, Pharmacy in Tsarist Russia (1985), 115–137.

95 'Iz muncipalizatsii aptechnogo dela v Petrograde', *Vestnik professional'nykh soiuzov* No. 1, 4 May 1918, 16

96 Ia. Iaroslav, 'K voprosu', 1918,44–45; *Izvestiia komissariata zdravookhraneniia Souiza kommun severnoi oblasti* No. 1, November 1918,131 and V. A. Bazanov, 'Organizatsiia zdravookhaneniia', 53.

97 See 'Besplatnye lekarstva dlia uchashchiksia, pedagogov i slushchaschikh v shkolakh', *Izvestiia Petrogradskogo Soveta*, 13 October 1919, No, 32, 2 and 'O besplatnom otpuske lekarstvu' *Izvestiia Petrogradskogo Soveta*, 1 November 1919, No, 249, 2.

98 L Kanetskii, 'Medikamentyi golod i mery bor'by s nim' *Izvestiia komissariata zdravookhraneniia Souiza kommun severnoi oblasti* No. 1, November 1918, 46.

99 'Massovoe izgotovlenie lekarstvu', *Izvestiia Petrogradskogo Soveta*, 13 October 1919, 2.

100 A. M. Kopylov, 'Bol'nichnoe delo v Petrograde v pervye gody Sovetskoi vlasti', *Sovetskoe Zdravookhranenie* 1962, No. 6, 78.

101 *Izvestiia komissariata zdravookhraneniia Souiza kommun severnoi oblasti* No. 1, November 1918, 141 and *Statisticheskii ezhgodnik 1918–1920gg* (Trudy TsSU, Moscow 1921), t. VIII, Vyp. 1, Ch. 2, 81.

102 On training see B. Sokolov, *Nauka v Sovetskoi Rossii* (Berlin 1921a), 42–43, 54–56. On the pre-revolutionary legacy see N. N. Alova, 'Podgotovka i ispol'ovanie farmatsevicheskikh kadrov (XIX-XX-XXI v.) na primere sankt-Peterburga', Avtoreferat Candidate degree in Pharmaceutical science, Sankt-peterburgskaia gosudarstvennaia khimiko-farmatsevticheskaia akademiia, 2004.

103 In a September 1919 meeting at the Military-sanitary administration it was noted that Petrograd lacked 200 pharmacists ('Nadostok farmatsevtov', *Izvestiia Petrogradskogo Soveta*, 2 September 1919, No, 197, 2. For more on shortages see L. Kanetskii, 'Medikamentyi golod i mery bor'by s nim' *Izvestiia komissariata zdravookhraneniia Souiza kommun severnoi oblasti* No. 1, November 1918, 46–47.

104 'S"ezd mediko-sanitarnykh otdelov Soiuza kommun Severnoi oblasti 2–7 noiabria 1918g v Petrograde', *Izvestiia komissariata zdravookhraneniia Souiza kommun severnoi oblasti* No. 2 December 1918, 87.

105 Ia. Iaroslav, 'K voprosu', 53.

106 'O nationalizatsii optovykh aptekarskikh skladov', *Izvestiia komissariata zdravookhraneniia Souiza kommun severnoi oblasti* No. 2–3 January–February 1919, 8.

107 M. Schaeffer Conroy, *In health and in sickness: Pharmacy, pharmacists and the pharmaceutical industry in late Imperial, early Soviet Russia*, Columbia University Press, New York 1994, 398–399.

108 'Soiuz aptechnykh rabotnikov', *Trud* 16 February 1920, 2.

109 A. Musatov, 'Konferentsiia medrabotnikov Petrogradskoi gub'. *Trud* 16 February 1920, 2; 'Pervaia gub. Konferentsiia rabotnits lechebno-sanitarnogo dela', *Trud* 11 October 1920, 2 and 'Gubernskaia konferentsiia Petrogradskogo gubotedela "Vsemediksantrud"', *Trud* 1 November 1920, 21.

110 'Gubernskaia konferentsiia', *Trud* 1 November 1920, 21.

111 Cited in W. Horsley Gantt, 'A medical review of Soviet Russia – II: Hospitals and Health conditions', *British Medical Journal* 23 August 1924a, 328.

112 B. Sokolov, 'Medicine in Soviet Russia', *The Lancet* 23 April 1921a, 876.

113 A. M. Kopylov, 'Bol'nichnoe delo v Petrograde v pervye gody Sovetskoi vlasti', *Sovetskoe Zdravookhranenie* 1962, No. 6, 76.

114 This was not a new venture because the Petrograd city Duma possessed its own hospital commission in August 1917. At that time however, it only contained 2 Bolsheviks (A. A. Ioffe and I. B. Rogal'skii), the rest being SRs, Mensheviks

and Kadets by affiliation (V. M. Kruchkovskaia, *Tsentral'naia duma Petrograda v 1917g* (Leningrad 1986), 131).

115 It was managed by a committee consisting of a senior doctor, a supervisor, a doctors' representative, sisters, nurses and junior medical personnel.

116 *God raboty Narodnyi komissariat zdravookhraneniia, 1918–1919gg* (Moscow 1919), 80.

117 Cited in Horsley Gantt, 'Hospitals and Health conditions', 328.

118 Examples here include the Yudevich acute parasitic infirmary no. 55 and the Ushakovsk and Rizhsk hospitals (*God raboty* 1919, 81).

119 Quoted in Horsley Gantt, 'Hospitals and Health conditions', 338.

120 Kopylov, 'Bol'nichnoe delo', 78. The nature of these 'mistakes' is not specified.

121 Bazanov, 'Organizatsiia zdravookhaneniia', 1969b, 58. For some indications of the variations in 1920 see *Statisticheskii sbornik po Petrogradu i Petrogradskoi gubernii* (Petrograd 1922), 314–315.

122 Kopylov, 'Bol'nichnoe delo', 77.

123 Ibid., 77.

124 *Izvestiia komissariata zdravookhraneniia Souiza kommun severnoi oblasti* No. 3–4 January-February 1919, 11

125 Kopylov, 'Bol'nichnoe delo', 78.

126 For a discussion of the pre-revolutionary legacy see T. G. Yakovenko, 'Okhrana materinstva i mladenchestva vo vtoroi polovine XVIII – nachale XX vv. (na materialakh Sankt-Peterburga)', Candidate degree in History, Sankt-Peterburgskii gosudarstvennyi universitet 2008. The maternity department and council liaised with the Ministries of Labour (Narkomtrud) and Justice (Narkomiust) over women's labour protection and legal rights. The Ministry of Social security was involved on welfare and maternity provision issues (A. M. Sluster, 'Kratkii ocherk deiatel'nosti Pod'otdela Okhrany materinstva i mladenchestva Petrogradskogo Otdela zdravookhraneniia za pervoe polugodie 1919g', *Izvestiia komissariata zdravookhraneniia Petrogradskoi Trudovoi Kommuny* No. 7–12 May–December 1919, 17 and *God raboty* 1919, 81).

127 A. M. Sluster, 'Kratkii ocherk', 18; P. V. Ivanov, 'Organizatsiia lechebno-profilakticheskoi pomoshchi detiam rannego vozrasta v Leningrade v pervoe desiatiletie Sovetskoi vlasti (1917–1927gg), Avtoreferat candidate degree medical science, Leningradskii pediatricheskii meditsinskii institute 1955, 8–9 and V. A. Bazanov, 'Organizatsiia zdravookhaneniia', 54.

128 A. Kollontai, *Sem'ia i kommunisticheskoe gosudarstvo* (Moscow: Gosudarstvennoe izdatel'stvo, 1920), 21

129 Semashko, *Health protection*, 17–19.

130 See Susan Gross Solomon, 'Soviet social hygiene and Soviet public health, 1921–1930' in Susan Gross Solomon and John F. Hutchinson (ed.), *Health and Society in Revolutionary Russia* (Indiana University Press, Bloomington and Indianapolis, 1990), 175–199.

131 Cited in I. G. Kochergin, 'Osnovye voprosy teorii Sovetskoi meditsiny i zdravoohraneniia v trudakh N.A. Semashko', *Sovetskoe Zdravookhranenie* 1965, No. 5, 25.

132 Quoted in Kochergin, 'Osnovye voprosy', 27.

133 A. N. Antonova, 'Neobkhodime reformy akusherskikh skhol v interesakh dela okhrany materinstva i mladenchestva', *Izvestiia Petrogradskogo gubzdravotela* No. 7–12, July-December 1920, 160–161. Similar factors are highlighted in contemporary studies of infant mortality rates see for instance C. Davis and M. Feshbach, *Rising infant mortality in the USSR in the 1970s*, US Department of Commerce, Census Bureau, Series P-95, No. 74, June 1980, Chapter 3.

134 For an example see 'Primernye chasy kormleniia grud'iu ot 6 do 12 mesiatsev' (Approximate times for breast-feeding from 6 to 12 months) at http://digital .nls.uk/74506106.

135 On this important issue see Natalia Chernyaeva, 'Childcare manuals and construction of motherhood in Russia, 1890–1990', unpublished PhD in Women's Studies, University of Iowa, December 2009.

136 According to Antonova, the 3 year courses combined theory and practice with placements in women's consultation clinics, refuges for pregnant women or maternity homes and the emphasis throughout was on the mother's right to be with and feed her child, on the need for adequate financial allowances and on the necessity for midwives to follow up or provide a check-up service for mothers (Dr A. N. Antonova, 'K voprosu o podgotovke srednogo personala po okhrane materinstva i mladenchestva' *Izvestiia komissariata zdravookhraneniia) Petrogradskoi Trudovoi Kommuny* No. 7–12 May–December 1919, 59–63 and Antonova, 'Neobkhodime reformy', 158–164).

137 See 'Reorganizatsiia dela rodospomozheniia', *Izvestiia komissariata zdravookhraneniia Petrogradskoi Trudovoi Kommuny* No. 5–6 March–April 1919, 156–157.

138 Bazanov, 'Organizatsiia zdravookhaneniia', 54–55.

139 Health educationalists played a major role giving lectures on children's health in schools or on women's health in their clinics (*God raboty*, 82).

140 *Statisticheskii materialy po sostoianiiu narodnogo zdraviia i organizatsii meditsinskoi pomoshchi v SSSR za 1913–1923gg* (Moscow 'Narkomzdrav' 1926), 82–84. For more on this see Ivanov, 'Organizatsiia', 10–14. These difficulties arose primarily because of financial constraints, despite 33.76 million roubles spent in 1920 on all these organisations (S. M., 'Zdravookhranenie i bor'ba s epidemiami s biudzhetnoi zreniia', *Petrogradskogo Soveta*, 7 September 1920, 2).

141 *Statisticheskii materialy po sostoianiiu narodnogo zdraviia i organizatsii meditsinskoi pomoshchi v SSSR za 1913–1923gg* (Moscow 'Narkomzdrav' 1926), 85–87.

142 Ivanov, 'Organizatsiia', 14; Sigal, 'Pervye gody', 53 and Bazanov, 'Organizatsiia zdravookhaneniia', 5.

143 A. I. Nesterenko, 'O rabote vrachebno-sanitarnogo otdela Petrograsdskogo komietea v oktiabre-dekabre 1917g', *Sovetskoe Zdravookhranenie* 1976, No. 11, 60. The Military health establishments were located in the Winter Palace, Central Telegraph Office and on Nevskii Prospekt (A. I. Nesterenko, *Bolsheviki – organizatsory sanitarnykh otriadov v revoliutsionnom Petrograde* (Leningrad 1969), 103. For a more detailed discussion see V. Malakhovskii, 'Sanitarnoe chast' Krasnoi gvardii v 1917g', *Proletarskaia revoliutsiia* No. 11, November 1927, 195–201; G. M. Popov, Voenno-sanitarnaia sluzhba Russkoi Armii pered oktiabr'skoi revoliutsii (Leningrad 1958), t. VII, 123–128 and A. I. Nesterenko, *Bolsheviki – organizatsory sanitarnykh otriadov v revoliutsionnom Petrograde* (Leningrad 1969), 118–122.

144 Bazanov, 'Organizatsiia zdravookhaneniia', 56.

145 *God raboty*, 22, 89.

146 Ibid., 22, 90.

147 Ibid., 87.

148 Ibid., 89–92 and V. A. Bazanov, 'Sanitarnoe prosveshchenie v Petrograde v pervye gody Sovetskoi vlasti', *Sovetskoe Zdravookhranenie* 1972, No. 3, 50–53. It was assisted in this work by the anti-epidemic commission founded in May 1919. The department opened 76 schools in its first year of existence and some 1,505 lectures were delivered (Z. G. Frenkel on hygiene, V. I. Svortsov on food hygiene and nutrition and others on government policy regarding parasitic and social diseases). These were attended by 180,000 people.

149 David F Hoffman, *Stalinist values: The cultural norms of Soviet Modernity, 1917–1941* (Cornell University Press, Ithaca and London 2003), 16.

150 Hoffman, *Stalinist values*, 58.

151 Victoria E Bonnell, *Iconography of power: Soviet political posters under Lenin and Stalin* (University of California Press 1998), 366–369.

152 Christopher Read, 'Values, substitutes and institutions: the cultural dimension of the Bolshevik dictatorship' in Vladimir N. Brovkin (ed.), *The Bolsheviks in Russian Society: The Revolution and civil Wars* (Yale University Press, New Haven and London 1994), 303–305.

153 Read, 'Values, substitutes and institutions', 306.

154 Ibid., 310–312.

155 *God raboty*, 87. Even though 16 million roubles was spent on dental establishments in 1920 (S. M., 'Zdravookhranenie i bor'ba s epidemiami s biudzhetnoi zreniia', *Petrogradskogo Soveta*, 7 September 1920, 2), state establishments were poorly equipped and staffed so some people relied on private dental care if they could afford it (in money or barter terms).These included the inter-departmental supply bureau, the extraordinary sanitary-technical commission, the medical supply centre and the medical provisions department (*God raboty*, 88–91)

156 These included the inter-departmental supply bureau, the extraordinary sanitary-technical commission, the medical supply centre and the medical provisions department (*God raboty*, 88–91).

157 This strategy seems to have been successful because 36 hospitals were built in Petrograd at a cost of 8 million roubles (*God raboty* 1919, 87). Budget allocations were frequently revised as new challenges or problems associated with infectious disease epidemics occurred.

158 *God raboty*, 88 and Bazanov, 'Organizatsiia zdravookhraneniia', 56.

159 *God raboty*, 35.

160 Ibid., 36.

161 S. Svarts, 'Strakhovye dekrety "raboche-krest'ianstvo pravitel'stva', *Strakhovanie rabochikh i sotsial'naia politika* No. 8, December 1917, 22–23.

162 'V strakhovom Sovete', *Strakhovanie rabochikh i sotsial'naia politika* No. 2–3, January – March 1918, 34.

163 Sally E. Ewing, 'Social insurance in Russia and the Soviet Union, 1912–22: A study of legal form and administrative practice', unpublished PhD in Sociology, Princeton University, 1984, 154.

164 On this see Smith, *Red Petrograd* 1983 Ye. L. Korbina and V. A. Korbin, 'Petrogradskie bol'nichnie kassy v bor'be za sozdanie zdravookhraneniia novogo tipa', *Sovetskoe Zdravookhranenie* 1969, No. 7, 73.

165 Ye. L. Korbina and V. A. Korbin, 'Petrogradskie bol'nichnie kassy v bor'be za sozdanie zdravookhraneniia novogo tipa', *Sovetskoe Zdravookhranenie* 1969, No. 7, 73.

166 According to one source, 29 kassy were merged between September–December 1917, adding 159,869 to the membership of the Petrograd medical funds (G. Baturskii, 'Po paklionnoi ploskoti (Biurokratizatsiia obshchegorodskoi kassy)', *Strakhovanie rabochikh i sotsial'naia politika* No. 5, April–May 1918, 17).

167 'Kak proizvedeny byli vybory v strakhovoi sovet', *Strakhovanie rabochikh i sotsial'naia politika* No. 1, January 1918, 29 and Ewing, 'Social insurance in Russia and the Soviet Union', 161.

168 Korbina and Korbin, 'Petrogradskie bol'nichnie kassy', 74.

169 Korbina and Korbin, 'Petrogradskie bol'nichnie', 74. Part of the reason for the large number of staff was the attractive wages offered. Kassy doctors received 5–6,000r a year (*Kak organovlas' Peterburgskaia obshchegoroskaia bol'nichnye kassa*, Vyp. 1 (NKT, Peterburg 1918), 58).

170 Korbina and Korbin, 'Petrogradskie bol'nichnie', 73–74 and Ewing, 'Social insurance in Russia and the Soviet Union', 168–173.

171 A. I. Vishnevetskii, *Razvitie zakonodatel'stva o sotsial'nom strakhovanii v Rossii* (2nd edition, Moscow 1926), 82 and Ewing, 'Social insurance in Russia and the Soviet Union', 173–174.

172 Vishnevetskii, *Razvitie zakonodatel'stva*, 86. On the background see Ewing, 'Social insurance in Russia and the Soviet Union', 174–179.

173 For a useful discussion of the pre-revolutionary system of offering anti-TB aid in St. Petersburg see V. F. Zhemkov, 'Nauchnoe obosnovanie sovershchenstvovaniia sistemy okazaniia protivotuberkuleznoi pomoshchi naseleniia krupnogo goroda v usloviiakh reformirovaniia zdravookhraneniia (na primere Sankt-Peterburga)', Candidate degree in Medical Science, Sankt-petersburgkii gosudarstvennyi meditsuinskii universitet 2005 and on Russian approaches as a whole see M. Z. David, 'The White plague in the Red Capital: Tuberculosis and its control in Russia, 19000–1941', PhD University of Chicago 2007. This overview is taken from Dr Nesline, 'The fight against tuberculosis in the RSFSR' in *La Lutte contre de la tuberculose dans la RSFSR* (Moscow-Leningrad 1934), 3.

174 *God raboty*, 87 and Roubakine, *La Protection*, 33.

175 Roubakine, *La Protection*, 33.

176 For reasons of space this issue cannot be discussed here see N. B. Lebina, *Povsednevnaia zhizn' Sovetskogo Goroda: Normy i anomaly 1920/1930 gody* (St. Petersburg, Kikimora 1999), 25–33; V. A. Popov, 'Bor'ba s narkomaniei i toksikomaniei detail i podrostkov v 20–30-e gody', *Sovetskoe Zdravookhranenie* 1989, No. 5, 67–70; S. Ye. Panin, 'Potreblenie narkotikov v Sovetskoi Rossii (1917–1920-e gody)', *Voprosy Istorii* No. 8, 2003, 129–134; P. Vasilyev, 'Medical Science, the State, and the Construction of the Juvenile Drug Addict in Early Soviet Russia', *Social Justice: A Journal of Crime, Conflict, and World Order*. Vol. 37. No. 4. 2012, 31–52 and P. A. Vasil'ev, 'Narkotizm v Petrograde-Leningrade v 1917–1929gg: sotsial'naia problema i poiski ee resheniia', Candidate degree in History, St. Petersburg Institute of History, RAN, 2013.

177 For reasons of space we cannot discuss child homelessness. See I. A. Yegor'kova, 'Bor'ba s detskoi besprizornost'iu i beznadsornost'iu v 1918–1935gg', Candidate degree in History, Vladimir gosudarstvennyi Gumanitarnyi universitet, 2011.

178 Nesline, 'The fight against tuberculosis', 5–12.

179 *God raboty*, 87 and Nesline, 'The fight against tuberculosis', 13.

180 A. P. Belova et al., 'Dostizheniia v okhrane zdorov'ia detei v Leningrade za gody Sovetskoi vlasi', *Zdravookhranenie Rossiiskoi Federatsii* 1977, No. 10, 18.

181 R. H. Bruce-Lockhart, *The Two Revolutions: An Eye witness account of Russia, 1917* (Bodley Head, London 1967), 45.

182 O. Ya. Budina, 'Voprosy byta i kul'tury Russkikh rabochikh na stranitsakh bol'shevistki pechati', *Ethnograficheskoe izuchenie byta rabochikh* (Moscow 1967), 171

183 P. A. Khromov, *Ekonomicheskoe razvitie v Rossii v 19–20 vekakh* (Moscow 1950), 507 and A. Vainstein, *Narodnyi pokhod Rossi ii SSSR* (Moscow 1969), 66.

184 P. Herlihy, *The Alcoholic Empire: Vodka and Politics in Late Imperial Russia* (Oxford University Press, Oxford 2002).

185 For attitudes towards alcohol in this period apart from Herlihy see J. F. Hutchinson, 'Medicine, morality and social policy in Imperial Russia: The early years of the Alcohol Commission', *Histoire Sociale* Volume 7, No. 4, 1974, 202–226; John F. Hutchinson, 'Science, politics and the alcohol problem in post-1905 Russia', *Social and East European Review* Volume 58, No. 2, 1980, 232–254 and R. E. F. Smith and D. Christian, *Bread and Salt: A Social and economic history of Food and Drink in Russia* (Cambridge University Press, Cambridge 1984), Chapter 8.

186 Prohibition cost the Tsarist government 900 million roubles or 28% of its national income at a time when money was needed to provide soldiers with weapons, the city with bread etc (Herlihy, *The Alcoholic Empire*, 145).

187 Herlihy, *The Alcoholic Empire*, 144.

188 These events are discussed in *Leningradskie rabochie v bor'be za vlast' sovetov 1917g* (Leningrad 1924), 111–112 and P. Ia. Kann, 'Bor'ba rabochikh Petrograda s p'ianymi pogrammi (Noiabr'-dekabr' 1917g)', *Istoriia SSSR* No. 3, May–June 1962, 133–136.

189 Kann, 'Bor'ba rabochikh Petrograda', 1962, 136; N. Weissman, 'Prohibition and alcohol control in the USSR: The 1920s campaign against illegal spirits', *Soviet Studies* Volume 38, No. 3, July 1986, 350 and the recent excellent work of V. I. Musaev, *Prestupnost' v Petrograde v 1917–1921gg i bor'be s nei* (RAN Institute of Russian History, St. Petersburg filal/Bulganin St Petersburg 2001), 46–69.

190 Lenin equated the riots with anarchism and hooliganism in a speech of 18 November 1917 see A. G. Parkhomenko, 'Gosudarstvenno-pravovye meropriyatiia po bor'be p'ianstvom v pervye gody Sovetskoi vlasti', *Sovetskoe gosudarstvo i Pravo* No. 4, April 1984, 113. On the general crime situation see McAuley, *Bread and Justice* 1991, chapter 4. The link between alcoholism and crime was nothing new see J. Neuberger, 'Stories of the street: Hooliganism in the St. Petersburg press', *Slavic* review Volume 48, No. 2, Summer 1989, 177–195.

191 *Pravda* 7 December 1917. There were an estimated 700 private alcohol stores in Petrograd at this time

192 Struggles between drinkers and anti-alcohol brigades at times resulted in pitched battles. Wade cites one such incident at the Petrov vodka factory in early December 1917 in which three Red Guards and eight soldiers were killed (Rex A. Wade, *Red Guards and workers' militsias in the Russian Revolution* (Stanford University Press, California 1984), 316.

193 Parkhomenko, 'Gosudarstvenno-pravovye meropriyatiia', 113–114. A Soviet state monopoly did not come into effect until August 1925.

194 Ibid., 113–114.

195 Ibid., 113–114. Both Parkhomenko and Weissman argue it was not actually a 'dry law' and no alcohol prohibition occurred (Parkhomenko, 'Gosudarstvennopravovye meropriyatiia', 114 and Weissman, 'Prohibition', 350). The main intention of the 1919 law was to prevent grain hoarding.

196 Weissman, 'Prohibition', 350.

197 This was because militsia staff were in short supply and on defence duties. On the militsia at this time see Ekaterina Potemkina, Avtoreferat 'Rol' informatsionnoi sluzhby militsii Petrograd-Leningrada v bor'be s prestupnostiiu, 1918–41gg' Candidate degree in History, MVD sankt-peterburgskii Universitet, 2001. However, some local councils also totally ignored such laws by formally fixing market prices for moonshine (*Izvestiia* 17 January 1919, 4), and so the Commissariat of State Control uncovered 30 places in the first half of 1919 where the sale of alcohol was legalised (Weissman, 'Prohibition', 350–351).

198 Semashko, *Health protection* 1934, 15. On this question see G. I. Il'ina, *Kul'turnoe stroitelstvo v Petrograde: Oktiabr' 1917–1920gg* (Leningrad 1982) and M. McAuley, 'Gentlemen versus Comrades: Culture in civil war Petrograd', CREES University of Birmngham, SIPS Seminar paper, February 1986.

199 Semashko, *Health protection*, 118.

200 'Bor'ba s venericheskim zabolovaniam v Petrograde', *Izvestiia Narkomzdrav* No. 9–10, 10 October 1918, 19; Sigal, 'Pervye gody', 1957, 56–59; Bazanov, 'Organizatsiia zdravookhaneniia', 1969b, 55 and V. A. Bazanov, 'Bor'ba s venericheskim zabolovaniiam v Petrograde v 1918–1919gg' *Vestnik dermatologiia i venerologiia* 1971, No. 4, 65–69.

201 Semashko, *Health protection*, 102.
202 GARF f. A-482 op 10. d. 1914, list 44. These figures refer to those who applied for medical aid to institutions (i.e. registered cases) and as such probably under estimate the real extent of the problem as the social stigma attached to sexually transmitted diseases meant that many went unrecorded. For a review of the situation as a whole see Laurie Bernstein, 'Yellow tickets and state licensed brothels: The tsarist government and the regulation of urban prostitution', in Susan Gross Solomon and John F. Hutchinson (ed.), *Health and Society in Revolutionary Russia* (Indiana University Press, Bloomington and Indianapolis, 1990), 45–65.
203 Z.G. Frenkel' (ed.), *Zdravookhranenie v Sovetskoi Rossii za X let (1917–1927gg)* (Leningrad 'Meditsina' 1927), 38.
204 'Bor'ba s venericheskim zabolovaniam v Petrograde', *Izvestiia Narkomzdrav* No. 9–10, 10 October 1918, 19; Sigal, 'Pervye gody', 57; Bazanov, 'Organizatsiia zdravookhaneniia', 55.
205 The Tsarist legacy in relation to prostitution is discussed in R. Stites, 'Prostitution and society in pre-revolutionary Russia', *Jahrbucher fur Geschichte Osteuropas* N.F. Band 31, 1983, 348–364 and L. H. Edmundson, *Feminism in Russia, 1900–1917* (Stanford University Press, California 1984), 143–147 whilst early Soviet approaches to prostitution are outlined in Z. Tettenborn, 'Zadachi Sovetskoi vlasti v bor'be s prostitutiei i nishchenstvom', *Zhurnal Narodnogo komissariata sotsial'nogo obespecheniia* No. 5–6, June–July 1919, 10–20 and A. Kollontai, *Prostitutsiia i mery bor'by s nei (Rech na III Vserossisskom sovershchenii zaveduiushchikh gubzhenotedlami* (Moscow 1921).
206 Semashko, *Health protection*, 108.
207 See R. E. Drumm, 'The Bolshevik Party and the organisation and emancipation of working women, 1914 to 1921 or A history of the Petrograd Experiment', unpublished PhD in Political Science, Columbia University, 1977, 489–490.
208 C. Williams, "War, medicine and revolution: Petrograd doctors, 1917–20', *Revolutionary Russia* Volume 4 (2), December 1991, 265.
209 B. Sokolov, 'Medicine in Soviet Russia', *The Lancet* 23 April 1921a, 876. The number of health workers in the city of Petrograd fell from 2,314 in 1913 to 1,168 in 1920 (or by 49.5%) whilst the number of secondary medical personnel declined from 2,370 in 1913 to 700 by 1920 (29.5%) (Williams, 'War, medicine and revolution', 265).
210 Barsukov, *Velikaia oktiabr'skaia sotsialisticheskaia revoliutsiia i organizatsiia Sovetskogo zdravookhraneniia (Oktiabr' 1917-iiul' 1918g)* (Moscow 1951), 86–88.
211 M. I. Barsukov and A. Zhuk, *Za sotsialisticheskuiu rekonstruktsiiu zdravookhraneniya,* (Moscow 1932), 13–14
212 Field, *Soviet socialised medicine*, 28, 55, 58.
213 V. I. Musaev, 'Byt gorozhan' in V. A. Shishkin (ed), *Petrograd na perelome epokh: Gorod i ego zhiteli v gody revoliutsii i grazhdanskoi voiny* (RAN, Institute of Russian History, St. Petersburg filal/Bulganin St Petersburg 2000), 119.
214 Other scholars concur see Peter Krug, 'Russian public physicians and revolution: The Pirigov Society, 1917–20', PhD in History, University of Wisconsin-Madison 1979, 311.
215 Cited in Semashko, *Health protection*, 39.
216 Quoted in Semashko, *Health protection*, 40.
217 S. Fitzpatrick, 'New perspectives on the civil war' in D. P. Koenker, W. G. Rosenberg and R. G. Suny (eds), *Party, state and society in the Russian civil war: Explorations in social history* (Indiana University Press, Bloomington and Indianapolis, 1989), 16.

218 Cited in John F. Hutchinson, 'Who Killed Cock Robin?' in Susan Gross Solomon and John Hutchinson (eds), *Health and Society in Revolutionary Russia* (Bloomington and Indianapolis: Indiana University Press, 1990), 10

219 N. Frieden, *Russian Physicians in an Era of Reform and Revolution, 1856–1905.* (Princeton University Press, Princeton 1981) 198–199.

220 Chernyaeva, 'Childcare manuals', 2009 includes tsarist propaganda and manuals on women and children's issues

221 Herlihy, *The Alcoholic Empire* 2002 includes examples of tsarist anti-alcohol propaganda

222 Peter Kenez, *The birth of the Propaganda State: Soviet methods of mass mobilisation, 1917–1929* (Cambridge University Press 2003).

223 *Tiddskift for den Norske Loegeforening* cited in 'The plight of Petrograd doctors', British Medical Journal 31 July 1920, 3. Although many died from disease, overwork or starvation, others died in the fighting (see S. F. Baronov, 'Lazaret na ptrednem krae' and 'A. M. Ivanov, 'Pervye voennye avtosanitarnye otriady' in *Pitersy na frontakh grazhdanskoi voiny: Sbornik vospominanii* (Leningrad 1970), 211–217 and 369–374 respectively).

224 By late 1920, the pay of doctors engaged in infectious diseases work was 80% higher than other groups and they also received rations on a Red Army scale (L. Haden-Guest 'Public health in Soviet Russia II – The medical services', *The Lancet* 11 September 1920, 566).

225 For more on medical education and research see Williams, "War, medicine and revolution', 270–275

226 For a discussion of wage policy in relation to the medical profession during the civil war see Williams, 'War, medicine and revolution', 268–270.

227 On private practice see Williams, 'War, medicine and revolution', 276.

228 On this see Williams, 'War, medicine and revolution', 277–278.

229 Krug, 'Russian public physicians and revolution', 274–275.

230 'Petrogradskie vrachei i kholera', *Izvestiia Narkomzdrav* No. 7–8, 25 August 1918, 22.

231 See Williams, 'War, medicine and revolution', 279–280.

232 'Spiski meditsinskogo personela NKZa RSFSR po sostoyannego na dekabr' 1921 goda' in GARF f. A-482, op. 2, d. 231 list 2 ob-3 ob. The sample included physicians, pharmacists, physiotherapists, feld'shers, midwives, therapists, surgeons, clinical psychologists, bacteriologists and sisters and junior nurses.

233 Z. I. Frenkel', 'Sanitarnoe blagoustroistvo i vrachebno-sanitarnoe delo' in *Petrogradskaia gorodskaia duma v 1913–1915gg* (Petrograd 1915), 168 and S. M., 'Zdravookhranenie i bor'ba s epidemiami s biudzhetnoi zreniia', *Petrogradskogo Soveta*, 7 September 1920, 2.

234 On this see G. Sec, *The Local budget system in the USSR: its development and functions* (Russian Research Program on the USSR, New York 1955), 2 and R. W. Davies, *The Development of the Soviet budgetary system* (Cambridge University Press, London 1958), 2. Malle estimates that the state budget deficit increased from two thirds of total expenditure in 1918 to more than four fifths of it by 1920 (Malle, *The Economic organisation*, 168).

235 These organisations were run by D. K. Zabolotnyi, A. A. Vladimirov, G. B. Khlopin, K. V. Karaffa-Korbutt, G. I. Dembo, N. F. Gamaleia, N. Ia. Iakovlev, N. R. Vasilevskii and S. I Gusev (*God raboty* 1919, 85–88; Sigal, 'Pervye gody', 56 and Bazanov, 'Organizatsiia zdravookhaneniia', 55–56).

236 *Krasnaia gazeta* 10 July 1918.

237 *Materialy po statistike Petrograda, Vyp. I* (Petrograd 1920), 104–105. In 410 cases the age was unknown.

238 *Materialy po statistike Petrograda, Vyp. I* (Petrograd 1920), 106–107.

239 For reasons of space, it is not possible to consider the role of the local council in depth, see Potekhin, *Petrogradskia trudovaia kommuna,* Chapters 2, 5 and A. V. Gogol'evskii, *Petrogradskii sovet v gody grazhdanskoi voiny* (Leningrad 1982), 129–137.

240 'Kholernaia epidemiia v Petrograde', *Izvestiia Narkomzdrav* No. 7–8, 25 August 1918, 16.

241 *God raboty* 1919, 88; V. A. Bazanov, 'Bor'ba s epidemiei kholery v Petrograde v 1918g', *Zhurnal mikrobiologii I immunobiologii* 1970, No. 9, 142–143; V. A. Bazanov, 'D. K. Zabolotnyi v krasnom Petrograde v 1918g', *Sovetskoe Zdravookhranenie* 1969c, No. 1, 81, 84).

242 'Kholernaia epidemiia v Petrograde', *Izvestiia Narkomzdrav* No. 7–8, 25 August 1918, 16 and M. N. Potekhin, *Petrogradskia trudovaia kommuna (1918–1919gg)* (Leningard 1980), 128.

243 'Kholernaia epidemiia v Petrograde', 16; N. F. Gamaleia, 'Intensivnyi metod prigotovleniia ospennoi vaktsiny', *Izvestiia komissariata zdraviookhraneniia Souiza kommun severnoi oblasti* No. 3–4, January–February 1919, 71, 74 and Bazanov, 'D. K. Zabolotnyi', 82.

244 *Izvestiia Petrogradskogo Soveta,* 25 September 1920; *Statisticheskii materialy po sostoianiiu narodnogo zdraviia i organizatsii meditsinskoi pomoshchi v SSSR za 1931–1923gg* (Moscow 'Narkomzdrav' 1926), 170–171. These vaccination points and units were run by 2 doctors, a disinfector and 3 orderlies.

245 B. S. Sigal, *Meditsinskie rabotniki Leningrada v gody velikoi oktiabr'skoi revoliutsii I grazhdanskoi voiny v SSSR* (Leningrad 1958), 46, 49.

246 *Materialy po statistike Petrograda, Vyp. I* (Petrograd 1920), 104–105 and *Materialy po statistike Petrograda, Vyp.IV* (Petrograd 1921), 116.

247 *Statisticheskii materialy po sostoianiiu narodnogo zdraviia i organizatsii meditsinskoi pomoshchi v SSSR za 1913–1923gg* (Moscow 'Narkomzdrav' 1926), 170–171.

248 GARF f. A-482, d. 231, op 10 d. 23 lists 76, 80.

249 See Council of Medical Board minutes in GARF f. A-482, op. 4, d. 31.

3   Health, class and the market under the NEP, 1921–27

With the introduction of the NEP in 1921, Russia's cities began to bustle again: by 1926, Leningrad was repopulated; housing was being built rather than disassembled (and) traders offered wares that had been unavailable in more troubled years.[1]

The purpose of this chapter is to construct a fuller picture of the impact of the introduction of the New Economic Policy (NEP) on the evolution and development of the Petrograd/Leningrad health service between 1921–27 than has hitherto been available. We will analyse the city's proletarian and migrant peasants, the demographic recovery and aspects of daily life in so far as they affected health conditions during the 1920s. We discuss the public health objectives pursued during the NEP as a whole, the issue of health budget reform and the financial constraints operating, and the impact on the organisation of health care. This chapter addresses the important question of the development of the medical profession and the slow party penetration of it and the public health sector as a whole in the mid–late 1920s and most importantly the overall state of the Leningrad Health Service on the eve of the First five-year plan. Particular emphasis is placed upon medical provision for the insured and the way in which it generated conflict at a central and local level. A final section presents conclusions on the nature of health, class and the market up to 1927 before Stalin was in power.

State, society and party in transition – the NEP

Russia emerged from the throes of Revolution and Civil War an exhausted and devastated nation. The Bolshevik leadership had managed to consolidate its military and political position, but only at great cost – hunger, disease, high male mortality, widespread migration from the cities to the countryside, railway stations full of soldiers and homeless children (*besprizornye*) and the closure of factories with a corresponding fall in industrial production. The civil war had had a devastating impact on the families and households of Petrograd. Class determined university admissions, the allocation of food rations and housing priority. The Revolution had sought to reverse the situation in which the bourgeoisie were seen as the 'haves' and poor peasants and industrial workers as the 'have not's' but this was not always possible and the industrial working-class had become fragmented and dispersed during the civil war. The new regime's initial economic strategy (requisitioning, nationalisation of industry, monetary management) was a response to wartime conditions and resulted in shortages of food, fuel, decent housing, poor industrial performance and meant, in E. H. Carr's view, that by early 1920, 'the burdens of war communism seemed no longer tolerable', so a change in policy was deemed necessary.[2]

The implementation of the New Economic Policy took place against the end of the civil war, its consequences and a background of revolts by armed groups, rebellious peasants and striking workers, especially in Moscow and Petrograd. These groups, whose actions were typified by the Kronstadt sailors' uprising,[3] firmly believed that the Party had become isolated from the rest of society and that the high ideals of the Revolution had already been betrayed. This situation speeded up the Party's willingness to accept the NEP because the Bolshevik leadership was concerned that it might serve as a rallying point for a popular movement against them. They, therefore, needed to implement a policy – the NEP – which would lead in the short term to greater stability, a sense of normality and a surge in support for the Soviet government and Communist Party.

The NEP, which was ushered in at the Tenth Party Congress held in March 1921, provided a breathing space and allowed Lenin and the Bolsheviks to resume their strategy of building the Soviet state and a socialist health service, which was disrupted during the civil war. Under the NEP, a mixed economy prevailed. The Bolsheviks retained control of the commanding heights (economy, foreign trade, finance, large-scale industry, private and communal trade) but after 1921 a market was established between the town (working class) and the countryside (peasants) so that the latter could supply the former with food and raw materials in exchange for industrial and consumer goods. This new policy meant that in agriculture, food requisitioning was abolished and a tax in kind introduced. The aim was to give the peasant the freedom to dispose of any surplus produce on the local market in Petrograd while having the security of land tenure. In industry, meanwhile, steps were taken to develop rural and small industry, to abolish producer's cooperatives and to foster the growth of large scale industry. Any restrictions on private trade and production were eliminated and the goal was to allow industry and agriculture time to recover so that labour productivity increased and living standards improved. In August 1921, all organisations were also required to operate on an economic or commercial accounting basis (the so-called *khozraschet* system), meaning that all organisations, including public health establishments and institutions, had to meet their costs.

All of these changes were aimed at developing a broad popular consensus and building a strong Soviet state without the need for the use of coercion (Red Terror) that had prevailed in the civil war period. This was an enormous task and a complex process. There was still some defensiveness, suspicion and of course, great wariness. During the NEP, Lenin and the government in Moscow, and Grigorii Zinoviev, who was the Party leader of Petrograd/ Leningrad from November 1917 until March 1926 (only to be replaced by Nikolai Komarov who remained in the post until January 1930), faced a number of challenges – the influx of demobilised Red Army personnel, the return of workers from the countryside and more newcomers such as peasant migrants – which put pressure on housing, social services, the health service and led to job competition under NEP.

In the initial period (1921–23) Soviet economic development was aided by the revival of agriculture and by industry nearly reaching pre-war levels, but the NEP favoured agriculture, so the rate of recovery was less pronounced in industry. While light industry was doing rather well, heavy industry lagged seriously behind. These changes were taking place at a time of hyper-inflation. To cure the latter, the banking system was re-organised and a monetary reform was introduced. The aim was to balance the budget and stabilise the rouble. As part of this policy, a new budgetary system was implemented in late 1921 under which the State retained control of the commanding heights of the economy, largely sectors of national importance, while the remaining sectors, including health, were placed in the hands of the local authorities.[4]

This situation caused local grievances over a possible 'retreat' from the original goals of the Revolution as well as over wages, dismissals and work norms that led to strikes, labour activism and to a newly reaffirmed 'proletarian' identity that produced renewed class antagonism and led to the development of a re-proletarianised communist Party in Petrograd and elsewhere.

The use of private trade and traders in Petrograd/Leningrad led to an improvement on the shortages and black market experienced under War Communism. These private retail shops, which were taxed and licensed by the state, were stocked with government products. By 1922, the private share of retail trade stood at around 80%,[5] with government and proletarian employees making around 40% of their purchases of goods (textiles, hardware, leather foods) and food (eggs, meat and fruit and vegetables) from private enterprises by 1925–26.[6] By late NEP, however, amidst worries about the private procurement of grain, and shortages, a campaign was launched against private trade in 1926–27 and the number of private traders fell from 590,000 in 1925/26 to 213,700 by 1928/29, so the number of nepmen were gradually being eliminated by 1928.[7]

As a result of the demobilization of 4.1 million soldiers and a February 1922 Commissariat of Labour decree which ensured that veterans should receive preferential treatment when seeking work, women and juvenile workers lost their jobs in early NEP. By 1922, 67% of the 27,000 registered unemployed were female.[8] Women as widows, orphans and divorcees, all the product of the civil war and changes in family policy, became economic dependants at this time. This was especially true of those women with children, some of whom had been abandoned by their husbands. The situation varied according to individual, family circumstances and background but some women in Petrograd became wage earners and found low paid and unskilled jobs in education and health care and alongside female migrants, local inhabitants, competed for work in handicrafts, textiles and food processing. Other women suffered from higher levels of unemployment, thus and on average, Petrograd males waited only five months before they found a job, whereas women waited 10 months in 1923.[9] This brought hardships, increased female vulnerability and affected their sense of security. Some adult and young females who struggled to find work (due to cost cutting, the closure of certain branches of industry, reduced spending on the state sector and discrimination) with no other sources of support to feed and house themselves, become prostitutes (see below). The paupacy of state resources meant that it was not always possible to provide the necessary child care facilities for those who worked. Furthermore, peasant in-migration (the product of an over populated countryside and a desire for better jobs and lives) into Petrograd/Leningrad was a source of social conflict between workers and peasants and between the sexes as they fought for jobs. All these issues put the health service and its staff under pressure once again.

Demographic recovery and the collective

Under the NEP, there was a population revival and the city's numbers increased from 830,000 in 1921 to 1,379,000 by 1925. This 66% increase almost offset the decline during the Civil War. There were, of course, massive differences in the growth in population in particular years. Between 1921–23, the yearly increase was around 130,000, then in 1924–25, it rose by nearly 160,000 p.a. Up until the mid-1920s then, the city of Leningrad was well on the way to a speedy recovery following the successful conclusion of the Civil War. The population of the city of Leningrad then rose from 1,535,000 in 1926, before reaching 1,627,000 by 1927, the year prior to the introduction of the First Five-Year plan. There were gains of 92,000 and 73,000 respectively meaning that by the end of this decade, the rate of growth was slowing down again. It was not until 1931 that the size of the city's population surpassed its pre-revolutionary total. This section analyses the reasons for this growth and how this affected the profile of the city's population and health conditions.

The birth rate recovered rapidly from the adverse effects of Revolution and Civil War. Two factors affected the birth rate, family size and family planning on the one hand, and variations in the proportion of women, changes in the age structure and the proportion of the population married, on the other. The number of marriages increased from 17,350 in 1921 to 24,369 in 1927 or by 40%. However, the tendency for the city's population to marry at progressively older ages during the early 1920s in comparison to the pre-First World War period, led to a decline in the overall marriage rate from 20.90 per 1, 000 in 1921 to 14.98 per 1,000 by 1927.[10] The birth rate fell to 34.4 per 1,000 in 1921 and fluctuated greatly thereafter. An improvement occurred in 1923 (29.2) but a decline then took place in 1924 (27.8). By 1925, the birth rate in the city of Leningrad stood at 27.8 per 1,000 and it remained constant in 1926 before declining to 24.7 in 1927, a level lower than in 1913 but higher than in 1920 (see Table 3.1).

Table 3.1 shows that there was a dramatic improvement in mortality rates compared with the Civil War period. The death rate declined by half in 1922 over its 1920 level (from 50.6 per 1,000 in 1920 to 25.3 in 1922), and it continued falling throughout the NEP reaching 16.0 per 1, 000 by 1927 or just under a third of its 1920 level. The net surplus of births over deaths for the period rose from 3,398 in 1922 to 14,209 by 1927. As a proportion of the net growth in population (667,000) only 5.2% was due to natural increase. Population growth was largely due to in-migration but two other factors: an excess of births over deaths, and falling morbidity and mortality also played their part (we shall discuss the latter further below).

A striking difference between pre- and post-revolutionary Petrograd was the sexual breakdown of the population. Under War Communism males either joined the military or left for the countryside and women filled their jobs. Petrograd families had fallen apart during the civil war which affected the birth rate. As Goldman notes:

> Years of war, civil war, and famine had undermined family and community ties. Peasant migrants to the cities abandoned older customs and traditions. Women joined with soldiers, strangers, and temporary providers in casual, short-term unions. De facto 'wives' flooded the courts seeking alimony and child support from the men who abandoned them. And for many, the new communist morality encouraged and justified looser forms of behavior.[11]

Table 3.1 Population of Petrograd/Leningrad, 1921–27

Year	Size of population	Number of births	Births per 1,000	Number of deaths	Deaths per 1,000	Rate of natural increase/decrease
1921	830,000	28,517	34.4	25,689	31.0	3.4
1922	960,000	24,252	25.3	27,650	28.8	-3.5
1923	1,093,000	31,906	29.2	17,482	16.0	13.2
1924	1,221,000	31,601	25.9	19,697	16.1	9.8
1925	1,379,000	38,402	27.8	20,102	14.6	13.2
1926	1,535,000	42,608	27.8	22,130	14.4	13.4
1927	1,627,000	40,219	24.7	26,010	16.0	8.7

Sources: *XV let diktatory proletariata: Ekonomiko-statisticheskii sbornik po gor. Leningradu i Leningradskoi oblasti* (Leningrad 1932), 135, 143

Civil marriages and divorce, made possible by the Code on Marriage, the Family and Guardianship ratified by the Central Executive Committee of the Soviet (VTsIK) in October 1918, impacted upon this situation. This move was seen as a means of ensuring female emancipation and no grounds for divorce were now necessary. The new Code provided for alimony for either gender, but support was limited to the disabled poor and both parties were expected to support themselves.[12] After the new law came into force, the divorce rates in Petrograd/Leningrad increased from 1,980 in 1921 to 16,008 by 1927 or from 128 to 657 per 1,000 population.[13] By 1927, half of the marriages in Leningrad were ending in divorce either as a sign of Soviet male lack of commitment to marriage or of independent women's desire to have more freedom than they had in the tsarist era and to avoid the constraints of patriarchal family structures.[14] These changes in family policy, relations between the sexes, attitude to marriage etc affected the birth rate in an adverse way. However, the recovery of the city's economy, to something like its pre-war level, generated an influx of demobilised Army personnel, encouraged workers to return home and peasant migrants to come back to the city, after 1921. This created a baby boom in 1922–23 and 1924–25. Better wages and job opportunities acted as a 'pull' whilst varying employment in the countryside and poverty were amongst the 'push' factors.[15] Some workers moved to Petrograd on a permanent basis attracted to job opportunities in metal-working, textiles, transport and construction. Other arrivals wished to retain their ties with the village and so came to the city on the long established seasonal basis to augment earnings from agricultural work. Migration from villages into the city of Leningrad stood at nearly 452,000 p.a. between 1925–27.[16] The decline in population growth by 1927 was probably due to the fact that those returning after the civil war had now already done so and rising unemployment and poor-quality housing (see below) probably discouraged some, though not all, seasonal workers from coming to the city. Those workers or peasants who arrived also faced possible health risks, which we shall now discuss.

The lifestyle adopted by some groups – excessive alcohol consumption, smoking, abortion, perceived promiscuous sexual behaviour (leading to VD), poor levels of hygiene and sanitation and a low protein diet – meant that the life expectancy of the working class was reduced in comparison to other social groups. These problems were, of course, compounded by high levels of infectious and social diseases. Whether these diseases were caused by the urban environment, the result of worker close ties to the villages or due to backward peasant traits and habits was widely debated by the Party and the medical profession during the NEP.

Table 3.2 presents archival data on morbidity from infectious diseases under NEP. Infectious diseases exhibited a cyclical behaviour pattern and certain civil war trends remained in early NEP but then overall levels started to significantly drop. A year by year breakdown reveals that in 1921 morbidity was greatest from relapsing fever (68.9 per 10,000), dysentery (34.6)

Table 3.2 Incidence of infectious diseases in Petrograd/Leningrad, 1921–1927 (rates per 10,000 population)

Type of disease	1921	1922	1923	1924	1925	1926	1927
Typhoid	32.3	9.8	4.5	10.5	19.3	14.8	17.2
Typhus	51.0	83.0	6.5	3.1	1.4	0.7	0.02
Relapsing fever	68.9	49.4	3.9	0.3	0.1	0.05	0.02
Smallpox	1.8	1.2	0.5	0.09	0.09	0.05	0.07
Measles	12.5	9.95	17.0	79.6	64.0	57.4	65.4
Scarlet fever	9.5	7.5	9.5	32.4	65.3	61.6	69.4
Diphtheria	6.9	2.5	6.7	6.0	6.2	7.5	9.0
Dysentery	34.6	24.6	9.1	17.0	10.0	7.4	3.4
Total	217.5	188.2	57.7	149.0	166.4	149.5	185.5

Source: GARF f. A-482 op. 10. d. 292, lists 26-28, 30-35

and measles (12.5). In 1922, typhus was more prominent (83.0), followed by relapsing fever (49.4), dysentery (24.8) and measles (9. 95), which was on the decline. In 1923, however, measles, scarlet fever and diphtheria were all on the increase (standing at 17.0, 9.5 and 9.1 cases per 10,000 population respectively). In 1924, the same diseases as well as typhoid (up from 4 5 to 10.5 per 10,000) posed the greatest problems for the local authorities. By 1925, mid-NEP, it was scarlet fever, measles (now on the decline) and diphtheria which were the main causes of ill health in Leningrad, with all other diseases becoming less prominent. Regarding infectious diseases trends between 1925–27, a number of points can be made. Firstly, morbidity from typhoid, typhus and relapsing fever was continuing to fall. Typhoid levels, for example, declined from 19.3 per 10,000 in 1925 to 17.2 per 10,000 in 1927; typhus fell from 1.4 to 0.7 and relapsing fever from 0.1 to 0.2 over the same period. Secondly, other diseases, such as smallpox and dysentery, showed similar patterns of decline with the former becoming negligible at 0.07 per 10,000 by 1927 while the latter dropped from 10 to 3.4 per 10,000 in the period 1925–27.

However, morbidity was greatest from children's diseases. Measles was by far the most prevalent disease increasing slightly from 64.0 in 1925 to 65.4 per 10,000 by 1927. Likewise, scarlet fever and diphtheria showed slight upward movements from 65.3 to 69.4 and from 6.2 to 9.0 respectively in late NEP. Rising morbidity occurred at a time of dwindling health service resources. Thus when the anti-scarlet fever campaign was launched in 1925–27, 10,000 inoculations were administered but a year later only 5,946 jabs were given and in only one district of the city because of a shortage of staff, needles and serum. In other districts no such campaign was launched at all. Greater success was had with smallpox, with the number of vaccinations remaining steady at around 33,000 between 1926–27 although the number of follow up vaccinations given declined from 80,459 in 1926 to 39,058 by 1927.[17] These reductions probably reflected budget constraints.

Poster 5 shows a 1921 poster from V.S. that encourages Soviet males to wash themselves in a public or factory steam bath in order to prevent them

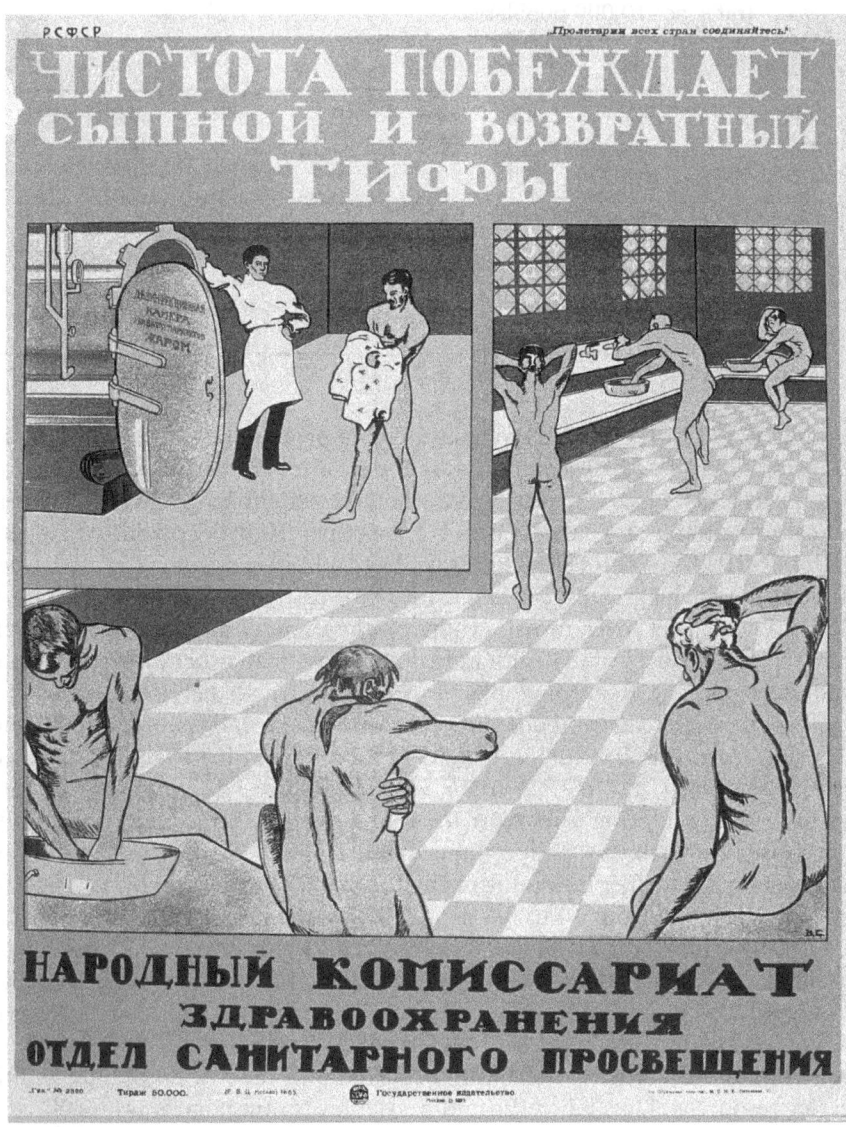

Poster 5 Cleanliness and combating typhus and relapsing fever

Source: 'Washing and cleanliness defeats typhus and relapsing fever'. Narkomzdrav, R.S.F.S.R. Department of Health Education poster, Colour lithograph by VS., Moscow 1921. Credit: Wellcome Collection, Wellcome Library, London (CC BY 4.0)

from catching typhus. It also depicts men in the background (in inset) taking off their clothes cleaned and putting them in a disinfection tank. Those who followed these instructions were less likely to catch typhus and this might account in part for the trends shown in Table 3.2.

Sexual diseases were also rife during the NEP. Morbidity from venereal diseases (VD) was initially relatively low in early NEP, with syphilis reaching nearly 3,000 cases and gonorrhoea only 656 cases in 1921. After this period of initial calm, the incidence of syphilis dramatically increased tenfold by 1924–25 reaching a peak of nearly 28,000 in 1924 whilst gonorrhoea reached its highest level at over 26,000 in the same year. This posed a significant challenge to the population and health service. VD levels fell after this point to 11,929 cases of syphilis and 13,866 cases of gonorrhoea by 1927. In overall terms, cases of syphilis doubled and gonorrhoea tripled per 10, 000 population under NEP.

The trend displayed in Table 3.3, created a fear of a VD epidemic, of a loosening of morals and above all the notion that those with VD were threatening not just their own health, but the collective health of the population of the city. This situation created, as Bernstein's excellent work shows, a concern on the part of the Party leadership and health officials that there was an unhealthy interest in sex and too much experimentation and casual sex happening during the NEP. As a result, there was calls from the medical profession to regulate sexual behaviour which Bernstein refers to as the new 'dictatorship of sex'.[18] This led to sexual health and hygiene campaigns to educate those deemed to be 'ignorant' or 'backward' and to attempts to instil a new sexual lifestyle (see below).

A detailed examination of the reasons for VD under the NEP falls beyond the scope of this study, but socio-economic factors, such as population movement, rapid economic development, co-educational schooling, greater urbanisation and industrialisation and increased alcohol consumption as well as cultural factors, such as a greater tolerance of certain types of sexual behaviour, a higher level of pre- and extra-marital sex, greater sexual freedom and a lack of sex education, which meant that patients might fail to recognise that they had been infected with VD and therefore continue to change partners and hence force the level of VD upwards, all contributed

Table 3.3 Morbidity rate from venereal diseases in Petrograd/Leningrad under NEP

Year	Syphilis		Gonorrhoea	
	a	*b*	*a*	*b*
1921	2,996	36.1	656	7.9
1922	2,408	25.1	542	5.7
1923	13,248	120.9	6,675	61.1
1924	27,710	226.9	26,010	31.7
1925	22,092	160.2	18,517	25.5
1926	16,460	107.2	15,131	96.0
1927	11,929	73.2	13,866	22.6

Notes: *a* Absolute numbers   *b* rate per 10,000
Source: GARF f. A-482 op. 10. d. 1914, list 44 and GARF f. A-482 op. 26, d. 18, list 5

to these patterns. Petrograd/Leningrad health personnel were expected to diagnose, treat and cure VD patients and health educationalists, through their posters,[19] reinforced this medical responsibility. In the process, women with VD were equated with prostitutes and often wrongly demonised, and portrayed as a threat to society and to the collective.

Although unemployment in Petrograd during early NEP was, in the main part, never quite as bad as it was during the Civil War, the situation was particularly acute among women nevertheless.[20] Facing impoverishment, some women turned to prostitution. As one Leningrad Women's department (*Zhenotdel*) meeting noted some unemployed women abandoned their children and got into crime or prostitution.[21] Although prostitution was illegal under Criminal Code Articles 155, 167 and 169–71, there were still 17, 000 prostitutes in Petrograd by 1921 and a year later, the number had jumped to 32,000 with most practising their trade on Nevskii Prospect and being in the age group 20–30 years.[22] As in earlier periods,[23] prostitutes were accused of being main cause of the upsurge in VD. Thus of the patients examined in Vasileostrovskii district's VD dispensary in early 1926, 45% had contracted VD during contact with prostitutes.[24]

From a public health perspective, poor standards of personal hygiene among the prostitutes increased the risk of infection, so male clients (ranging from nepmen, privileged officials and foreign specialists or students or workers on a business trip) were said to be more likely to contract VD.[25] The enormous increase in the number of divorces in Leningrad resulted in armies of deserted and destitute women roaming the streets. From mid-1926 onwards a campaign was launched to close illegal brothels (*pritonoderzhitel'stva*) and a tougher line was taken against the criminal elements guarding the women looking for clients on the Ligovka and Nevskii in Leningrad.[26]

The approach taken in relation to prostitution was one which emphasized re-education through advice to the Soviet masses on the unacceptability of this practice, the eradication of unemployment, the use of VD dispensaries or prophylactoria to treat patients and visits to rehabilitation centres to cure prostitutes and enable them to return to work. In this context, the number of urban VD dispensaries in Leningrad increased from 115 in 1925–26 to 159 by the end of 1927; while the number of rural ones increased from 66 in 1925 to 144 by 1926. The number of patient visits increased from 76,547 to 156,369 over the same period.[27] By 1926, hospital bed spaces for VD patients in Leningrad totalled 802, a fall in comparison to the year before [840], but by 1927, the number of beds increased to 860.[28]

The aim of the Soviet regime was to change the *byt* or everyday life or lifestyle of males and females and create a new Soviet person who transcended the traditional and old bourgeois ways of conduct and behaviour. This was captured by the central Bolshevik notion of the collective and idea of collectivism which emphasised, according to Kollontai, that a person's private life (*lichnaia zhizn'*) cannot be separated from that of the collective.[29] Thus everyone's behaviour, in this case sexual, whether a member of the Party or not, was a concern to the state. The idea of the collective was centred on the importance of class, revolution, Party and socialist regime and focused upon the development of a new form of social-ist morality and consciousness, which destroyed the pre-1917 exploitative society and the sources of exploitation. Such a transition was represented in Soviet discourse as a significant cultural advance over pre-revolutionary times.

One 1923 poster entitled 'After the destruction of Capitalism – the proletar-iat will abolish prostitution the scourge of humanity', is in line with this belief and shows that if men and women in the new NEP society worked together, then they will not only smash capitalism and the capitalists (depicted here as being trodden on and defeated by the working class), but also eradicate female exploitation and rid Soviet society of prostitution. The desire for unity and equality is symbolised in this poster by the male worker extending his hand to his female comrade. The Soviet leadership assumed that any 'backwardness' amongst the new population could be overcome by enlightenment (increased class consciousness) provided by schools, trade unions, the Komsomol, Party etc.[30] However, creating such a new byt was not easy to realise in the 1920s. Failures were attributed to the NEP 'retreat' as it was alleged that class ene-mies were corrupting 'pure' communists with decadent, bourgeois tendencies, ensuring the old habits and ways of behaviour still persisted. This situation was referred to by Michael David Fox as 'NEPification'.[31]

Despite the well-meaning message of 'After the destruction of Capitalism – the proletariat will abolish prostitution the scourge of humanity' 1923 poster, it was hard to change male attitudes. Peter Konecny points out how, for instance, during one debate among Petrograd students in 1923 which called for such respect and males and females sharing any hardships, some male students attending replied that work and food were more significant than the so-called 'women's question'.[32] Thus this 1923 poster, which targets the most conscious proletarian ideal of masculinity, was meant to act as a means of urging all men during the NEP (and beyond) to treat women as equals.

This visual discourse was part of the gendered and context-based use of imagery in public health posters which drew subtle distinctions between urban/rural contexts and different categories of women. This involved mixed, contradictory images. Soviet women were sometimes portrayed as negative, such as prostitutes, those having abortions or peasant midwives (*babki*) performing illegal abortions; and sometimes; and on other occasions as positive such as when depicted as mothers, women encouraging men not to drink etc. Thus despite all the legislative changes and collective rhetoric from Lenin to Stalin, the Soviet regime maintained prescribed clear gender roles to males and females, as part of its goal to eliminate so called deviant practices or officially designated 'bad' health habits. This is evident in the posters included in this book.

Generally speaking, the high mortality rate from TB emerged out of the bad conditions prevailing during War Communism and became, according to Dr Neslin and his colleagues, a major cause of the high death rate in Petrograd during early NEP.[33] Even though the mortality rate was down in 1921 compared to the year before (38.5 as against 55.7), TB was more prominent in 1922 (41.0 per 10,000). Thereafter TB levels fell, averaging at around 26.1 for the period 1923–25. While, such a decline is impressive in comparison to pre-revolutionary times, in 1925 Leningrad (22.43) had more TB related deaths than other major European cities, such as Vienna (22.0), Berlin (12.0), London (11.0), Brussels and Copenhagen (both 10.3). Only Paris with 28 deaths per 10,000 had a higher mortality rate from TB.[34] Mortality from TB in Leningrad, a major killer striking all age groups, had reached, 21.6 by 1926 before rising to 24.1 by 1927.[35]

Soviet medical practitioners viewed TB as a 'workers' disease' and classified it as a social disease because it was the result of human contact and had a clear correlation with social class.[36] Housing was seen as the main cause in Soviet medical discourse, either because of overcrowding, which increased the risk of infection, or as a consequence of poor hygiene and sanitation, which lowered people's resistance to TB. During the civil war, a decline in the housing quality, poor hygiene and sanitation, malnutrition and a lack of basic amenities resulted in TB mortality being higher than it was in 1913. Under the NEP, the population was expanding and overcrowding was becoming more of a problem but there was only some improvement in the level of public hygiene and sanitation (see below).

The USSR followed German experience in favouring the use of the sanatoria because housing conditions were said to preclude domiciliary treatment. TB patients were encouraged to seek treatment in either sanatoria or specially created TB dispensaries. Although the total number of visits to TB dispensaries in the city of Leningrad increased from 70,991 in 1922 (of which 18,526 were primary) to 295,409 (of which 39,335 were primary) by 1925, this represented a decline in real terms from 73.9 visits to 28 5 per 1,000 population over the same period.[37]

In Leningrad's case, TB sanatoria were the product of three things: first, an attempt to satisfy workers' demands for health care institutions which operated in their interests; second, a consequence of a health policy under the NEP which favoured the insured; and, third, they stemmed from the medical profession's assumption that TB was curable and the best place to treat the sick was in sanatoria or dispensaries. All three, of course, overlap with one another but the first two variables are a product of prevailing ideology, whereas the third reflected physician's view of causation and was also part of their professional interests and their attempt to play a leading role in public health affairs and medical policy. One indication of priority is the expenditure on these establishments (sanatoria, rest homes, health resort facilities) which rose from 2,191,900r in 1924/25 to 3,481,300 by 1926.[38]

A key role in fighting this disease was assigned to the Leningrad TB Institute which was created in 1925 and continued to expand throughout the period under discussion. By late 1926, for example, it had a wide range of facilities: two clinics, an experimental-biology department, an X-ray unit, various polyclinics, dispensaries and social pathology and hygiene sections as well as a thriving medical training division responsible for educating future TB specialists. The emphasis in its work was on treatment of the insured using calcium therapy or in more radical cases, surgery.[39]

The tendency to treat these patients in sanatoria, rest homes and convalescent homes continued throughout this period, with much the same results as before, namely the outward appearance of success and growing evidence of the State paying attention to 'workers' needs', while in reality having little impact on this lethal disease. There appears, however, to have been a gradual acknowledgement that they were far from successful with the number of sanatoria falling from 920 in 1922 to 315 by 1925 before reaching 240 in 1927.[40]

Poster 6 depicts a woman in blue pointing to the benefits of a clean, park open area setting for those with TB accompanied by a young girl with a chequered top and doll. Children are shown the background playing and sitting in the park attended by staff. An industrial city can be seen in the background in the top right. This image suggests that clean, healthy environments rather than polluting cities (as symbolised by the smoke from factory

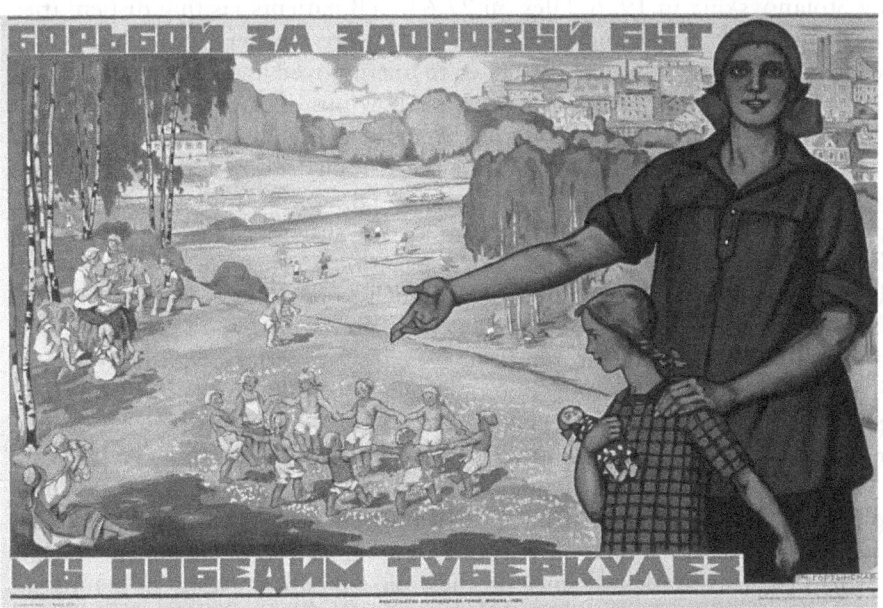

Poster 6 Combating tuberculosis

Source: 'Fighting for a healthy existence. We will conquer tuberculosis' Narkomzdrav poster 1926. Courtesy of the U.S. National Library of Medicine, Bethesda, Maryland, USA

chimneys) are good for the health of children and prevent them from becoming TB patients. The other message is that State care and fresh air aids their rate on recovery.

Those not allocated places in these institutions were treated in special TB dispensaries. The number of visits to TB dispensaries in city of Leningrad totalled 291,836 in 1926 of which 13,735 were primary visits. Visiting figures to TB dispensaries were down slightly on the previous year, which is not surprising as TB mortality had declined between 1925–1926.[41] According to one source, the day sanatoria had used up 26,771 bed-days and the night ones 23,883 bed-days in 1926.[42]

This was a time of rapid population expansion and cut backs instigated during the 'regime of economy'. Attempts were nevertheless made to expand facilities. On 1 October 1926, a night sanatorium was opened in Moscow-Narva district with 100 beds and another one in Volodarskii district with 75 beds. A Special dietary unit was also created at a cost of 200,000r and 8–10 more new TB dispensaries were planned in the near future.[43] During the first quarter of 1927, visits to existing TB dispensaries already totalled 111,914, of which 9,587 were primary, reflecting an upsurge in cases and deaths from TB. This amounted to 7,085 bed-days in the day and to 5,177 bed-days in the night sanatoria over the same period.[44]

A high degree of overcrowding was said to be a cause of TB in Soviet medical thinking at this time. This point is emphasised in a study made by Stoianovskaia in 1926. Files on 22,643 TB patients visiting dispensaries were analysed and of the patients, 87.1% were workers and white-collar workers and their families; 11.0% were unemployed and/or pensioners and 1.9% came from other undisclosed social groups/occupations. The level of TB recorded varied between districts. Petrograd side district had the highest number followed by Vasilevostrovskii, then the city centre and finally Vyborg district. The reason cited for contracting TB was housing. Stoianovskaia points out that 72.1% of the sample of TB sufferers lived in unsanitary housing conditions, 11.2% had poor ventilation and 19.4% lived in poverty hence the upkeep of their dwelling left much to be desired'.[45] Most patients lived in crowded accommodation, in damp conditions, with both bad light and poor ventilation.[46] In addition, the large majority of patients ate an inadequate diet.[47] All in all, Stoianovskaia concludes 'unsanitary housing, poor diet and low levels of personal hygiene' were found to be the main reasons for TB in Leningrad at this time.[47]

With the benefit of hindsight, such faith in a medical solution seems misplaced and money would have probably been better spent on improving housing provision and nutrition rather than on staffing sanatoria, as the latter had no discernible influence on the course of TB mortality in Leningrad during early NEP. Such a conclusion was never drawn, so similar approaches still prevailed in the second half of the 1920s and early 1930s. Furthermore, the local authorities cut TB bed provision at a time when TB was posing the greatest threat to health status in Petrograd/Leningrad and relied instead on the sanatoria.

Although the insured had the necessary coverage to enable them to seek early treatment and even undergo after-care, the non-insured patients did not have such financial backing and did not present themselves for treatment until their condition was intractable. In such cases, TB could not have been tackled institutionally. The available evidence suggests that medical intervention only played a small part in reducing TB mortality in Leningrad by isolating infectious cases.[48] It was declining poverty and better nourishment which helped; though arduous working conditions complicated things. Smith, Bryder and McFarlane argue that institutional treatment of respiratory TB was ineffective prior to the introduction of streptomycin and the advent of effective chemotherapy in the late 1940s.[49] Medically, Soviet strategy was not very helpful, though politically it was a greater success as it indicated how the Soviet State cared for its workers.

Under the NEP, the per-capita consumption of beer increased from 17.52 litres in 1922–23 to 49.78 litres in 1925 reaching 54.46 litres by 1926; while vodka consumption doubled from 7.1 litres in 1925 to 14.2 litres in 1926.[50] The public health leadership continually emphasized in the city's medical journal and the Party also stressed the dangers associated with alcohol abuse in its health education posters.

Poster 7 says 'Every river begins from a small stream' at the top and 'I became an alcoholic from sipping a small glass' at the bottom. The front of the poster shows a young worker downing a glass of spirits/vodka while a shadow behind either depicts an older worker downing a bottle of spirits/vodka, so acting as a bad role model, or it refers to the same person at a later stage becoming an alcoholic. Posters such as this pre-date the Soviet temperance movement, but demonstrate state and medical profession concern with alcoholism especially among workers, as excessive drinking can cause death. In this context, the death rate from alcoholic poisoning was down on the First World War period (when partial prohibition was in force), plummeting from 31.1 per 100,000 in 1921 to 2.6 per 100,000 in 1924. Mortality was on the increase again to 6.2 per 100,000 a year later and the figure virtually doubled between 1926–27 rising from 10.9 per 100,000 to 18.0 per 100,000.[50] Deaths from acute alcoholic poisoning were, therefore, only marginally below their pre-revolutionary level by the end of NEP. This trend was caused by excessive consumption and brewing moonshine illegally, which contained toxic impurities.

Most of those dying from alcoholism came from the working class. Thus according to Didrikhson, the death rate from alcohol stood at 9.7 per 100,000 in 1926 among those living in the Petrograd side of Leningrad and at 11.7 per 100,000 among those residing in the Moscow-Narva district. This compared with a mortality figure of only 5.5 per 100,000 among city-centre residents.[51] Even allowing for the fact that the NEP

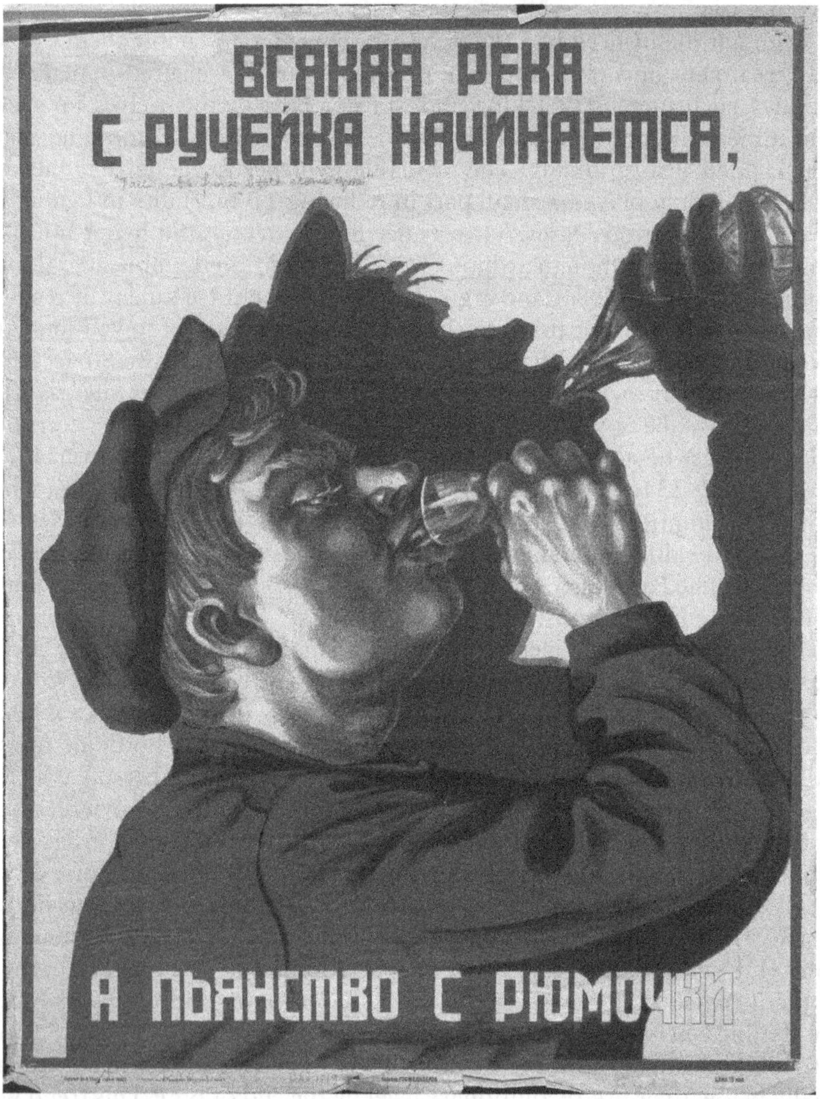

Poster 7 Anti-alcohol poster

Source: 'Every river begins from a small stream.... I became an alcoholic from sipping a small glass'. Poster ca. 1930. Courtesy of Soviet Poster Collection, Swarthmore College Peace Collection.

resulted in greater residential mixing and therefore significantly reduced the sharp discrepancies between districts, it still remains true that mortality due to alcoholism was greater among 'workers' than other social groups. Thus, five times more male workers were dying from alcoholic poisoning than their white-collar counterparts in Leningrad in 1926–27.[52]

The introduction of the anti-alcohol legislation described below failed to stem the rising tide of drunkenness, so the central and local governments stepped up their anti-alcohol campaigns in the mid-late 1920s. The basic approach taken besides administrative measures,[53] involved the use of the militsia to make mass arrests. In Petrograd/Leningrad's case, the number of police arrests for being drunk and disorderly increased from 2,058 in 1922 to 32,954 by 1925.[54] Fiscal considerations probably also influenced government action. The local authorities expressed concern over economic losses and absenteeism due to alcoholism.[55] Poster 8 depicts a graph on Soviet productivity. Labour productivity increases but a drunken male, swigging from a vodka bottle, reduces productivity by their drinking (symbolised by him holding onto the end of the graph). It illustrates the dangers of alcohol to a person's health, economic policy and labour productivity and encourages temperance.

The tax on alcohol was high, with the price of a bottle of beer increasing from 10k before the First world war to 30k in 1925 (or 50k in restaurants[56]), and so a 'fiscal dilemma' probably existed during the NEP.[57] Nikolai Semashko, the RSFSR Health Minister, vigorously denied any such suggestion declaring 'In this question (anti-alcohol enforcement) fiscal considerations in no way dominate over the interests of the health status of the population or socialist development'.[58]

In the mid-late 1920s, the use of administrative measures to combat this problem was less common and the emphasis instead was placed on cultural and medical solutions.[59] As argued elsewhere, in 1926 the RSFSR Criminal Code made persons liable for making home brew with intent to sell; the price of State produced vodka was increased by 50% and a Sovnarkom decree of 11 September 1926 enabled Narkomzdrav to organise compulsory treatment facilities for chronic alcoholics.[60] Finally, in March 1927, a ban was placed on vodka sales then in May 1927 local anti-alcohol commissions were set up.[61] In addition to this, and prompted by the alcoholism research of Narkomzdrav's Institute of Social Hygiene, which began in 1925–26, local health services began emphasising the use of health education. This involved the use of posters and films to get the anti-alcohol message (danger to health, high probability of divorce, loss of friends and workmates) across.[62] It was probably too soon for the above vodka ban to take effect, so levels of consumption continued to climb and by 1927 of all the towns surveyed by Didrikhson, Leningrad was second closest to tsarist drinking patterns.[63]

As sales and consumption of alcohol in Leningrad increased, so did the number of detentions made by the militsia, resulting in people's placement in sobering-up stations which rose from nearly 33,000 in 1925 to somewhere between 110–113,000 by 1927.[64] Poor law enforcement, engendered partly by the 'regime of economy' policy in 1926 which meant that the militsia had less money and staff and so assigned this problem less priority, resulted in alcoholism still being widespread. A change in government attitudes towards

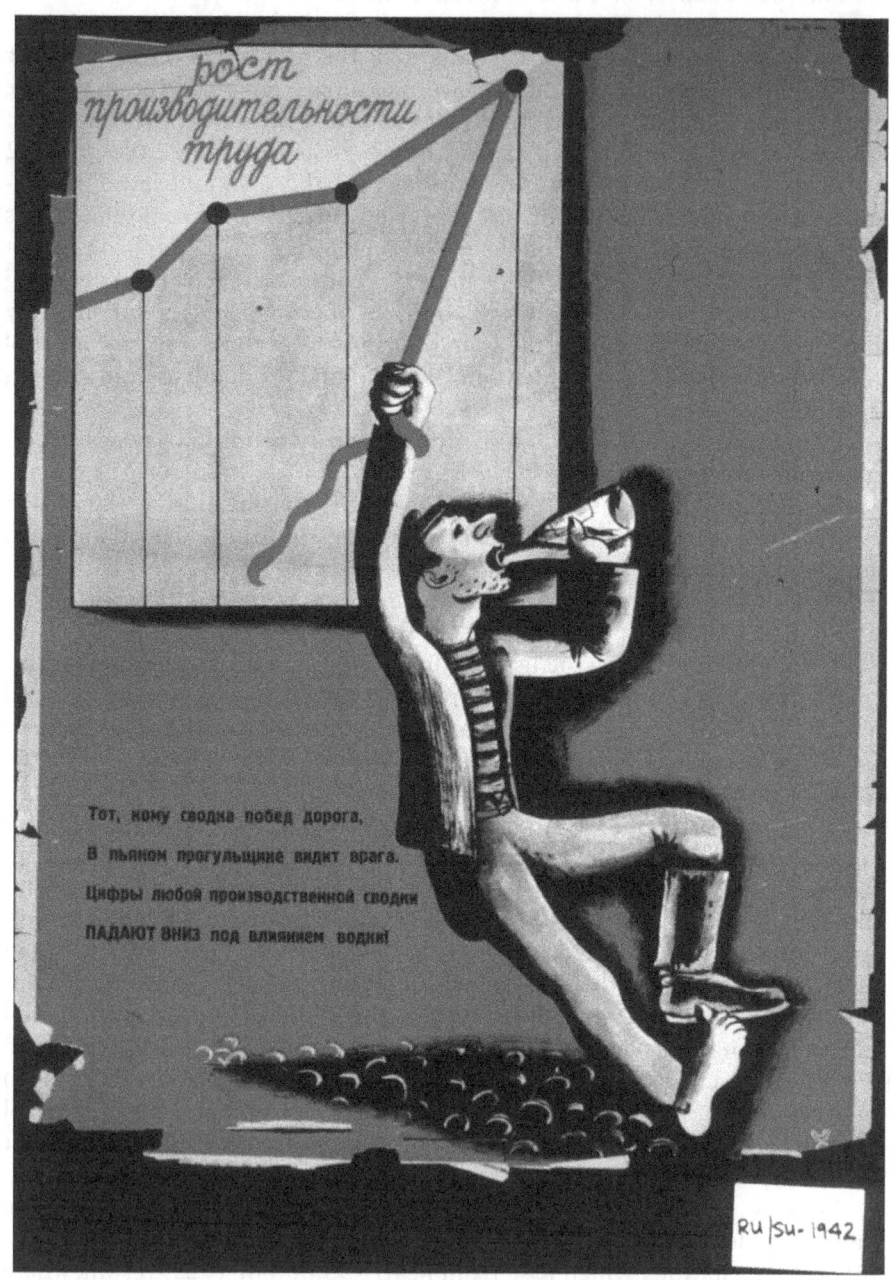

Poster 8 Alcohol and labour productivity

Source: 'Those who seek a winning road see drunk absentees as the enemy'. Poster Collection, Poster ID# RU/SU 1942, Hoover Institution Archives.

alcoholism occurred in late 1927 as the negative impact on labour productivity became clear.[65] This explains the importance of Poster 8. But it was not until the industrialisation and collectivisation drives got underway and the First five-year plan was being implemented, that a Temperance Movement emerged. Its impact on Leningrad is discussed in Chapter 4.

Phillips concludes that in Soviet official dialogues on drinkers 'Backward' or 'rank and file' workers were said to inhibit 'a coarse and bawdy world – a world of heavy drinking, brawling, womanizing and cursing were common' whereas 'conscious' or 'advanced' workers instead 'valued sobriety, clean language, neat dress, sexual restraint, political involvement and educational improvement'.[66] One 1926 poster entitled 'Who is smart, and who is the fool! One for the book and the other in the tavern' fits this assumption. It was meant to generate additional political and culturally conscious males, symbolized by the educated reader, who were able to control their alcohol consumption and abstain from it, whereas the peasant 'other', a possible migrant to Leningrad during NEP, was seen to be weakening socialism by heavy drinking and uncultured habits.[67] Drink was therefore seen as endangering the collective as a whole.

Another reason for the varying birth rate under the NEP were trends in the infant mortality rate (IMR) which increased from 18.9 in 1921 to 23.3 in 1922, then fell to 14.3 in 1923 and increased again to 17.3 in 1924. The IMR declined again to 15.4 per 1,000 by 1925, well below its pre-First World War level. The IMR rate finally reached 17.2 in 1927, which is marginally below its 1921 level.[68]

Poster 9 'Protect your child' by the artist A. Komarov was produced in 1921, at the start of the NEP by the mother and child protection department. It shows an infant in a small boat alone, implying danger. The child is at sea surrounded by rocks with the labels indicating different reasons why infants can die including 'poor care', 'filthy conditions', 'feeding cows milk' etc and advises mothers to provide a 'warm room' the right food (such as grain or oats) up to 6 months and so on. As we saw in Chapter 1, urban conditions were extremely unhealthy and the health care available was limited before 1917. The Soviet government assigned more priority to children and women's health in the civil war but the circumstances hindered developments. The Soviet regime then expanded the number of women and infant facilities which probably contributed to improving the situation overall under NEP.

The main cause for infants under one year dying was typhus, smallpox, measles, scarlet fever, diphtheria, whooping cough, dysentery and pneumonia in early NEP. Shuster-Kadyshev argues that heavy drinking among women in Petrograd 1921–23 not only affected their health, but also that of the newborn in terms of size.[69] There was also little improvement in the food supply of mothers whose inability to purchase milk together with an inadequate diet also lead to an increase in the IMR.[70] Other factors influencing this trend, include pregnant women's lifestyle (eating, smoking, drinking

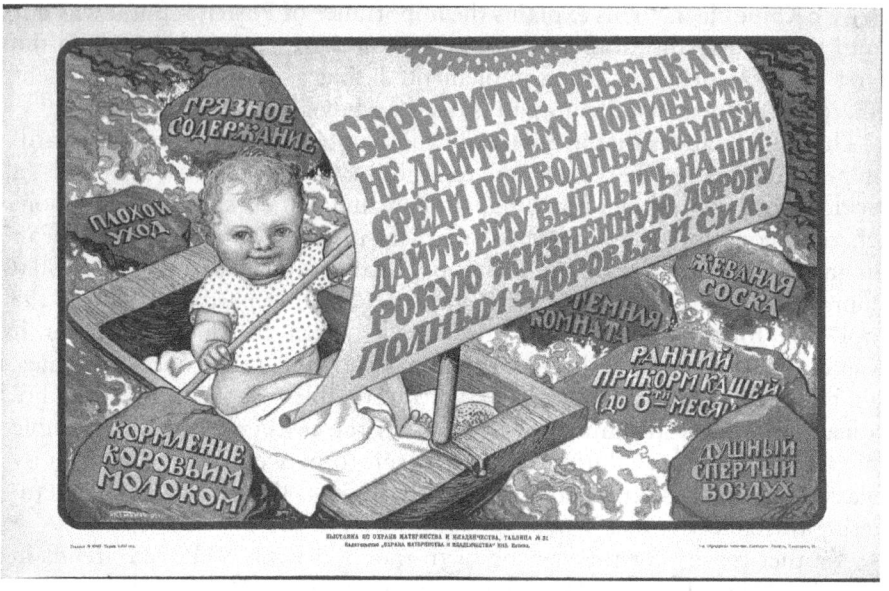

Poster 9 Babies in the collective

Source: 'Beregitie rebenka' (*Protect your child*). Artist A. Komarov. 1921 Poster. Courtesy of Soviet Poster Collection, Swarthmore College Peace Collection.

habits, employment etc.) and illness during pregnancy, repeated abortions (see below)[71] underutilisation of health facilities, poor housing, lack of hygiene and sanitation, widespread environmental pollution and finally inadequate child-care facilities.[72]

Poster 10 by A. A. Ioffe illustrates Narkomzdrav's and doctors' views (via a department of mothers and infants) poster on the causes of IMR by the mid-1920s in Leningrad. Panel 1 in the top left shows a pacifier (dummy) made of chewed bread, kasha and dirt, which is not good for the baby's health. It suggests that some mothers do not know how to care for their very young children. This implication is that ignorance causes many babies to die in the remote villages of Leningrad Oblast. Once again, the 'modernisation of motherhood' agenda is evident. Panel 2 states 'the more literate a mother, the fewer children will die'. Mothers are urged to educate themselves, by reading medical advice literature (symbolised by the book on the left of panel 2 top right) rather than let their children die out their ignorance (the right-hand side of panel 2 shows a mother in despair). Panel 3 (bottom left) has women dressed in different national costumes and compares the IMR per 100 births by country. Thus Switzerland had a rate of 9%, England, 14%, Italy, 17%, Germany, 20% and the USSR, 26%. Thus this 1925 poster is honest enough to say that Russia's IMR is the highest of all

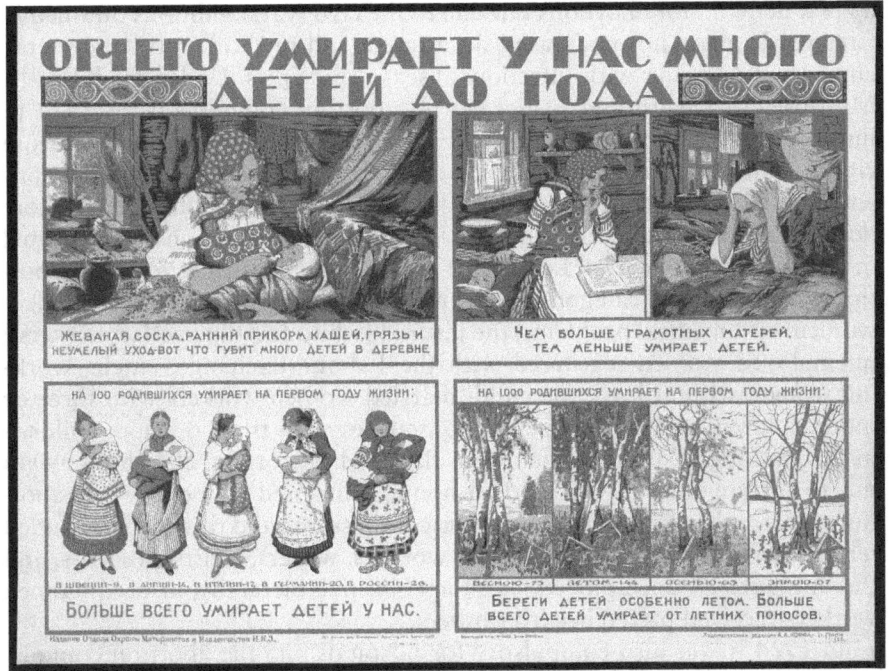

Poster 10 Advice to mothers on causes of infant mortality

Source: 'What kills many babies under one year old'. Department for the Protection of Motherhood and Infants poster, Leningrad, Soviet Union, 1925. O. Griun. Credit: Wellcome Collection, Wellcome Library, London (CC BY 4.0).

these countries. Finally, panel 4 (bottom right) informs the female viewer that IMR levels vary according to time of the year – spring, 73; summer, 144, autumn, 63 and winter, 67. It is urging mothers to pay attention to their young ones all year round, but especially in the summer when under one-year-olds are susceptible to diarrhoea.

Abortion was legalised on 18 November 1920. It was to be provided free, performed by a doctor (only). Any nurse or midwife found guilty of performing an abortion could be struck off and tried by the People's Court and any doctor carrying out an abortion for personal gain in their private practice could also be referred to the People's Court.[73] According to Goldman

> prevailing opinion on abortion rested on three basic tenets: first, that poverty drove women to seek abortion, and that better material circumstances would thus obviate the need for it; second, that the decision to bear a child was not personal but social; third, that society's reproductive needs ultimately took primacy over an individual woman's desires.[74]

As with other health issues the collective came first. The 1920 decree led to a great demand for abortions but due to the civil war conditions outlined in Chapter 2, many hospitals were devastated, and medical staff were preoccupied with dealing with infectious disease epidemics. Under the NEP, the Ministries of Health and Justice set up abortion commissions in 1924 to improve the situation. They consisted of a doctor and representatives from city's women and infants' department and the Zhenotdel. The commissions emphasized the risks of abortion and its negative impact on society before deciding who would receive an abortion.[75] These commissions were located in urban centres such as Leningrad and allocated permits for 'free abortions' where certain categories of women met state criteria. These included: women with medical problems; the insured (white and blue-collar workers); unemployed women registered with the Labour Exchange; single, working women with at least one child; married women workers with three or more children; and working-class housewives with three or more children in this ranking. Peasant women were classified as working-class housewives due to carrying out unpaid work at home. Uninsured women seeking abortions were to be reviewed last by these commissions and this group included female students, servants, handicraft workers, writers, artists, peasants, and the unregistered unemployed.[76] In the collective hierarchy, insured women workers received preference over others.

In 1924 it was also compulsory for hospitals and the abortion commissions to complete abortion cards (*kartochki ob aborte*).[77] Data from these cards allows us as historians to analyse the frequency of abortions, who was having an abortion and their motivation. But the cards are not without their problems. They do not cover those who failed to get a permit from the abortion commissions. These women had to have illegal abortions performed by unqualified peasant midwives outside hospitals or by doctors working in the private sector. The only other choice these women had was paying for an abortion, a source of income for local authorities at a time when money was urgently needed for women's medical facilities. The number of legal (i.e. hospital based) abortions in Petrograd/Leningrad increased from 3,060 in 1923 (or 2.8 per 1,000 population) to 35,523 (or 21.8 per 1,000) in 1927[78] whereas the number of illegal abortions increased from 1,285 (or 1.17 per 1,000) in 1923 to 8,384 (or 5.15 per 1,000) in 1927.[79] The number of deaths following abortions was 3.9 per 1,000 births in 1922; 3.5 in 1923, 2.7 in 1924 and 2.4 in 1925 but increased to 2.7 in 1926 and then fell slightly to 2.3 by 1927.[80]

Poster 11 by S. Iaguzhinskii emphasises the adverse consequences of abortions. It suggests to the female viewer that any kind of abortion can be dangerous. To the uneducated midwives (*babki*) who performed these illegal abortions (panel one top left), it implies that they are guilty of committing a crime and could ultimately cause the death of their misguided client (bottom panel 3). This public health department of women and infants sanctioned poster demonises the peasant babki who are seen as 'backward'

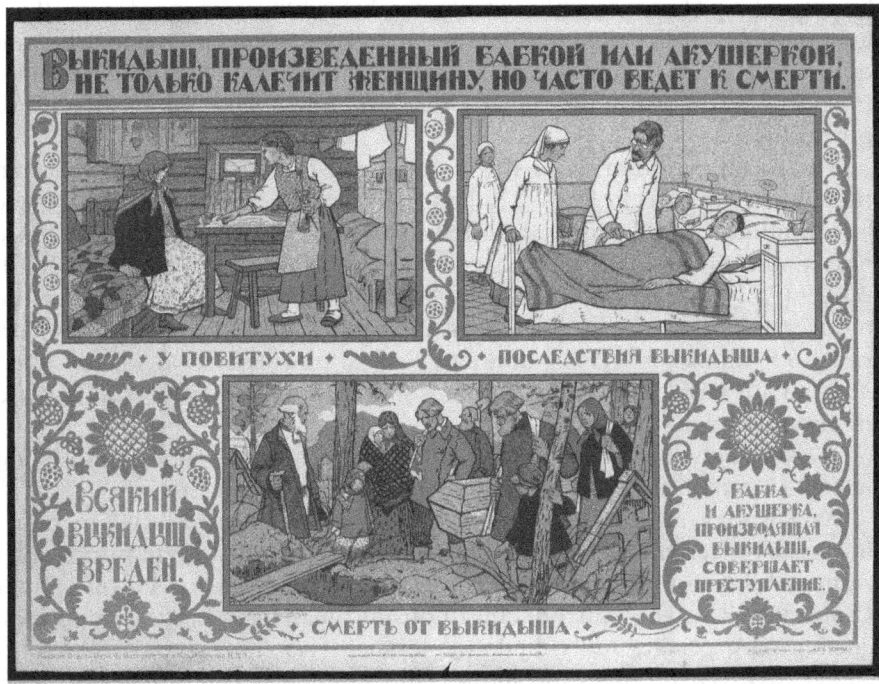

Poster 11 Anti-abortion poster

Source: 'Abortions performed by a babka or a midwife not only injure women but often lead to death'. Department for the Protection of Motherhood and Infants poster, Leningrad, Soviet Union, 1925, Artist S. Iaguzhinskii, Credit: Wellcome Collection, Wellcome Library, London (CC BY 4.0)

(hence the primitive rural setting). This is contrasted with Leningrad health service doctors who are shown working in a clean modern, urban setting, implying that they are more advanced and working in a 'safer' context from a women and unborn babies health point of view (panel 2 top right). Enlightened new Soviet women are explicitly being advised to consult licensed doctors rather than ignorant midwives in cases of an abortion. This poster also appeals to the conflict between city and countryside, building upon a similar theme explored earlier in relation to alcohol that existed by the end of the NEP which negatively contrasted the ignorant peasant with a modern city worker. In the case of Poster 11, this indirectly criticises peasants (symbolised by the babki) because of their opposition to the Family Code. Finally, Poster 11 depicts members of the medical profession – led by the male doctor and followed by two women nurses – as a key part of the modern advanced socialist public health service of Leningrad under the NEP and as acting in the collective's best interest by trying to protect and preserve women's health. Thus reproduction is favoured over abortion in Soviet policy. However, although the city's health service prided itself on guaranteeing special facilities for women and children, with the express aim of reducing the IMR and abortions, financial constraints and rapid population growth resulted in the demand for staff and facilities outweighing supply during late NEP.[81]

The social composition of the women who received abortions reflected the city's urban base. In 1926–27, the social class/economic situation of those having abortions in Leningrad is shown in Table 3.4. The age range of those having abortions was 15–17 years (2.0 per 1,000 women); 18–19 (20.5); 20–29 (75.7); 30–39 (50.0) and 40–49 years (8.7 per 1,000).[82] Among the motives, the main reasons for having an abortion were poverty/money worries (46.9%); illness (7.9%); desire to conceal pregnancy (0.5%); still nursing (6.3%); large family (9.1%), do not want another child (12.6%) and motive unknown (16.7%).[83]

We shall now consider how far housing and diet and standard of living impacted upon health conditions under NEP.

As Sosnovy argues, there were radical changes introduced in housing policy after the Civil War. These policies included giving occupants responsibility for their own dwellings; leasing houses via co-operatives (*Zhakty*) or trusts; introducing housing managers and committees; encouraging private individuals or nepmen (via preferential treatment) to get involved by investing money and building single houses or large apartments; embarking upon a limited de-nationalisation programme; increasing government control over housing by various means (increased investment, greater capital repairs or simply transferring housing over to government use) and so on.[84] The general aim of government policy at this time was to improve the provision of basic amenities, such as running water, and to extend the water supply and sewage network.[85] As a result of extensive purification programmes by the end of 1921, the Petrograd sewage network covered a distance of 636km and 800,000 barrels of rubbish were taken from the streets and 900,000 barrels from the Neva.[86] Many houses were still in a poor condition, with the large majority made of wood.[87]

Table 3.4 Abortions by economic situation/social class in Leningrad, 1926–27

Socio-economic category	Number of abortions
Worker	22,125
White-collar worker	14,756
Unemployed	6,329
Housewife	1,280
Other	9,800

Source: V V Paevskii, 'K voprosy o rozhdaemosti v Leningrade' in *Statisticheskii sbornik Leningradskogo oblastnogo otdela zdravookhraneniia za 1928 god* (Leningrad 1929), 71

By the time of the 1923 census, the quality of housing had improved, with 9,163 (51.8%) of the city's 17,685 houses having running water and 8,661 (48.5%) a functioning sewer system.[88] However, rapid population growth was putting a strain on the housing supply. Thus, whereas in 1920, 9.3% of the city's dwellings had more than two persons per room, by 1923 the figure had already increased to 22.3%.[89] This was largely because the number of rooms had only increased by 1% between 1920–23 whereas the population increased by 48% in the same period.[90] In 1923, per-capita housing space stood at 13.3m² with dwelling space being lower in traditionally working-class areas by the mid-1920s, where amenities were also fewer.[91]

To rectify the housing shortage, the local authorities launched various programmes including more repairs and increased housing finance. One 1924 survey of 2,314 Leningrad homes revealed that only 21% were in a satisfactory position; 51% were well-below standard and 22% found unsatisfactory. This was the case even though 6.5 million roubles had been spent on repairs in that year. In addition, 4.5 million roubles was spent on new housing to alleviate shortages.[92] According to Kabo, by the end of 1925, per capita expenditure on housing (repair, construction etc) was 6r 64k,[93] but this did little to eradicate these difficulties, as underscored by another 1925 survey.[94] By mid-NEP, then, the majority of the quality of housing was still poor and as a direct consequence of population growth, Leningrad citizens were forced to live in close proximity to one another. This situation made Party claims of progress and the benefits of socialism seem rather farfetched.

Overcrowding also spread disease. There was an urgent need to provide accommodation for the rapidly expanding urban population, especially factory workers. As one April 1926 Party resolution put it:

> The Party and the State must in the immediate future attach great significance to housing construction, in view of the fact that industrial growth, labour productivity and better living conditions for the masses are hampered by the housing crisis.[95]

According to 1926 census data, there were 257,658 apartments in Leningrad, of which 249,740 were occupied and 7,938 empty.[96] Of this stock, 54.5% was made of wood; 43.5% of stone; 1.9% of a mixture of both and 0.1% of other materials.[97] Drawing upon the successful use of housing cooperatives in 1924–25, decrees issued in October 1926 and November 1927 called for the construction of large apartment houses by public enterprise using public finance. Of the 19,764 already built, the pattern of ownership was as follows: 3,140 – State; 7,640 – cooperatives; 5,128 – privately owned and 3,856 were in local community hands.[98]

The housing cooperatives were therefore playing a major role in house building in Leningrad at this time. But building was slow. Even minimum sanitary norms could not be fulfilled. As the housing question grew more acute, the product of a 27% decline in housing space in Leningrad between 1923–26[99], it threatened the very basis of local industrial growth as the situation was extremely bad in industrial districts. Thus, Shtreis notes: 'There was an acute housing crisis in workers' districts, when the norm is 5–6m^2 or less per person'.[100] Thus the health of key members of the collective was under threat.

To alleviate these problems, pressure was brought to bear on housing contractors. As a result, new housing construction increased from 33,000m^2 in 1924–25 to nearly 41,000m^2 in 1926, before finally reaching 141,000m^2 by 1927.[101] However, this was still not enough to meet demand due to inadequate investment in housing. By 1927, only 12 million roubles was invested in new construction.[102] It was not just a shortage of money; residents' attitude towards the upkeep of the places where they lived left much to be desired.

Attempts were made during late NEP to improve the water supply, which was undergoing renovation in 1927 and water purification stations were also being set up. By 1927, Leningrad's water supply network covered 784km, as compared to only 102km in 1917.[103] Similarly work on the new sewage system, started in 1925, was continuing and major repairs to the old system were carried out in 1926–27. All in all, the sewage system had expanded from 50km in 1917 to nearly 600km by 1927. These were significant improvements, but problems still remained, such as the dumping of garbage in the Neva, so incinerator stations were set up in Vasilevskii-Ostrov and Leningrad city centre districts.[104] Finally, more repairs were to be carried out, with funding for the latter rising from 14 million roubles in 1926 to a planned 17 million by 1927.[105]

The housing crisis impinged on worker productivity, undermined labour force stability and, most of all from the point of view of this book, its inferior quality endangered health as our previous discussion of TB and infectious diseases suggested. On the eve of the First five-year plan, then, the demand for housing still exceeded supply and families were forced due to communal living to share what basic amenities existed. Such shortages of housing increased the likelihood of illness, women asking for abortions and put severe strains on family life.

Another factor that made daily life in Leningrad difficult in the 1920s was food and diet during the NEP. After the economic collapse and deprivations of War Communism, the living standards of workers in Petrograd started to gradually improve. There was a transition from barter to money wages between 1922–24, although wages were sometimes delayed. Average wages by 1926 were reaching their pre-First World War level. Workers in the city spent at least half their wages on food and slightly more, if they were better paid. This had an impact on the amount of foods purchased and workers daily calorie intake levels in the city of Petrograd which initially increased from 2,615 calories in April 1921 to 3,379 calories by October 1922. Thereafter levels declined to 3,627 calories in February 1923 and fell still further to 3,489 calories in February 1924. Calorie levels in Leningrad then rose again to 3,636 in February 1925, finally settling at 3,521 calories in June that year.[106]

Working-class families were eating meat, fish and dairy products as well as rye and wheat, vegetables and potatoes. Daily protein availability also rose from 72.2g in April 1921 to 119.0g by June 1925 as did animal protein intake from 13.0g to 51.6g respectively over the same period.[107] There was in Stephen Wheatcroft's view a 'remarkable improvement' in nutritional levels after the 1922 harvest when working class families suddenly began receiving 11% (more calories) per head in Petrograd.[108] It was at this point that mortality levels fell and the first period of demographic crisis was over. This situation was certainly aided by a dramatic fall in the retail price of rye flour in Petrograd from mid-1921 until early 1923.[109] The severe food production supply and consumption problems experienced during War Communism abated during early NEP as rationing was replaced by workers' ability to purchase food from state stores, cooperatives and in the private markets.

However, in mid–late NEP, the food supply situation changed and the per capita consumption of foodstuffs declined. Table 3.5 shows that the food supply situation had become grave by late 1926–early 1927. Consumption was low with the population of Leningrad having to rely on meagre diets for their survival. Thus, with the exception of meat and fish, the per-capita consumption of which increased by 10.8% and 6.0% respectively, consumption of all other products declined as follows: rye and wheat flour by 4.2%; butter by 22.3%; fruit and vegetables by 10% and potatoes by 13.3%. However, the fact that meat and fish intake was considerable, providing more protein and vitamins, probably prevented a more marked decline in health status among Leningrad inhabitants. Price reductions in the cost of butter to 2–3r and meat to 29k per 400g in March 1927 as well as a fall in the price of bread in April 1927 undoubtedly helped to increase consumption and this may have meant an improvement in diet at the end of this

Table 3.5 Per-capita consumption of various products by the urban population of Leningrad in late NEP, 1925-27 (in kilogrammes)

Foodstuffs	1925–26	1926–27
Rye and wheat flour	148.2	142.1
Meat	60.3	66.8
Butter	9.4	7.3
Eggs	14.3[a]	14.3[a]
Fish	16.7	17.7
Sugar	31.5[a]	31.5[a]
Fruit and vegetables	6.0	0.6
Potatoes	6.0	0.8

Notes: *a* Average of both periods

Sources: A. Iakobi, 'O poteblenii gorodskogo naseleniia', *Statisticheskoe obozrenie* No. 1, January 1929, 65-68 and I. Miliavskii, 'Natural'nye balansy kartofelia, ovoshchei i bakchevykh kul'tur za 1924-1928gg', *Statisticheskoe obozrenie* No. 3-4, March-April 1930, 31

period.[110] The steady improvements witnessed in the early 1920s, now gave rise to uncertainty over food.

In 1927, the country faced a war scare and peasants, especially kulaks, were accused of hoarding their produce. According to Carr and Davies 'By the autumn of 1927, shortages of food in the cities had become widespread and chronic. ... The failure of grain collections in the winter of 1927–28 deepened the crisis and brought the threat of worse privations to come'.[111] As a result, according to Shreis, the food situation became very difficult in Leningrad:

> There was a rapid decline in the quality and quantity of food on offer to the population of Leningrad throughout 1926 and up until early 1927. Attempts were made by food technologists to increase the number of inspections and thereby reduce the level of poor foodstuffs marketed.[112]

Leningrad, by the end of 1927, was facing unemployment, overcrowded housing, the birth rate was falling and death rates and social diseases were increasing. More importantly, workers' standards of living were starting to fall. The question we must now explore is how the health service coped with these challenges.

The NEP and public health policy

The Russian civil war had weakened progress towards a socialist health service. At the Third All-Russian Congress of Public Health Departments held between 27 October–1 November 1921 a special document 'Concerning the organisation of medico-sanitary aid during the course of the NEP' was discussed. This indicates what impact the NEP was to have on the medical system and it also illustrates Congress delegates and public health specialists' dissatisfaction about the way in which the medical system had developed during War Communism. The essence of this document can be summarised in a number of points, which we will examine in turn.[113]

First, delegates expressed their dissatisfaction with the 'class restrictiveness' (*klassovost'*) of Soviet medicine. Here medical professionals were pointing out that some of the capitalist traits of Tsarist medicine had not yet been eliminated. The Bolsheviks, as we saw in the previous chapter, were concerned not with 'equal access' for all, but with positive discrimination in favour of workers and poor peasants, key components of the collective. Delegates emphasised that in the medium term such class discrimination was inevitable. Universal provision was not spoken off except in reference to some far off socialist society. As I shall demonstrate, the introduction of the NEP did not solve this issue because urban/rural inequalities and differences in access to health care between the insured/non-insured persisted throughout the 1920s and the implementation of a 'class line' at this time merely exacerbated this problem.

Second, delegates wished to see the NEP encourage greater participation of the masses in public health affairs. Ever since October 1917, this was seen as a vital element in the emerging Soviet philosophy of medicine. For the leadership it was seen as an essential pre-requisite for the success of its new, and revolutionary, social policies, while for the working class it was evidence that this new 'workers' state' was functioning in their interests. As the proletarianisation of Soviet medicine got under way, it was hoped that the working class could influence their own lives by acting either as decision-makers in hospital or other establishments or by influencing health policies at a more grass roots level via the local soviets (councils), trade unions or factory committees. But as in the previous point, delegates were quick to emphasise that such a situation only existed on paper. They urged the People's Commissariat of Health (Narkomzdrav or NKZ for short) to take immediate steps to rectify this problem.

Third, the document mentions that under the NEP a special subscription was to be paid by enterprises so that medical facilities could be provided for the workforce. This point relates to medical care for the insured, namely insurance medicine, and it shows that from the very start the NEP meant priority being placed on the provision of medical facilities for the insured worker. Hence the notion of access to health care for all social groups, even as a theoretical ideal, was not in place at this time. As severe financial difficulties were in place, the existence of facilities for certain socio-economic groups, such as the Army and high-ranking party officials as well as dominant industrial groups, such as the factory and railway workers, became increasingly important.

Fourth, delegates at this 1921 Congress drew attention to proposals concerning the opening of private or personal medical facilities. This tendency was to be *tolerated* but the exploitation of users was not. This change in policy might at first sight appear contradictory, especially in view of the fact that we are supposed to be talking about a 'socialist state', because the very term private medicine has petty bourgeois overtones and one visualises a situation in which despite the October Revolution those able to pay for health care via their enterprises still received the best care and attention available. Thus a decree entitled 'Concerning the opening of private medical establishments and pharmacies', which was issued after the third Congress finished on 9 January 1922, included a clause which stated that if state health care patients visited any of these places, then they must be rendered care or given drugs free of charge.[114] Delegates viewed this clause as necessary in order to prevent any retreat into the evils of Russia's capitalist past.

Finally, the last point in this 1921 document highlighted that special taxes were to be paid by specific groups in return for medical care. Those involved in independent work (handicraftsmen or artisans) as well as those with unearned incomes (traders, landlords or entrepreneurs) had to pay a tax (*nalog*) to be given medical treatment. Unlike the insured workers, this did not mean that they then received preferential treatment, rather it meant they simply gained access to medical facilities. Generally speaking, it was still the insured workers who were given priority throughout the 1920s.

Hence in the health sector under the NEP there was a distinct lack of firm adherence to socialist principles of health care because of: the prevailing economic and political constraints; the introduction of fees for medical services; the continued existence of private medicine though on a small scale; the introduction of rationing via the implementation of a 'class line' in the health sector; greater inequality in access to health care both between social groups and within and between regions; problems in securing adequate finance; greater priority being assigned to insurance medicine; and, finally, some deterioration in the quality of the services offered despite an improvement in health conditions and an increase in most quantitative indicators of medical provision.

In order to explain why this was the case, it is necessary to examine the budget reform of 1922 and the 1926 'regime of the economy', both of which affected the general question of health service financing during the NEP.

Health care cuts: the 1922 budget reform and 1926 'regime of the economy'

It is necessary to remember, first of all, that financial constraints had for many decades hampered the work of the municipal authorities trying to improve local health and sanitation. This problem had existed in tsarist times (as we saw in Chapter 1) and it still remained after the revolution. As explained in the previous chapter, the health service had had to operate during the Civil War period under extreme pressure not only because of adverse changes in demographic trends and health conditions, but also because of the political situation and lack of financial resources.

Nikolai Semashko expressed his concern about the impending public finance reform in a paper entitled 'The NEP and public health work' as did many of the delegates attending the Third All-Union Congress of Public Health Departments. This change, he argued, would mean that although in theory the State was supposed to play a dominant role by being the main source of revenue, in practice it would now cease to perform this role with responsibility for raising public health funds being placed in local government hands.[115]

A debate on this issue followed. Many Congress delegates saw the need for such a reform pointing to the collapse of the rouble in 1918–19, increasing inflation and the enormous budget deficits which were a characteristic feature during the period 1918–20. Other delegates, meanwhile, pointed to the negative aspects of this proposed reform by arguing, for instance, that certain unique features of the Soviet health service night disappear, such as infant care.[116] Concern was also raised about possible closures and reductions in medical facilities and about the well-known fact that medical resources were already seriously depleted as a result of years of world war, revolution and Civil War.[117] Furthermore, delegates did not want to see private medicine thrive in a workers' state because they believed that if it was permitted to do so, then some of the principles on which Soviet health care was based, especially the notion of free access to medical facilities, irrespective of one's ability to pay, might be sacrificed.[118] A month or so after these debates had taken place, some of the medical professions original fears were realised.

On 10 December 1921 Lenin and Kalinin signed a Sovnarkom decree approving the transition from central to local funding in most sectors of the economy.[119] 'Every quarter' expressed concern about the catastrophic impact which this change would have on health care,[120] but it did not take long for this decision to be implemented in the health sector. On 1 May 1922 responsibility for financing medical services was passed initially from All-Union down to Republican level and finally onto the local authorities.[121] In Petrograd it was not long before the full impact of this reform was being felt.

The rest of this section assesses, first, the impact of the 1922 budget reform and second, the financial difficulties facing the health service in Petrograd/Leningrad during early NEP. Table 3.6 presents data on the extent of cut-backs in medical services taking place at regional level, excluding the city, between 1921–22. In only five out of the 13 categories listed was there any increase in the level of facilities available. In the remaining eight cut-backs occurred with the severity varying in each case ranging from a 14.2% cut in the number of mothers and infants homes to an 80.1% reduction in the number of dentists in Leningrad gubernia between 1921–22.

Table 3.6 Cut-backs in the Leningrad gubernia health system, 1921–22

Indicator	1921	1922	Percentage change (%)
Number of out-patient points	124	42	-66.1
Dental out-patient points	14	8	-42.8
Number of medical uchastok	82	89	+8.5
Doctors	302	207	-31.4
Feldshers	214	232	+8.4
Number of feldsher points	82	115	+40.3
Dentists	131	26	-80.1
Pharmacists	205	76	-62.9
Number of pharmacies	110	116	+5.5
Number of hospitals	118	136	+15.3
Number of hospital beds	5180	5269	+1.8
Women's consultation clinics	21	11	-47.6
Creches	35	20	-42.8
Homes for mothers and infants	21	18	-14.2

Source: *Statisticheskie materialy po soistoianiiu narodnogo zdraviia i organizatsii meditsinskoi pomoshchi v SSSR za 1913–1923gg* (Moscow "NKZ" 1926), 28–29, 32–33, 86–87, 120–121, 352–353

These developments adversely affected the organisation of the health service with the cuts occurring at a time when the population was on the increase and recovering from the negative impact of the Revolution and Civil War.

Attempts were made to try and the limit the damage of these cuts, for example by increasing the number of feldshers by 8.4%, thereby partially offsetting a 31.4% cut in the number of doctors, some of whom had already probably entered private practice.[122] Many areas of the health services were badly affected. For instance, the protection of the health of mothers and infants was threatened as the number of women's consultation clinics fell by 10 (47.6%) and the number of crèches by 15 (42.8%). Leningrad fared badly compared to other regions. Thus after the 1922 budget reform, Leningrad gubernia had one of the lowest per-capita rates of expenditure on public health.[123]

Such cuts were not made, however, until all attempts to raise revenue had failed. This included the introduction of charges for medical care in March–June 1921.[124] This was clearly against the new regime's declared socialist principles and certainly endangered part of the collective's access to health care which was partly based on ability to pay. This was probably viewed as a temporary measure, in view of the financial constraints operating. In this instance, according to the Leningrad regional public health bulletin, medical charges totalled 2,516, 562r in the year 1922–23 or 0.5% of the regional public health department's budget.[125] Unfortunately medical charges remained after the 1922 reform and became a permanent feature. The existence of large deficits (199,806r in the year 1922–23 at regional level)[126] also hampered the ability of the health service to resist such cuts, as government subsidies were removed, and Lenin and his government sought to restore economic growth and allocate labour, machinery and capital in a more efficient and rational manner. Economies clearly led to fewer resources being available and to a reduction in the level of services on offer in some cases.

As Davis has pointed out, health care was financed in four basic ways: the state budget, local budget, the medical assistance fund (or as it was commonly known in Russian as *fund meditsinskoi pomoshchi* (FMP for short)) which was based on employers' contributions, and special means.[127] Finance continued to be one of the problem facing the health service throughout the NEP. In relation to Table 3.7, it is crucial to remember that all expenditure is given in current prices, so changes in price levels have not be taken into account. As the period under discussion was one of significant price inflation this reduced actual levels of health expenditure.[128]

Table 3.7 shows that the State or Narkomzdrav contributed little money to enable the city health service to meet the local population's medical needs in the light of the challenges outlined above. Revenues raised in this way constituted 3–4% of the overall total. Local and FMP contributions together made up over three quarters of the total health care budget. In the period, 1923–27, local expenditures dominated. By the mid-1920s, however, the gap between the former and the FMP had narrowed with the FMP

Table 3.7 Expenditure on public health budget in Petrograd/Leningrad, 1923-1927

Source of budget expenditure	Size of public health expenditure in roubles				Increase/ decrease
	1923–24	*1924–25*	*1925–26*	*1926–27*	
State budget	503,605	1,057,847	1,125,245	1,362, 200	+2.7
Local budget	9,142,244	11,167,576	11,727,850	13,601,500	+1.5
FMP	4,151,666	9,892,887	12,136,411	16,591,300	+4.0
All-Russian reserve fund	48,760	354,500	361,508	-	+7.4
Other insurance funds	111,000	240,000	-	69,800	-62.9
Special means	-	1,107,301	1,866,672	3,008,700	+2.7
Total	13,956,275	23,783,111	27,236,686	37,518,000	+2.7

Source: GARF A-482 op. 10 d. 1026, list 16 ob; *Zdravookhranie v g. Leningrade i gubernii* (Leningrad 1927), 15; *Otchet Leningradskogo oblastnogo ispolkoma Noviabr' 1927g – Aprel' 1929g* (Leningrad 1929), 141

making a greater contribution by the end of the NEP in 1926–27. Finally, mention should be of the category 'special means' which includes payments by individuals (for medicines) or organisations (for places in health resorts) for health services.[129] This made up 5–6% of the budget revenue and was greater than Narkomzdrav's contribution.

Ginzberg argues that the relatively small amount spent on health care reflected the low priority assigned to it by the local government.[130] However, such a view needs qualifying. The fact that public health expenditure as a percentage of the overall budget of the city of Leningrad increased from 32.4% in 1923/24 to 39.3% by 1924/25 (from a third to two-fifths) suggests that it was by no means a totally neglected sector.[131] Nevertheless, Dreisin argues that per capita expenditure on health care in Leningrad gubernia in 1925/26 as a percentage of real 1913 levels was only 82%.[132] Thus, although Leningrad had a better record than Smolensk, Vladimir, Tambov and Saratov, pre-revolutionary spending on St Petersburg was nevertheless still higher than that of the Soviet regime by the mid-1920s.

The reason for this was because the priority sectors under the NEP were agriculture and industry, so in relative terms public health fared badly. For example, one Leningrad Soviet and Party executive committee document of 1925 demonstrates that as a proportion of the fulfilled (*ispol'nenii*) 1923–24 budget for the city of Leningrad, public health received 756 million roubles.[133] Whilst in the Stalin era public health declined as a state priority even further, the origins of neglect of health and welfare pre-dates Stalin's rise to power, a fact not always acknowledged by historians. There was a decline in the share of the city's overall budget given over to public health from 27,224,010r (or 38%) in 1925/26 to 31,494,780r (or 28.5%) by 1926–27.[134] This was probably as a result of the negative impact of the 1926 'regime of economy' campaign – a renewed drive to make more economies and conserve resources.

The 'regime of economy' policy was launched on 23 February 1926 with the aim, according to Carr and Davies, of cutting costs, rationalising production and increasing labour productivity.[135] Narkomzdrav then issued circular No.76 in its Bulletin specifying how such a policy could be approached in the health sector. Economies were to be made on heating, lighting, research (fewer business trips), food (while retaining 'quality and suitability'), medical supplies (via the elimination of duplication, drug assortment), office administration and equipment (number of forms, bureaucratic registration procedures, use of telephones, telegrams, postage).[136] However in an article entitled 'Regime of economy in public health work' Semashko cautioned that 'With regard to the regime of economy every possible economy on expenditure and management activities is to be made but *not at the expense of patients*'.[137]

Kul'vanovskii provides details on what types of economies were favoured by the 21 public health departments surveyed up to February 1927. The results reveal that 16 favoured cut backs in medical supplies; 12 in administrative expenditure; 12 reorganised pharmacy management (spending less on advertising, the packaging of drugs, assortment, quantity dispensed); 10 made cutbacks in food and fuel; seven reduced the number of hospital referrals for specialist treatment and three curtailed the role played by the VKK in referring patients for medical treatment.[138] Thus despite the good intentions, these cuts still affected patients and their care. This policy had two key aspects: economy and rationalisation. With regard to the first, it had little success because it was badly coordinated; central directives were few and far between and information on the aims infrequent, with only three articles published in *Biulleten' NKZ* . On the second aspect – rationalisation – little was done to eradicate bureaucratic inefficiency and waste as well as arbitrary central intervention in local public health affairs, so this failed too, with local public health departments rapidly abandoning the 'regime of economy' policy.[139]

Golubeva's article on 'Mass economic work in medical establishments in the city of Leningrad' shows that although this policy was widely debated, with the number of meetings discussing economic issues rising from 98 in January 1926 to 128 by July 1927, health administrators and other officials dragged their feet and shuffled papers when it came to implementing proposals. Thus the percentage of directives fulfilled fell from 61.7% in 1925 to 48.5% in 1926 and still further to 46.7% by mid-1927.[140] Narkomzdrav issued a special circular to the regional and local public health departments requesting they toe the line in economic policy by responding to central directives. Nevertheless, 'the results were still very disappointing'.[141] The reason was that greater rationalisation of labour had taken place, but more maintenance and repairs had been carried out and expenditure on administration was higher than ever before.[142]

Thus local staff in Leningrad tried to limit the impact of budget cuts on the health service and its patients in the mid to late 1920s. Having dealt with finance, we are now able to examine how changes in demographic and health conditions, on the one hand, and financial constraints on the other, affected the organisational development of the health service during in Petrograd/Leningrad during the NEP.

The organisation of health care under the NEP

Each department was ascribed the same roles as in 1918–20 but, of course, by 1923, Petrograd, like the country as a whole, had returned to a relative state of equilibrium. The NEP was in place and the epidemics of infectious diseases and hunger had subsided. The local medical system had also sta-bilised after the budget cuts. Karanovich's analysis shows that the health service under the NEP was a very slimmed down version of what it had been under War Communism.[143] There were fewer main departments – nine in 1921,[144] six in 1923[145] and four by 1924[146] as well as fewer sub-departments which fell from 10 in 1921[147]to eight in 1923[148] to five in 1924.[149] At city level, the number of departments within the health service initially increased from 24 in 1917–18 to 33 by 1921, but then fell to 19 by 1925 to only seven by 1928.[150] This was partly because of the rationalisation caused by financial constraints, but it was largely as a result of the crisis free situation.

From 1923 onwards the health system was rebuilt meaning that despite being plagued by financial restrictions, all categories of medical personnel

Table 3.8 Number of medical personnel in Petrograd/Leningrad, 1921–1927

Year	Doctors		Dentists		Dental doctors		Pharmacists		Secondary medical personnel	
	i	ii	i	ii	i	ii	i	ii	i	ii
1921	1,047	11.4	28	0.4	302	3.7	611	7.4	21	0.3a
1922	-	-	-	-	-	-	-	-	-	-
1923	1,248	11.4	-	-	-	-	1,396b	12.8	199a	1.9
1924	2,033	29.5	286	4.9	-	-	835	-	597c	41.0
1925	2,429	-	347	-	-	-	1,065	-	825c	-
1926	4,929	32.1	714	4.65	-	-	1,533	9.98	12,457d	81.2
1927	3,921	24.1	513	3.2	-	-	1,512	9.3	5,062d	31.2c

Note: i absolute numbers   ii rate per 10,000
a feldshers only
b includes dentists, dental doctors, midwives and pharmacists
c all categories i.e. feldshers, midwives etc
d includes c as well as nurses, orderlies and technicians
Sources: GARF f. A-482, op. 10, d. 36, list 70; GARF f. A-482, op. 10. D. 292, list 93; *Statisticheskii materialy po sostoianiiu narodnogo zdraviia i organizatsii meditsinskoi pomosh-chi v SSSR za 1913-1923gg* (Moscow "Narkomzdrav" 1926), 116–117, 120–121; *Vseoiuznaia perepis' naseleniia 17 dekabria 1926 goda. Kratkii svodki, Vyp 9: Sotsial'nyi sostav i zaniatiia g. Leningrada* (TsSU Soiuza SSR, Moscow 1928), 28

expanded: doctors increased from 1,047 in 1921 to 3,921 by 1927; dentists from 28 to 513 and secondary medical personnel (feldshers, midwives etc) from 597 in 1924 to 5,062 in 1927. There were more of some types of personnel per head of population (doctors increased from 11.4 per 10,000 in 1921 to 24.1 by 1927 and dentists from 0.4 to 3.2 between 1921–27) but fewer of other staff (secondary medical personnel fell from 41.0 in 1924 to 31.2 in 1927). The number of hospitals, however, fell from 77 in 1921 to 66 in 1927, with the number of beds in them also declining from 21,444 to 15,766 over the same period. Thus there were fewer of both per head of population (0.93 to 0.40 and 258.4 to 97.0 per 10,000).[151] (see Table 3.8) The overall trend under NEP, therefore, was one of a partial gradual revival of the health service from the adverse effects which it had experienced during War Communism, but it was still not in its best position to combat death and diseases.

As we saw earlier, social diseases (TB, alcoholism and VD) posed more of a problem during NEP, so a special department was created to combat VD. Previously, only TB and alcoholism had their own sub-sections. Medical expertise and control departments also existed. Reflecting the priority assigned to insurance medicine, a new department dealing with the insured was set up (see below). Generally speaking, though, for such a major industrial city Leningrad had a rather streamlined health service by 1927.

Medical care for the insured: a key part of the collective

It is against this background that subscriptions were introduced. Medical care was financed by employers' contributions. Minkoff notes:

> all social insurance funds were derived from an earmarked tax levied on the wage bill and paid by the institutions and persons employing labour. The tax rate, therefore, was varied according to the degree of health and accident hazard believed to be inherent in enterprises of various types. Of course, the State provided for modifications of the principle to facilitate the attainment of primary economic and political goals.[152]

Medical care was paid for by employers, who gave a proportion of their wage fund to the local authorities in return for them granting the insured industrial workers preferential access to health service facilities. A special fund, 'G', was set aside by the local authorities to provide medical care for insured workers. The health service was then held accountable by employers and workers for the service it provided.

There were four categories of enterprises paying these social insurance contributions during the NEP. In order of risk of danger and health hazard, and following the German system of occupational disease classification, they ranged from trade and agriculture, the least dangerous, to textiles then the chemical and rubber industry through to the most dangerous of all, namely the timber industry and those firms manufacturing explosive materials.[153]

The level of tax imposed was based on the number of workers employed and the level of risk involved. Levies from employers were collected by the trade unions (*profsoiuzy*) and insurance agencies (*gosstrakh*). These taxes varied over time and, according to geographical area, but in general they were determined in accordance with central directives. In 1922, for instance, they stood at: 21% of the wage fund in trade and agriculture; 23.5% in textiles; 26% in the chemical and rubber industry; and, finally, 28.5% in timber and enterprises involved in manufacturing explosives.[154]

Following problems with the collection of these taxes, levies were reduced in April 1923 to 16%, 18%, 20% and 22% respectively for the four categories, with a special rate of 16% being introduced for the fuel and metallurgical industries as well as state transport and communications.[155] An Insurance Council was set up in 1924 to monitor developments and regulate tariffs and a further revision of the tariff took place in February 1925, when the system of four separate risk categories was abolished and the following tax levels set: 10% for mining, metallurgy, machine tools, electrical and war industries; 12% for state transport and 14% for the timber industry producing for export.[156] Although the costs of medical care were to be met using these funds up until 1936, the following situation applied according to Minkoff:

> free medical aid, as a legal right, was limited to insured persons and to the following dependents ... spouse; children, brothers and sisters under 16 years of age, or 18, if they are students, or regardless of age if they had become incapacitated before their sixteenth birthday.[157]

Some appreciation of the attitudes adopted during the debate on medical care for the insured is important because the Soviet state considered this group a vital part of the collective. Under War Communism there was institutional rivalry between the Ministries of Labour and Health after Narkomzdrav set up special workers' medical departments (*rabmedy*). However, due to the demands of Civil War these departments were abolished in February 1919 with medical provision for the insured now the responsibility of the general insurance kassa.[158] Later in the same month, these kassy were eliminated in favour of a unified Soviet medicine.[159] These differences resurfaced under the NEP as a result of concern about falling labour productivity and the debates on the scientific organisation of labour and the role of the trade unions.[160] Following the re-introduction of the social insurance system in November 1921 and with it the provision of sickness benefits, invalidity pensions and unemployment benefit a decision was taken to provide medical care for the insured.[161] For example, Semashko' s paper on 'The work of Narkomzdrav, RSFSR and the plan for its future activities' delivered at the Fourth All-Union Congress of Medico-sanitary Departments held in December 1922, urged all health departments to devote 'greater attention to this matter by using all the means at their disposal to achieve this objective'.[162] This view was shared by delegates who believed 'insurance medicine to be one of the most progressive areas of Soviet medicine and a vital part of the overall class struggle'.[163] As we saw earlier, insurance medicine was paid for by employer's contributions to the local authorities, and under this arrangement the insured were allowed preferential access to health facilities.[164]

The People's Commissariat of Social Security (NKSO) was initially responsible for insurance medicine. However, it tended to be bureaucratic and was frequently criticised for failing to meet the needs of the collective and so, on 21 December 1922, responsibility for the insurance kassy was transferred from the Ministry of Social Security to the Ministry of Labour (NKT).[165] During the NEP, Narkomzdrav (NKZ) advocated a policy which would mean that health care for the insured was simply one aspect of its overall health strategy; NKT wished to see insurance medicine under its jurisdiction arguing instead that insured workers and their families, as important economic groups, should be given preferential treatment by ensuring that fund 'G' was used for and by the insured only. However, it was the Ministry of Health, not Labour, who had ultimate control over fund 'G' and it could decide when, where and on whom it was to be used.

Table 3.7 shows that there was a four-fold increase in the FMP in Petrograd/Leningrad from 1923/24 to 1926/27. This occurred because local trade union and social insurance agencies sought to provide adequate medical facilities for their members, which almost doubled from 224,089 to 433,189 between December 1922 and October 1925, together with some degree of protection against financial constraints imposed after 1922.[166] The city responded rapidly to meeting the needs of the insured. In 1922–23, for example, 132.5 million roubles was spent on insurance medicine in Leningrad gubernia.[167]

In order to secure health facilities for insured workers, pressure was brought to bear in a variety of ways by local NKT agencies, such as the Insurance three-man Commission (*Strakhovaia troika*) which was formed in October 1923. Although it had a wide remit, health insurance was a priority with the aim being first, to ensure that the special fund 'G' was used for its original purpose[168] and second, to provide a wide range of medical establishments (hospitals, maternity homes, out-patient clinics and so on) for the insured worker.[169]

A sub-department responsible for medical aid for the insured was established in late 1923-early 1924 and attached to the Leningrad regional public health department. Its aims were: to improve the food supply for insured patients; to increase the level of medical supplies, equipment and drugs; to restore X-ray facilities and physiotherapy equipment together with raising the quality of treatment offered; to conduct more research on the development of prosthetic appliances; to carry out regular repairs and maintenance work on medical establishments; to organize frequent meetings to discuss changes in policy and other important matters; to ensure better relations with the localities; and to increase the wages of medical workers so that staff of the right calibre could be enticed in sufficient numbers to work in medical establishments catering for the insured.[170] In this way, then, the insured worker plus their family would hopefully be provided with the best care and attention available, meeting Semashko's demands.

To achieve the above objectives, nearly 1.5 million roubles was spent on insurance medicine between October 1923–March 1924 alone. Of this sum: 222,000r was spent on food (or 16% of the total); 154, 000r on repairs (11%); 399,000r on medical supplies (29%); 21,000r on rendering specialist treatment at Narkomzdrav institutions and 372,000r on staff wages (27%). The size of the insured as a group and the Ministry of Labour's strong institutional base largely explains this, but concern over the health status situation was also a prominent factor.[171] This was necessary as Beleliubskii found the following situation in Leningrad between June–December 1923: 8.2 workers per 1,000 suffered from influenza; 4.8 had acute gastric infections; 4.7 diseases of respiratory organs; 1.3 nervous diseases; and 4.5 per 1,000 had been injured at work. When a follow up study was made six months later between January–June 1924, the situation had worsened because there were 9.3 cases of influenza per 1,000 workers every month, 7.1 cases per 1,000 workers of acute gastric infections, 8.0 cases per 1,000 workers of respiratory disease, 4.1 cases per 1,000 workers of nervous disease and 12.5 workers per 1,000 had been injured at work.[172] Another study carried out in 1924–25 discovered that insured workers in Moscow-Narva district had lost 137.2 days per 100 workers due to illness while those in Vasilevostrovskii district had lost 153.3 days. The highest morbidity levels recorded in the Vyborg district where 199 days were lost per 100 workers.[173] To combat these problems greater priority was assigned to insurance medicine.

In the early NEP, the insured in Petrograd received the lion's share of resources. The non-insured, meanwhile, had to endure shortages of medicines, long queues, treatment by overworked staff and generally put up with a fall in the quality of care being given. Although this was not true in all instances, by early 1924, insured workers in Leningrad gubernia had access to 440 out of the 549 beds; 24 out of the 30 out-patient clinics and to 17 hospitals with 3,571 beds. Thus the insured had access to nearly half the hospitals (47.2%) and beds (42.6%).[174] By June 1925, according to Rubinshtein, facilities were being targeted at providing care for the insured at home. Thus there were 37 housing based medical points (*punkty kvartirnoi pomoshchi*) staffed by 210 doctors in Leningrad, together with a wide range of out-patient facilities and 40 hospitals and maternity homes equipped with 9,982 beds.[175] During the first half of 1925, 420,000r was spent on medical aid for the insured at home; 3,528,000r on out-patient care; 450,000r on enterprise medical points; 7,257,000r on maintaining an in-patient service and 600,000r on carrying out repairs to medical establishments catering for the insured.[176]

Thus, despite the rhetoric of 'free' services and services for 'all' not all members of the new collective were as important or treated the same as others in terms of access to medical care.

Petrograd was said to run a superior service during the NEP. Establishments were staffed by reliable, caring and highly qualified personnel, who were well-respected practitioners setting an example for the rest of Russia to follow.[177] Enterprises and certain occupational groups had their own individual health sub-system within the general medical framework. One such enterprise, the 'Treugol'nik' factory, possessed its own out-patient clinic with 40 beds and a pharmacy. The majority of those treated came from the ranks of the insured.[178] Furthermore construction and transport workers in the city of Leningrad each had a 120-bed hospital at their disposal.[179]

A great effort was made to expand the health service, despite shortages of income, in order to meet the needs of certain groups in the collective, such as the insured. But the cut backs instigated in 1922 were being felt by all. Although the non-insured suffered most; the insured also complained about the services on offer. The health service was accused of utilizing the special fund 'G' for its own ends meaning that there had been 'no noticeable real improvement in medical provisions for the insured in mid-NEP'.[180]Although this is clearly an exaggeration, there were still local anxieties about this. For instance, one article in *Vestnik Truda* in May 1923 argued that funds were not sufficient to cover first aid services and drug supplies, let alone adequate enough to provide a specialised health care for the insured.[181] In a similar vein, it was pointed out that FMP funds were inadequate for two reasons: first, because contributions as a proportion of the wage fund had declined significantly due to growing unemployment and second, because Medsantrud, the medical workers' union, was constantly faced with budget deficits, meaning that it sometimes used fund 'G' for other purposes.[182]

Other scholars blamed institutional rivalry for this situation. Thus Dr Abramov declared in *Questions of Insurance* in September 1923 that

> At present, medical provision for the insured is far from satisfactory due to the intense conflict between the regional public health department and the insurance kassy over the question of who has responsibility for their health. This is having catastrophic results – medical supplies and other provisions are totally inadequate and patients are not being given good medical care by qualified medical practitioners. Nurses are having to substitute for doctors, pharmacies are only open irregularly and doctors are allowing workers time off work for dubious reasons.[183]

It was the role of Medical Control Commission (*vrachedno-kontrol'nye komissii*) or the VKK and VEK's (Medical Expert Commissions), set up by Sovnarkom decree on 23 January 1923, to undertake regular examinations of the insured; to assess changes in their health status and to define who was sick and who was healthy. Petrograd' s VKK staff numbered between

13–19,000, were highly qualified, long serving individuals with 10–12 years' experience by the 1920s.[184] Nevertheless, the VKK in Petrograd were accused of failing to keep insurance payments within the bounds of available resources and of not giving the insured priority or denying them access altogether to health care facilities. During increased workers' unrest in the NEP period, VKK staff were under great pressure and accused of approving malingering claimants (*simulantov nichlozhno*).[185] The secretary of the Putilov factory, N. K. Kovolev, declared in February 1925: 'There are up to 8,500 malingerers in various enterprises in Leningrad who seek to avoid work and who do not have a serious attitude to it. Instead they are faking illness'.[186]

By late 1925, malingerers allegedly made up 24% of those visiting Leningrad clinics. An additional 12% were 'faking' at home and 2% not living at the address declared on the medical form.[187] Abramov notes that 'other groups' (nepmen, the non-insured etc.), often took up beds designated for the insured which led to their failure to be treated. This occurred in the Pervykin hospital in Petrograd side of the city, for instance, while the Petropavlovsk was 'off limits' altogether.[188]

The Ministry of Health had allegedly used fund 'G' resources in a wasteful and inefficient manner and its duplication of many of the functions performed by the Ministry of Labour was against workers' interests as it was preventing medical staff from combating industrial accidents, social diseases and from providing the insured with adequate medical supplies of drugs, instruments, staff and so on.

The number of industrial accidents in Leningrad increased from 692 in the first half of 1922 to 8,210 by 1924. In the first half of 1925, 7,865 cases had been recorded.[189] Most of the accidents occurred in heavy Industry. There were 66 industrial accidents per 1,000 metal-workers in Leningrad in 1922 with the number falling to 31 per 1,000 by the first half of 1924.[190] The main causes of these accidents were no safety precautions (50%); violation of labour protection rights by factory administration (15–20%); unsanitary conditions (5%); occupational risk (7–8%) and other reasons (5–10%).[191] Other scholars add poor awareness of technical instruments among unskilled and unqualified peasants and the rudimentary labour protection system operating in early NEP[192] or attribute the situation to the demands for higher labour productivity which caused accidents to rise.[193] Leningrad's Institute of Occupational diseases did not open until November 1924, so had little impact until a later stage.[194] Those who were unable to return to work were classified as invalids (catogories I-II were 60% incapacitated; III – 45–60%; IV – 30–44%; V between 15–29% and those in category VI less than 15% incapacitated).[195]

Poster 12 from 1927 urges workers to support government industrial health measures and graphs show significant improvements by mid-NEP 1925 in comparison to the period 1897–1913 in the level of labour protection. For instance, the reduction in working hours from 11.5 hours a day in 1897 to 7.6 hours a day by 1925; the provision of rest homes and more

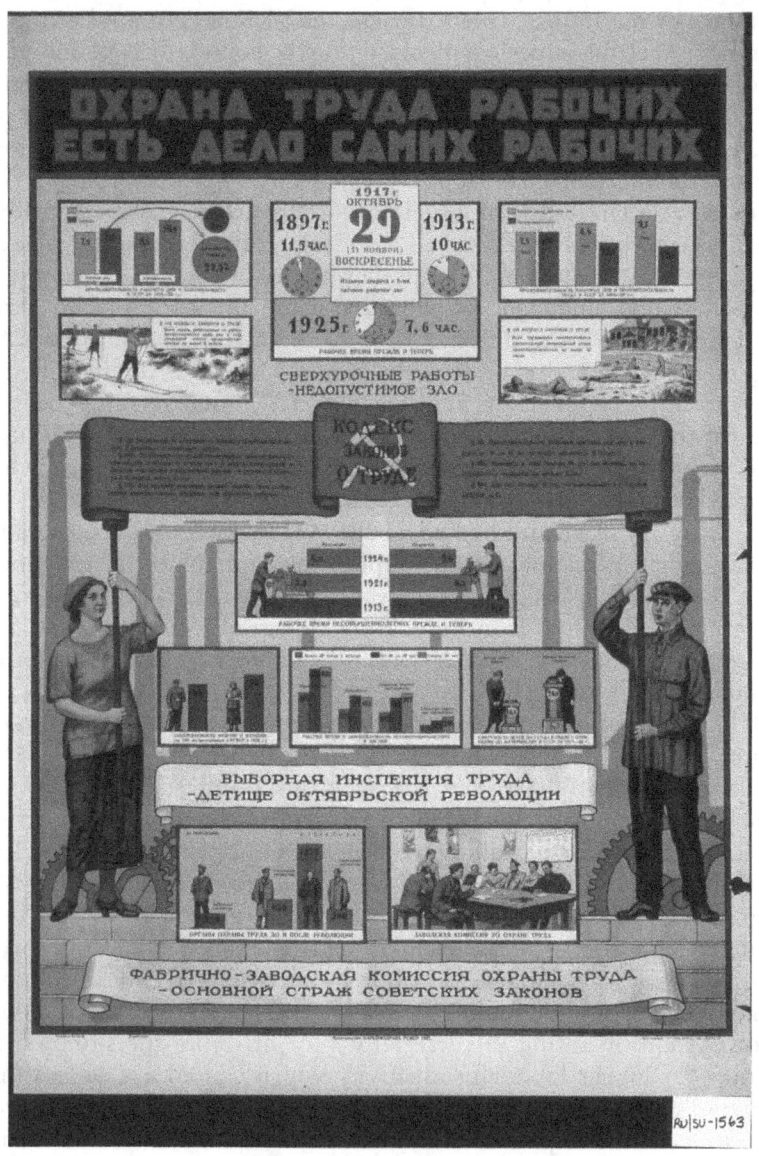

Poster 12 Progress on labour protection – comparison of 1897, 1913 and 1925

Source: 'Labour protection is the work of the workers themselves ... the election of labour inspectors on the anniversary of the October Revolution ... the factory labour commission – the basic guardian of Soviet Labour laws' 1927 Poster. Poster collection, Poster ID# RU/SU 1563. Hoover Institution Archives.

leisure facilities; the increase in the number of labour protection organs and how the USSR compares favourably with England in its treatment of workers.

Such improvements were not easy to achieve. Despite increased wages for staff dealing with the insured, many became dissatisfied with their working conditions so labour turnover was high and workloads increased. Some doctors and nurses found that they could not cope with the demand and so insured workers received increasingly inadequate care and attention.[196] The Ministry of Labour also urged NKZ to use fund 'G' in a selective and discriminatory fashion in order to solve medical supply problems, carry out repairs, reduce wafting lists and ease the pressure on staff and patients.[197] No miracles were achieved but gradually there were outward signs of recovery. Hence the number of visits made by the insured to out-patient clinics in the city of Leningrad rose from 2,536,099 (or 56% of the total) in 1924 to 4,691,352 (or 62%) by 1925.[198] These figures imply that the non-insured were being squeezed in favour of more insured workers treated in Soviet medical establishments during this period. The main reasons were an increase in the number of insured; concern regarding the insured workers' health status and greater financial provision via the FMP.

Table 3.9 shows that when the Medical Control Commission or VKK doctors carried out investigations in the city of Leningrad 1924/25, the large majority of insured workers were incapacitated as a result of respiratory disease, which prevailed in nearly half of the sample. Next came infectious diseases, closely followed by diseases of the nervous system and of other illnesses including those occurring at work. Workers, provided they

Table 3.9 Incapacity among insured workers in Leningrad, 1924–25

Type of disease	Number of insured who are sick
Influenza	2,185
TB of lungs	25,884
TB of other organs	757
Venereal diseases	1,224
Malaria	594
Other infectious diseases	2,104
Industrial accidents	9,047
Non-industrial accidents	3,991
Neoplasm	320
Anaemia	10,551
Diseases of the nervous system	15,930
Blood or lymph disorder	6,248
Respiratory diseases	56,269
Gastro-intestinal organs	8,907
Urinary diseases	1,504
Diseases of the sexual organs	7,685

(continued)

Table 3.9 Incapacity among insured workers in Leningrad, 1924–25 (*continued*)

Type of disease	Number of insured who are sick
Brian diseases	1,632
Hearing difficulties	10,269
Bone disease	7,627
Skin disease	4,054
Other diseases of various kinds	4,112
Total	124,113

Source: M. N. Rubinshtein, 'Rabota vrachebno-kontrol'nye komissii g. Leningrade', *Leningradskii meditsinskii zhurnal* No. 5, 1927, 104

could prove they were not malingerers, went to rest homes[199] sanatoria or health resorts to recuperate. For example, 20,000 Leningrad workers visited such establishments in 1924 and their number had increased to 30,000 by 1925.[200]

By the mid-1920s, insurance medicine was firmly entrenched in Leningrad. Expenditure on medical aid for the insured in the city of Leningrad increased from 9.4 million roubles in 1924–25 to 17.8 million roubles by 1927–28 or from 27r 39k to 31r 29k per capita over the same period.[201] Expenditure was highest on insured workers and they also consumed a disproportionate share of the medical services available. As a sizeable group, the insured exerted influence on the development of insurance medicine through the trade unions and local councils, primarily via employer contributions to the health budget (through the FMP). Medical care for the insured was financed by employers through the levying of taxes on the wage bill with levels ranging from 17.2% to 28.6% depending on size of workforce, health hazards and geographical region.[202]

Despite, the 1922 health reform and the 'regime of economy' policy, the amount spent on the insured rose from 16r 08k in 1923–24 to 29r 06k in 1926–27 per capita as compared to a small rise on the non-insured from 10r 73k to 13r 44k over the same period.[203] By 1926–27, there were 32 out-patient units, seven dental polyclinics, 43 enterprise first aid points, seven infants homes, 21 women's consultation clinics, eight children's out-patient units, five children's sanatoria's, one psychiatric sanatorium, one Bacteriological Institute, one Serological Laboratory, eight epidemics units, 11 TB dispensaries with 325 beds, three TB sanatoria's with 351 beds, eight VD dispensaries, a malaria station and an Occupational Diseases Institute with 25 beds, all catering for the needs of the insured in Leningrad.[204] But despite this impressive range of facilities, Vainshtein concludes that 'they were insufficient to meet the requirements of the insured in Leningrad'.[205]

This situation occurred because the construction of new medical facilities failed to keep pace with demand; there were few first aid points in the gigantic factories that had mushroomed on the city's landscape; the medical equipment utilised was obsolete and money allocated for insurance medicine was being squandered on other items by NKZ.[206] Another difficulty was what Ewing terms 'bureaucratic formalism', that is a failure to quickly process workers' applications for benefit or in order to receive treatment.[207] Red tape in social insurance agencies in Leningrad led to invalidity benefits taking two months to process by 1926.[208]

Even though fewer economies were made when the 'regime of economy' policy was implemented in 1926 than the centre desired, this still resulted in some deterioration in the quality of services offered. There was a drive in late NEP to revitalise insurance medicine with the trade unions encouraging more insured workers and their families to use the Leningrad health system. Of the patients coming to doctors' waiting rooms in Leningrad guberniia in 1926 – 75.1% were insured and 24.9% non-insured workers.[209] At a time when the health service and municipal authorities were short of cash, and trying to resist central pressure to make further cut backs, there was some concern about such large sums of money being spent on the insured to the detriment of other parts of the collective, such as the non-insured. The above figures certainly support the argument that the non-insured were being squeezed. Local health and government officials had little success reducing the degree of difference in health expenditure on these two groups. Thus whereas the per-capita public health expenditure gap between the insured/non-insured was only 5r 85k in 1923/24, it had already risen to 22r 10k a year later before narrowing again to reach 15r 46k by 1925/26 ending at a bigger gap of 15r 62k in 1926/27. Narkomzdrav were seemingly powerless to reverse this trend after the mid-1920s.[210]

During late NEP, the health service came under fire for not effectively monitoring its VKK staff who were still allegedly issuing medical certificates to 'malingerers', so responsibility for assessing temporary incapacity cases was passed over to the Ministry of Labour (via the social insurance agencies) in late 1926, a move which was officially sanctioned on 4 March 1927 when the rabmedy were abolished. After the late-1920s, NKT was controlling the VKK and ascribing the roles to be performed by its staff. Leningrad now gave even greater priority to insurance medicine. According to Vainshtein's calculations, Leningrad spent 40k on out-patient facilities and medicines, 2r 80k on hospital beds and 1r on home visits to the insured every day in early 1927.[211] Much had clearly changed since early NEP.

Consequently, any decline in health status under NEP, as detailed in this chapter, was probably more pronounced among the non-insured because they had put up with a severe reduction in the quality and quantity of medical services offered to them. This was all the result of a situation in which the Leningrad authorities gave greater priority to the insured and health care for this part of the collective throughout the NEP.

It is now time to consider what role the medical profession played in dealing with the aforementioned challenges and changes and if it was now fully incorporated into the new Soviet social order.

The medical profession and health service staff under the NEP

As noted in Chapter 2, the majority of the Petrograd medical profession readily cooperated with the Soviet regime after the Revolution. Throughout the War Communism period a number of conciliatory gestures were made to meet some of the demands and satisfy the interests of doctors who wished to play a key role in public health affairs. With the advent of the NEP, the need to rebuild a shattered economy, and within it the dilapidated health service, the cooperation of the old specialists was still as important as ever. Although by early NEP, this group was a fraction of their pre-revolutionary size and stature, there was still a desire, as we saw in the previous chapter, to see their professional goals implemented. However, senior figures within the medical profession, such as Semashko, were worried about the impact of certain groups within the medical profession. For instance, one letter sent by Semashko to the Politburo discussed the All-Russian Congress of Medical Doctors and the alleged influence of Kadets, Mensheviks and Social-Revolutionary personnel who were said to be against Soviet medicine, praising zemstvo and pre-1917 insurance medicine and not getting involved in worker movements.[212] The letter also mentioned that the Pirogov Society was carrying out anti-Soviet propaganda.[213] In the ensuing discussion, I. S. Unshlikht suggested to Stalin that any remnants of the zemshchina be eliminated and other proposals included preventing setting up autonomous groups in medical unions and using the GPU to remove members of opposition parties from this Congress.[214] Lenin asked Dzerzhinsky and Semashko to draw up a plan of measures and to report back to the Politburo. This approach was supported by Stalin, Trotsky, Kamenev, Rykov and Molotov, with Tomsky abstaining.[215] In the end, it was decided that meetings of specialists (*spetsy*), including the doctors' Congress, required NKVD consent.[216]

Partly to placate opposition to zemstvo specialists and to assure their loyalty, the Party began in early NEP to train its own proletarian medical cadres and to place Party appointees in health service positions. Of course, such control had started to be established during the Civil war, but due to the prevailing circumstances it had not been approached systematically. Now Party members were located in leadership positions, allowing the infusion of Soviet trained personnel and via the launching of a re-education programme for tsarist staff.[217]

Most of the Leningrad health service staff in post by the time of the 1926 census were trained in tsarist times and had been promoted since the Revolution, while others had graduated from Petrograd's medical establishments in the post-revolutionary period and were now in lower, junior posts but gradually working their way up the career ladder. For example, the 1926 census data detailed in Table 3.10 suggests that over half (59.3%) of Leningrad's 19,799 strong medical profession were born before 1905, and of these 27.9% were in senior, 17% in middle and 11.5% were in junior positions within the Leningrad health service. The remaining 40.7% of the profession were probably born after the Revolution but unfortunately, no data is furnished on this group. The Leningrad Party had, therefore, succeeded in fully incorporating the tsarist medical profession into the new social order by 1926, with political officials willing to give the spetsy, senior positions based on professional competence and experience, on the understanding that they would not embark upon counter-revolutionary activity.

The number of university medical establishments increased from four with 2,961 students in 1913–14 to five with 6,147 students by 1919–20. Under the NEP, the number of establishments remained stable until 1920–21 but the number of students fell to 4,245.[218] During the NEP, student enrolments in higher education increased 3-fold, as demobilised young Army veterans returned to the city and some entered university as Petrograd now had 26 universities with 45,000 students in December 1921. However, the financial cutbacks after 1922, led to the closure of six higher education institutions and the merger of several others into larger institutions.[219]

The aim of Party policy was to see working-class groups enter the profession to inject a more proletarian basis to its social composition and medical

Table 3.10 Age breakdown of medical personnel in Leningrad according to 1926 census

Age group	Position in health service hierarchy					
	Senior staff		Middle level		Junior staff	
	a	b	a	b	a	b
Under 20	–	2044	218	1760	221	1826
20–24	197	649	862	372	924	117
30–34	1274	387	1447	188	1006	55
35–39	1043	277	1231	175	1054	36
40–44	775	206	937	111	845	27
45–49	555	239	660	132	716	27
50–54	425	243	427	141	385	28
55–59	268	225	221	150	159	33
60–64	146	248	81	133	44	23
65–69	74	210	22	130	6	21
70+	39	345	6	122	2	12
Age unknown	3	2	4	–	3	–
Total	5809	5523	7549	3665	6634	2283

Notes: a Self-employed   b State employees
Source: *Vseoiuznaia perepis' naseleniia 17 dekabria 1926 goda. Kratkii svodki, Vyp 9: Sotsial'nyi sostav i zaniatiia g. Leningrada* (TsSU Soiuza SSR, Moscow 1928), 66

profession cadres. So-called workers' faculties (*Rabfak*) were created to prepare them for entry into Institutes or University as either doctors, feldshers or other medical personnel. As a result of a policy favouring the working class and the peasantry, the percentage of students from these social backgrounds in the medical establishments increased. For instance, in the Military-Medical Academy the number rose from 62% in 1920 to 84% in 1921 before reaching 93% by 1922.

Table 3.11, using the Leningrad medical institute[220] as an example, shows the changing nature of the city's student community under the NEP. There were a high proportion of females entering the medical profession from the end of the civil war (86.1%) and this trend continued until the end of the NEP (still at 66.8%), with the proportion of males more than doubling from 13.9% in 1920–21 to 33.2% by 1926–27. Also at this time, priority was given to working class and peasant students so the social composition altered, with the proportion of students from working class backgrounds increasing from 17.4% in 1924–25 to 25.4% in 1927–28 whilst the number from peasant backgrounds entering the Leningrad medical institute saw a five-fold increase from 4.1% to 20.1% over the same period.

Poliakov's survey of 1,351 Leningrad medical students in 1924 found that their living conditions, health and diet were poor and the halls of residence tended to be noisy and fellow students rowdy. Those who did not live locally had to travel two hours to and from university classes. Students also had three to four hours' political duties, labour brigade work or were required to serve in social organisations on a daily basis.[221]

In overall terms, during the latter half of the 1920s, although there was a gradual hardening of Soviet policy towards the old tsarist staff, coercion or disciplinary procedures were hardly necessary because the medical profession cooperated with the state, as they shared a similar desire to resolve health crises, similar medical philosophies (a belief in community medicine, that the environment was a cause of ill-health (now a key part of social hygiene approach) and saw the development of the above state institutions, and their role within them, as a means to gaining professionalization. As a

Table 3.11 Gender and social composition of Leningrad medical institute, 1921–28 (in percentages)

Gender	1920–21 (%)	1924–25 (%)	1926–27 (%)	1927–28 (%)
Male	13.9		33.2	
Female	86.1		66.8	
Social status	*1920–21 (%)*	*1924–25 (%)*	*1926–27 (%)*	*1927–28 (%)*
Worker		17.4		25.4
Peasant		4.1		20.1
Other		78.5		54.5

Source: P. Konecny, *Builders and Deserters: Students, state and community in Leningrad, 1917–1941* (McGill-Queens University Press 1999), 67

result, most of the medical profession in Petrograd/Leningrad continued to cooperate with the Soviet state in the 1920s.

The Petrograd Party Regional Committee (*Gubkom*) agitprop department was nevertheless still assigned responsibility for the ideological education of medical students during the NEP. Using the Komsomol (YCL) and the journal Red Student (*Krasnyi student*), the curriculum at Medical Institutes had a heavy political bias emphasising politics, historical materialism, Marxism-Leninism, the theory of proletarian revolution and economics alongside medical topics. In the first half of 1923, YCL members set about re-educating 300 non-Party students at the Medical Institute and 150 at the Institute of Medical Knowledge by introducing them to the above themes using guest Communist Party speakers. The flavour of these political meetings was distinctly anti-Trotsky and the Workers Opposition, given the power struggles at this time. By 1924, there were nearly 100 Party activists in higher education medical establishments (VUZy). Eventually over 40 members of the Institute of Medical Knowledge became candidate Party members. By spring 1925, 1,400 student medics were involved in political education circles in Leningrad.[222] Attempts to transmit a communist value system to VUZy medical students continued after 1925. According to Kurepin, 9% of the student intake in the Leningrad – Medical Institute were communists in 1927.[223] Kurepin argues that Party penetration was high (via political control over curriculum content, research activity and so forth) whereas Gantt believes that the degree of Sovietization was actually low. In 1924 he stated that

> control is normally in the hands of the Communists. However, the nominal control does not make so much of a difference as one would expect. I have never known of an efficient (public health) man ejected unless he is suspected of being counter-revolutionary.[224]

The available evidence in relation to Petrograd/Leningrad supports Gantt's conclusion. The relatively few conflicts involving medical workers[225] and the fact that there were also many white-collar members in the public health section of the regional party executive committee (*Gubispolkom*) – 243 in October 1923 and 156 in April 1924 suggests at least pragmatism, if not more.[226]

Furthermore, medical staff were no longer faced with constant anxiety about food and fuel so they could resume their scientific work[227] and during the first phase of the NEP, medical education facilities expanded, with an increased number of institutes offering medical courses of various kinds. Social hygiene flourished:[228] a Pharmaceutical and medical Research Laboratory was founded in 1922; a TB Institute in 1923; and a scientific Research Institute for Mothers and Babies was set up in 1925.[229] All of these establishments, helped by a more flexible approach by the State on medical education and training[230] played a key role in enabling tsarist doctors and medical specialists to research particular medical problems and to devise the appropriate policies to curtail them.

The wages of medical staff also increased significantly from between 7–18r on average in January 1923 to 64r 50k by 1925/26 before reaching 130r by 1927. More specifically, doctors' pay in Leningrad rose from 93r in 1926 to 103r by 1927, feldshers' wages from 45r to 64r and that of nurses from 29r to 33r over the same period.[231] The aim of these increases was to maintain the low level of disputes which had characterised most of the 1920s and to encourage more people to enter the medical profession.

This does not mean that everything was harmonious by 1927. First, there was Party dissatisfaction with the continued existence of private medical practitioners. Thus according to census data, there were 334 in Leningrad in 1926, made up of 90 doctors (including vets); 186 dentists and 58 feldsher/ midwives.[232] Many of these personnel were in fact pre-revolutionary medical staff who had retained their commitment to private practice. In addition, of the sample of nearly 12,000 mentioned in Table 3.10, 29.3% of senior, 38.1% of middle and 33.5% of junior medical personnel were defined as self-employed by 1926. Second, the Party wished to bring the health service in line with developments in the economy as a whole in readiness for the drive towards rapid industrialisation and forced collectivisation. Material on this aspect of Soviet medical policy in Leningrad is presented in the next chapter. In the charged political setting and power struggles of the mid-late 1920s, the medical profession and its allies were nevertheless sometimes seen as obstacles to progress and socialist construction (a view still reflected today), but this is not completely accurate in Leningrad's case.

During the NEP, former Tsarist medical staff had successfully occupied multiple identities – blending traditional with revolutionary (Soviet) values. This enabled them to adapt to an ever-changing, sometimes very stressful, political environment. As a result, some decided to 'accommodate' the new regime and adapt themselves to the Soviet context. Consequently, certain members of the old medical profession were able to speak 'Soviet' in a public health context (using the correct terminology, procedures and processes) to their and the new state's advantage. Through these 'accommodation' and 'assimilation' tactics, former zemstvo personnel worked with the Soviet regime to build a socialist health service and modernise and change the medical landscape so that train stations, public parks, clubs, factories and houses in Petrograd before 1924 and Leningrad after 1924 were as hygienic and clean as possible, and they helped the health system face its challenges. Whilst some members of the medical profession were perceived of as 'enemies', others were viewed as 'allies' and important to protecting the health of the collective. Trying to achieve socialist medicine at a time of financial constraints was extremely difficult and the state clearly needed a scapegoat for its failures and their adverse effects. As a result, members of the tsarist medical profession was deemed to be part of the so called 'bourgeoisie' and as such they were perceived by Party hardliners, as an enemy in the mid-late 1920s. Eventually, members of the pre-revolutionary medical profession gradually came under siege in the 1930s. These developments are considered in Chapter 4.

The Leningrad health system on the eve of Stalin's rise and the First five-year plan

We saw earlier in this chapter that the city's health system was affected by health finance cuts but by 1926 there were still nearly 5,000 doctors and almost 12,500 secondary medical personnel. With the exception of pharmacists, the growth of the most other health service staff increased faster than the population. Thus, the population increased by 25.7% between 1924–26 while the number of doctors increased by 36.9% and secondary medical personnel by 49.2%. In real terms, there were more doctors, feldshers, midwives, nurses, orderlies and technicians per head of population in 1926 over 1923–24. In 1927, the situation changed dramatically. While the population rose by a mere 6%, all Leningrad health service staff dwindled: doctors declined by 20.4%; dentists by 28.2%; pharmacists by 1.4% and secondary medical personnel by an enormous 59.4%. The same trend prevailed in the hospital sector where the number of hospitals only increased by one between 1925–26/27, although the number of beds rose by 28.4% to 15,728 over the same period. In per-capita terms the hospitals were becoming more overcrowded, as there were only 0.40 hospitals per 10,000 population in 1927, with patients competing with one another for beds.

In many ways, the Leningrad health service was more poorly equipped on the eve of industrialisation than it was immediately after the 1922 budget reform. The overall trend by 1927, therefore, was one in which the health service had failed to expand sufficiently in readiness for a shift in policy (the impending Stalinist rapid industrialisation and collectivisation drives). It was not in a much better position to combat death and disease than it had been up to the early 1920s. Of course, as in previous years, the organisation of the health service, evolved and developed in response to variations in health conditions, as we saw above. The health system was hindered by a lack of finance, having gone through cuts in 1922 then more proposed cuts in 1926, and was to a certain extent unable to meet some of the health needs of key parts of the collective. This fact, plus the deterioration in housing, food and basic hygiene and sanitation, explains the decline in health conditions and the evidence of growing morbidity and mortality among the population of Leningrad during late NEP.

To make matters worse further turmoil was yet to come as the 'Revolution from above' was approved by the Stalinist leadership. Badly-equipped to meet this change in economic and political strategy, the Leningrad health service and its leadership could do nothing, as we shall see in the next chapter, but sit and watch as health conditions deteriorated once again.

Conclusion

By the end of the Civil War in 1920, medical facilities in Petrograd were at an all-time low and worker discontent was widespread. The NEP was aimed at dealing with the crisis situation and, like most of industry, the health service remained in state ownership, but in order for the proletariat to retain its faith in the leadership, some relaxation took place giving rise to a limited private medical sector. Many of the socialist principles devised during War Communism were watered down or abandoned altogether. The State retained overall responsibility for public health, but local authorities were now expected to finance health initiatives themselves. Medical care was available but at a price and there was still an emphasis on preventive approaches. The gap between theory and practice had started to broaden.

Up to 1922, demographic and health conditions were still unfavourable, but the situation changed between 1923–25, when the population rapidly expanded, aided by a sharp decline in the death rate, and a rising birth rate. Although in-migration was largely responsible for population growth, falling mortality and morbidity from infectious diseases was also key. Social diseases (TB, VD, alcoholism) now became the major challenges. Mortality levels varied according to age, sex, social group and district; but residential mixing was now diminishing the degree of difference between various parts of the city. It was the elderly, weak and the very young who succumbed most. Slight improvements in basic sanitation and hygiene as well as food supplies, rather than better housing quality, were responsible for improved life expectancy in 1923 in comparison to 1910 and 1920, but by European standards it was still very low.

The financial constraints following the transition from central to local funding after 1922, hindered health service recovery and led to a more streamlined organisational structure. Although rationalisation had reduced the size of the health service, new departments to deal with social diseases and the insured were added during early NEP as were new institutes, such as that specialising in Occupational Diseases under Vigdorchik's leadership. During early NEP, the process of integrating the 'bourgeois' medical profession into the new social order started during the civil war continued. Moreover, new proletarian doctors and medical cadres of all types now existed and had gradually started occupying junior and middle, and some leadership, positions.

By the mid-1920s, the Leningrad health service had recovered from the adverse effects of war, Revolution, Civil War and financial reform. But the birth rate was on the decline, while the death rate increased. Although infectious diseases had now become negligible, the level of children's and social diseases were a cause of concern for the Party and medical profession. Morbidity was higher in 1927 than in 1923–25, with the latter varying according to age, sex and district – with the death rate still highest in the traditionally working-class districts of Leningrad by 1926. The main causes of the city's high level of illness were inadequate housing, an impure water supply, an imperfect sewer system and a lack of basic amenities.

The local municipal and medical authorities must be given great credit for tackling, and to a limited extent, mitigating problems at this time despite a lack of adequate finance following the 1922 budget reform and the 'regime of economy' campaign of 1926. Every effort was made, as we witnessed above, to resist this policy, by not adhering to central guidelines. To a certain extent this paid off, but some economies still took place. With fewer resources, the Leningrad health service was not equipped to deal with declining health conditions, let alone be in a position to prepare itself for the impending industrialisation drive and forced collectivisation.

Medical care for the insured and the industrial proletariat remained key policy objectives. This was evidence of the new regime's 'workers' policies in action. This generated a conflict between the Ministries of Labour and Health over who should have responsibility for this medical policy and part of the collective. At the end of the first stage, despite constant criticism about a poor-quality service, Narkomzdrav managed to hold its ground. But the Ministry of Labour succeeded by 1927 in having Narkomzdrav's department for the insured closed down.

The insured, of course, had always been a sizable group in the city and as their numbers expanded rapidly between 1926–28, they had a decisive influence on the shape and direction of public health policy. As a result, the lion's share of dwindling public health resources went to them thus squeezing out the non-insured, not without consequences in terms of declining health. There was an impressive rise in the FMP, and growing attempts at Party control over medical affairs. With regard to the former, increased productivity was essential to the revitalisation and growth of Leningrad's industry, but this was only achieved at the cost, namely a rise in the number of industrial injuries. The Party, of course, had always pursued a policy which in the short term exploited the talents of the tsarist medical profession to combat adverse health conditions while in the medium term aiming to integrate bourgeois specialists into the new 'socialist society'. Through a policy of state support and the fact that old and new medical profession had shared beliefs on the importance of medicine and serving the community, there was broad cooperation by 1927. However, hardliners in the Leningrad Party were growing anxious about the key role which the former zemstvo specialists were playing in public health affairs. The move from persuasion to coercion was, therefore, not very far off.

In theory, the focus was on rendering medical care to the workers using specially trained doctors and other medical personnel, but in practice a political dimension crept in. 'Illness' and 'entitlement' were both defined in ideological terms by the mid-1920s. Health coverage was mainly geared towards the insured or to those able to work and pay. Other sections of the population were labelled 'scroungers' and excluded from coverage. By the late 1920s, eligibility conditions for medical treatment were being tightened even more.

Leningrad's medical staff and the health service as a whole were ill-prepared, because of severe economic and political constraints, on the eve of the First five-year plan, for the implementation of a new Stalinist health policy. What consequences this move and a new leader, Stalin, had for the service, its staff and its patients in the period 1928–41 will be explored in the next chapter.

Acknowledgments

Earlier versions of parts of this chapter have been published in 'Old habits die hard: Alcoholism in Leningrad under the NEP and some lessons for the Gorbachev administration', *Irish Slavonic Studies*, 12, 1991, pp. 69–96.

Notes

1 Laura L. Phillips, *Bolsheviks and the Bottle: Drink and worker culture in St. Petersburg, 1900–1929* (Northern Illinois University Press: Dekalb 2000), 29.
2 E. H. Carr, *The Russian Revolution from Lenin to Stalin, 1917–1929* (Macmillan, London 1979), 28.
3 See P. Avrich, *Kronstadt 1921* (Norton/Princeton Univ. Press, London 1983).
4 J. E. Pickersgill, 'Hyper-inflation and monetary reform in the Soviet Union, 1921–26', *Journal of Political Economy* Volume 76 No. 5, September-October 1968, 1037–1048.
5 A. Ball, 'Private trade and traders during NEP' in S. Fitzpatrick, A. Rabinowitch and R. Stites (eds), *Russia in the Era of NEP: Explorations in Soviet society and culture* (Indiana University Press, Bloomington and Indianapolis, 1991), 94.
6 Ball, 'Private trade and traders during NEP', 94.
7 Ibid., 100, footnote 48, 105.
8 V. L. 'Vlianie novoi ekonomicheskoi politiki na byt trudashchikhsia zhenshchin', *Kommunistka* 3–5 (1922), 15. There was more to this than returning males and new laws, women faced prejudice and harassment because they were said to be incapable of heavy physical labour.
9 *Materialy po statistike truda*, Vyp. 15 (Petrograd 1924), 199.
10 *XV let diktatory proletariata: Ekonomiko-statisticheskii sbornik po gor. Leningradu i Leningradskoi oblasti* (Leningrad 1932), 143. These trends were slightly offset by an increase in the number of remarriages and by a rise in the index of legitimate births (See J. Coale, B. Anderson and E. Harm, *Fertility in Russia since the Nineteenth Century* (Princeton University Press, New Jersey 1979), 21; 39 and W. Berelowitch, "L' evolution de la fécondite légitimite a Saint-Petersbourg-Petrograd-Leningrad (1860 – 1926)', *Annales de Demographique historique* Paris 1982, 250).
11 Wendy Z. Goldman, *Women, the State and revolution: Soviet family policy and family life, 1917–1936* (Cambridge University Press 1993), 109.
12 Ibid., 51, 65.
13 W. Berelowitch, 'L'evolution de la fecondite legitime', 261.
14 M. Kaplun, 'Brachnost' naseleniia RSFSR', *Statisticheskoe obozrenie* 7 (1929), 95–97.
15 These migration concepts are taken from R. B. Johnson, *Peasant and Proletarian; The working-class of Moscow in the Late Nineteenth Century* (New Brunswick/Rutgers 1979), 28–42; J. Bradley, *Muzhnik and Moscovite; urbanisation in Late imperial Russia* (University of California Press, California 1985), 29–32.
16 *XV let diktatory proletariat* 1932, 146.
17 V Bronner, 'K Tret'emu Vsesoiuznomu s'ezdu po bor'be s venericheskim bolezniami', *Leningradskii meditsinskii zhurnal* 1929, No. 5, 5. According to Gorbovitskii, Wasserman tests were carried out from 1920 onwards. For example, the number of tests conducted by Leningrad's Serum Laboratory totalled a mere 1,034 in 1920 but then reached 12,787 by 1923 before rising to 113,216 in 1926 indicating the importance of VD (S. Ye. Gorbovitskii, 'K desiatiletiiu bor'by s venbolezhniami v Leningrade', *Leningradskii Meditsinskii Zhurnal* 1927, No.8–9, October-November, 137).

18 Frances Lee Bernstein, *The Dictatorship of Sex: Lifestyle advice for the Soviet Masses* (Northern Illinois University Press: Dekalb 2011).

19 For an example see the anti-syphilis poster figure 4.2 in Bernstein, *The Dictatorship of Sex*, 107.

20 At the time of the 1923 census, men made up 9.8% of the city's unemployed and women 11.9% (L. E. Mints, 'Dvizhenle bezrabotitsy', *Ekonomicheskoe obozrenie* Vyp. 12, December 1923, 1383) with unemployment at the start of 1924 being highest in Leningrad followed by Moscow (A. Isaev, *Bezrabotitsa v SSSR i bor'ba s niei (za period 1917–1924gg)* (Moscow 1924), 441).

21 Zhenotdel meeting held on 1 November 1927 (TsGAIPD SPb, f.16, op.13, d.13293, list 55). Other women went into prostitution to feed and clothe their children so not all women should be stereotyped in this way. On the Zhenotdel's attitude towards prostitution see Michelle J. Patterson, 'Red 'Teaspoon's of charity': Zhenotdel, Russian women and the Communist Party, 1919–1930', unpublished PhD in History, University of Toronto 2011, 96–137.

22 R. Stites, *The Women's liberation movement in Russia: Feminism, nihilism and Bolshevism, 1860–1930* (Princeton University Press, New Jersey 1978), 372; L. Fridland, *S raznykh storon: Prostitutsiia v SSSR* (Berlin 1931), 65.

23 See Laurie Bernstein, *Sonia's Daughters: Prostitutes and Their Regulation in Imperial Russia* (Berkeley: University of California Press, 1995).

24 'Polozhenie o bor'be s prostitutsei', *Gigiena i zdorov'e rabochei sem'I*, July 1926, No. 13, 11.

25 Dr A Sakhovskaia, 'Prostitutsia, prichiny ee puti raboty s neie', *Gigiena i zdorov'e rabochikh sem'I*, No. 19, 7 October 1924, 6 and Fridland, *S raznykh storon* 1931, 149.

26 Fannina W. Halle, *Women in Soviet Russia* (Routledge, London 1933), 218–267; Sakhovskaia, 'Prostitutsia' 1924, 6 and 'Chto my dolzhny delati v bor'be s prostitutsiei', *Gigiena i zdorov'e*, October 1928, No. 20, 48.

27 S. Ye. Gorbovitskii, 'K desiatiletiiu', 1927, 13 and V. Bronner, 'K Tret'emu Vsesoiuznomu s'ezdu po bor'be s venericheskim boleznami', *Leningradskii Meditsinskii Zhurnal* 1929, No. 5, 5.

28 *Zdravookhranie v g. Leningrade gubernii: K dokladu zavediaiushchego Leningradskom gubzdravotdelom na plenume Leningradskogo Soveta 29 iiulia 1927g* (Leningrad 1927), 44, 55.

29 See A. Kollontai, 'Pis'ma k trudiasheisia molodezhi – kakim dolzhen byt' kommunist', *Molodaia gvardiia* no. 1–2 (April–May 1922), 136–144. I am grateful to the late Prof. James Riordan for pointing out this source.

30 See Second poster in Christina Kiaer, 'Imagine no possessions: The Socialist objects of Russian Culture', *News from the Harriman Institute*, Fall 2005, 1.

31 Michael David Fox, *Revolution in the Mind: Higher learning among the Bolsheviks, 1919–1929* (Studies of the Harriman Institute, Cornell University Press, Ithaca and London 1997), 104.

32 P. Konecny, *Builders and Deserters: Students, state and community in Leningrad, 1917–1941* (McGill-Queens University Press 1999), 203.

33 Dr Nesline et al., *La lutte contre le tuberculose dans la RSFSR* (Moscow-Leningrad 1934), 25.

34 *Zdravookhranenie v g. Leningrade i gubernii* (Leningrad 1927), 18.

35 *Estvestvennoe dvizhenie naseleniia soiuza SSSR 1923–25* t. 1. Vyp. 1 (TsSU, Moscow 1928), xxxiii.

36 This view is typified by N. Semashko, *Proletarskaia bolezn': Tuberkulez* (Moscow 1920).

37 GARF A-482 op 10. d. 36, list 135; GARF A-482 op 10. d. 889, list 35 and *XV let diktatory proletariat* 1932, 144.

38 *XV let diktatory proletariat* (1932), 118–119.
39 Dr. Ia. Krizhevskii, 'Leningradskii tuberkuleznyi nauchnyi institut', *Gigiena i zdozov'e rabochei sem'i*, No.22, November 1926, 10.
40 A. M. Bramson, 'Dostizheniia i nedochety protivotuberkuleznogo dela i Leningrade', *Leningradskii Meditsinskii Zhurnal* 1927, No.8–9, October-November, 122.
41 *Zdravookhranie v g. Leningrade gubernii, plenum*, 40.
42 Ibid.
43 Dr. Rychkin, 'Rabochaia obshchestvennost' v bor'be s sotsial'nymi bolezniami', *Gigiena i zdozov'e rabochei sem'i*, No. 18, September 1927, 12.
44 *Zdravookhranie v g. Leningrade gubernii plenum*, 40.
45 V. L. Stoianovskaia, 'Rabota obsledovatel'skikh. Institute Leningradskikh tub-dispanserov (Po ochetam 1926g), *Leningradskii Meditsinskii Zhurnal* June–July 1928, No.6, 59.
46 Levels of overcrowding varied from 66.8% among Vyborg district residents to 80.4% among Vasiloestrovskii patients; 19.5% of Vyborg housing was damp and cold compared to 48.2% of Petrograd side buildings. Bad ventilation was uncommon in Vasileostrovskii (0.8%) but more widespread in Petrograd side (16.8%) (Stoianovskaia, 'Rabota obsledovatel'skikh', 1928, 60). No official norm for overcrowding is given.
47 Of the sample, 56.3% of Vyborg patients; 40.3% of city-centre; 60% of Vasileostrovskii and 27% of Petrograd side district patients lacked proper food and nourishment (Stoianovskaia, 'Rabota obsledovatel'skikh', 1928, 61).
48 Stoianovskaia, 'Rabota obsledovatel'skikh', 63.
49 Linda Bryder, *Below the Magic Mountain: A Social history of tuberculosis in Twentieth Century Britain* (Clarendon Press, Oxford 1988), 239; Neil McFarlane, 'Hospitals, housing and tuberculosis In Glasgow, 1911–51', *Social History of Medicine* Volume 2, No. 1, April 1989, 60 and F B Smith, *The Retreat of Tuberculosis. 1850–1950* (Croom Helm, London 1988), 167.
50 A. A. Mendel'son, 'Alkogolizm v sovremennom Leningrade', *Gigiena i Epidemiologiia* 1924, No.6, 51 and B. F. Didrikhson, 'K voprosy o bor' be s alkogolizmom v Leningrade', *Gigiena i Epidemiologiia* 1928, No. 1, 64
51 *Statisticheskii spravochnik po Leningradu* (Leningrad 1930), 36.
52 Deaths from alcoholic poisoning were as follows in 1926–27:

Occupation/social group	1926	1927
Workers	46	89
White-collar workers	13	31
Unemployed	17	31
Handicraft & Trade	15	26
Public figures	4	43
Peasants	2	2
Unknown	70	70

(F. Didrikhson, 'Alkokolizm Leningrada v 1927 godu', Leningradskii Meditsinskii Zhurnal 1928, No.7, August-September, 62)

53 The measures taken during NEP were contradictory to say the least. Despite a commitment to curtailing alcoholism, a series of decrees resulted in the alcoholic content increasing from 24° proof in January 1920 to 80° proof by October 1925; in the sentence for samogon related crimes being reduced from 5 to 3 years for professionals and to one year for amateurs in 1922; in the courts favouring fines instead of imprisonment, with samogon offences eventually being viewed as

minor and finally, in a State monopoly not being introduced until August 1925 (Helena Stone, 'The Soviet government and moonshine, 1917–1929', *Cahier du Monde Russe* XXVII (3–4), Juil-Decembre 1986, 359–80).

54 Mendel'son, 'Alkogolizm v sovremennom Leningrade', 1924, 51 and Didrikhson, 'K voprosy' 1928, 65.

55 The number of days lost per worker due to alcoholism in Leningrad increased from 5.1 in 1923/24 to 6.1 1925/26 (Didrikhson, 'K voprosy'1928, 70).

56 Mendel'son, 'Alkogolizm v sovremennom Leningrade', 51.

57 Expenditure on alcohol totalled 19,054,844r in 1923 and 33, 549, 534r in 1924, so state revenues were liable to be considerable (M. A. Shuster-Kadysh, ' K izuchenie dannykh i detskoi smertnosti i rozhdaemosti v Leningrade', *Leningradskii Medtsinskii Zhurnal* 1926, No. 6, June-July, 31). The notion of a 'Fiscal dilemma' whereby revenues outweigh other considerations, is taken from V. G. Treml, 'Alcohol in the USSR: a fiscal dilemma', *Soviet Studies* Volume 27, April 1975, 161–68.

58 *Izvestiia* 8 October 1922, 21.

59 A. G. Parkhomenko, 'Gosudarstvenno-pravovye meropriatiia po bor'be s p'ianstvom v pervye gody Sovetskoi vlasti', *Sovetskoe gosudarstvo i pravo* April 1984, No. 4, 115.

60 C. Williams, 'Old habits die hard: Alcoholism in Leningrad under N.E.P. and some lessons for the Gorbachev administration', *Irish Slavonic Studies* 12, 1991, 78.

61 Didrikhson, 'K voprosu', 70; A. Mendel'son, 'Dekret protiv p' ianstva', *Gigiena i zdozov'e rabochei sem'i*, No. 24, December 1928, 12.

62 A. P. Shishkin, 'Institut sotsial'noi gigieny i izuchenie problem alkogolizma', *Sovetskoe Zdravookhranenie* 1971, No.5, 66–67. For an example of one such 1926 poster 'Nabor'bu s p'ianstvom' (Battle against Drunkenness), 1926. see C. Williams, '"Lets Smash it" Mobilising the masses against the demon drink in Soviet era health posters' *The Pleasures and Problems of Drink* Special Issue of *Visual Resources*, Volume 28, Number 4, December 2012, 367.

63 Didrikhson, 'Alkogolizm Leningrada v 1927' 1928, 54.

64 Sobering up station detentions in Leningrad were as follows in 1926–27:

District	Number of detentions		Increase in number of detentions
	1926	*1927*	*(%)*
Volodarskii	18,343	20,155	9.9
Moscow-Narva	22,211	26,596	19.8
City-centre	28,455	34,677	21.9
Vasileostrovskii	9,049	9,429	4.2
Vyborg	9,635	9,973	3.3
Petrograd side	9,778	12,295	25.8
City as whole	94,791	113,120	19.3

(F. Didrikhson, 'Alkogolizm Leningrada v 1927' 1928, 57)

65 Both gubernia statistical department and trade union data confirm that absenteeism, due to alcoholism was on the increase from 5.1 per 1,000 on 1923–24 to 6.4 per 1,000 by 1925–26 (Didrikhson, 'K voprosu', 70)

66 Phillips, *Bolsheviks and the Bottle* 2000, 35.

67 This poster is given in C. Williams, '"Lets Smash it" Mobilising the masses against the demon drink in Soviet era health posters', *The Pleasures and Problems of Drink* Special Issue of *Visual Resources*, Volume 28, Number 4, December 2012, 365.

68 Z. G. Frenkel', *Petrograd: perioda voiny i revoliutsii: sanitarnye usloviia i kommunal'noe blagoustroistvo* (Petrograd 1923), 21 and *XV let diktatory proletariat* 1932, 144.
69 M. A. Shuster-Kadysh, 'K izuchenie', 32.
70 Shuster-Kadysh, 'K izuchenie', 31. An indication of how widespread female drinking was the number of females dying from alcohol poisoning which increased from 21 in 1926 to 38 by 1927 (F. Didrikhson, 'Alkogolizm Leningrada v 1927', 1928, 62).
71 Shuster-Kadysh, 'K izuchenie', 40.
72 C. Davis and M. Feshbach. *Rising infant mortality in the USSR in the 1970s* (U.S. Dept of Commerce, Census Bureau, Series P-95, No.74 June 1980), Chapter 3.
73 L. A. and L. M. Vasilevskie, *Abort kak sotsial'noe yavlenia: Sotsial'noe-gigienicheskoe ocherk* (Moscow-Leningrad 1924), 104. A translation of the November decree is available in R. Schlesinger (ed), *The Family in the USSR: Documents and readings* (RKP, London 1949), 44.
74 Goldman, *Women, the State and revolution*, 257.
75 Ibid., 261.
76 Ibid.
77 For an example of this card see L. V. Ul'iamovskogo, 'Abort i dekret 20 noiabria 1920 goda', *Zhurnal Akusherstva i Zhenskikh Boleznei* tom XXXIX, kniga 2, 1928, 186.
78 *Biulleten' Leningradskogo gubzdravotedel* No. 1, June 1924, 36; Dr Aduevskii, 'Doklad Leningradskogo oblastnogo otdela zdravookhraneniia' in *Biulleten' Leningradskogo oblastnoi otdel Soiuz 'Medsantrud'* 1928, No. 1, 16; 'Aborty v Leningrade', *Gigiena i zdorov'e rabochei sem'i* No. 23, December 1930, 16.
79 Dr. A Roubakine, *La protection de la santé publique dans L'URSS (Principes et resultants)* (Paris 1933), 82.
80 N. A. Semashko, *Health protection in the USSR* (London, Gollancz 1934), 86 and V V Paevskii, 'K voprosy o rozhdaemosti v Leningrade' in *Statisticheskii sbornik Leningradskogo oblastnogo otdela zdravookhraneniia za 1928 god* (Leningrad 1929), 63.
81 Thus although the number of maternity beds increased from 3,136 in 1926 to 3,521 in 1927, that is by 12.3% and faster than the growth of the population, the number of health points at which women could be treated had remained constant at 21 since 1924 and the number of visits made to various women's establishments had fallen by 73.4% from 511,426 in 1926 to 135,896 a year later (*Zdravookhranie v g. Leningrade gubernii* 1927), 18, 32–35).
82 Paevskii, 'K voprosy o rozhdaemosti v Leningrade', 66. Of the abortions performed in 1926: 52% were performed free and 48% for a fee, which was a dramatic increase over 1924–25. The background of non-fee paying patients was as follows: 61.8% – housewives; 17.3% the unemployed; 5.5% white-collar workers; 0.25% members of the free professions; 3.4% students and 11.6% were from undisclosed origin (*Zdravookhranie v g. Leningrade gubernii* 1927, 35).
83 Paevskii, 'K voprosy o rozhdaemosti v Leningrade', 79–80.
84 T. Sosnovy, *The housing problem in the Soviet Union* (Research Program on the USSR, New York 1954), 21–28, 40, 42, 45–48.
85 P. V. Novikov, 'Vodosnabzhenle' and M. S. Slenin, 'Kanalizatsiia' in *Gorodskoe khozyiastvo i ustroitel'stvo Leningrada za 50 let* (Leningrad 1967), 151 and 161 respectively.
86 *Statisticheskii sbornik po Petrogradu i Petrogradskoi gubernii* (Petrograd 1922), 222 and Sosnovy, *The housing problem in the Soviet Union*, 38.

87 By 1921, Petrograd had 32,692 houses made of wood and only 1,200 of concrete (Statis*ticheskii sbornik po Petrogradu i Petrogradskoi gubernii* (Petrograd 1922), 222.
88 'Doma i kvartiry Leningrada i Leningradskoi gubernil po dannyzn perepisi 15 marta 1923 goda', in *Materialy po statistike Leningrada i Leningradskoi gubernii, Vyp.6* (Leningrad 1925), 265.
89 'Zhilishchnyi vopros v Leningrade', *Vestnik Finansov,* 1925, No. 6, 227.
90 Ibid., 228. The number of rooms rose from 189,891 in 1920 to 194,004 by 1923.
91 The dwelling space figure is taken from Sosnovy, *The housing problem in the Soviet Union* 1954, 107
92 Sosnovy, *The housing problem in the Soviet Union,* 232.
93 Ye. O. Kabo, 'Kvartirnaia plata i rabochei budzhet', *Statisticheskoe obozrenie* No. 8, August 1927, 65. This was much lower than in other cities, such as Moscow (7r 03k), Ivanovo-Voznesensk (16r 59k); the Urals (18r 72k) and Kiev (15r 29k).
94 See G. S. Velen'skii-Belinskii, 'Zhilishchno-bytovye usloviia Leningrada i nabodnenie 1925g', *Gigiena i Epidemiologiia* 1926, No. 1, 15–25.
95 *Direktivy KPSS i Sovetskoe gosudarstva po khozyiasnym voprosam, 1917–1957gg* (Moscow 1957–58) t. 1, 57.
96 *Vseoiuznaia perepis' naseleniia 17 dekabria 1926 goda. Predvaritel'nye itogi,* Vyp 2: Goroda i naseleniia gorodskogo tipa (TsSU Soiuza SSR, Moscow 1927), 8.
97 *Vseoiuznaia perepis' naseleniia 17 dekabria 1926 goda. Kratkii svodki, Vyp VI: Zhilishchnyi fond SSSR* (TsSU Soiuza SSR, Moscow 1928), 6.
98 E. H. Carr and R. W. Davies, *Foundations of a planned economy, Volume 1* (Pelican, Harmondsworth, Middlesex 1974), 654.
99 *Vseoiuznaia perepis' naseleniia 17 dekabria 1926 goda. Kratkii svodki,* Vyp VI: Zhilishchnyi fond SSSR (TsSU Soiuza SSR, Moscow 1928), 34.
100 Per-capita housing space had fallen to 9.8m^2 by 1926 compared to 13.3m^2 in 1923 (A. I. Shtreis, 'Osnovye etapy razvitia sanitarnogo dela v Leningrade', *Leningradskii Meditsinskii Zhurnal,* 1927, No. 8–9, October-November, 112).
101 A. I. Shtreis, 'Osnovye etapy', 1927, 112. There were, of course, large variations in the extent of new building, as the following data from 1923–27 shows:
New construction in Leningrad according to district (in m^2)

	1923	1924	1925	1926	1927
Vasileostrovskii	158	6,117	9,116	5,210	21,803
Volodarskii	200	927	11,921	10,024	38,975
Vyborg	258	93	487	13,034	13,998
Moscow-Narva	-	314	9,206	11,860	18,207
Petrograd side	1,071	436	4,875	1,140	17,418
Smolnyi-October	227	1,057	4,063	11,399	31,321
Total	1,914	8,944	39,038	40,454	140,758

(*XV let diktatory proletariata*, 73)

102 *XV let diktatory proletariata,* 173.
103 A. I. Shtreis, 'Osnovye etapy', 1927, 109–110. According to another source, there were 75,516 main water stations and 18,154 river bank stations in Leningrad in 1927–28 (*XV let diktatory proletariata* 1932, 177).
104 '22 mil. rub. na remont i postroiku domov', *Krasnaia gazeta* [evening edition] 4 April 1927, 3.
105 A. I. Shtreis, 'Osnovye etapy', 110.

106 Wheatcroft. 'Famine and factors affecting mortality in the USSR: Appendices', 31.
107 Ibid.
108 Wheatcroft. 'Famine and factors affecting mortality in the USSR', 15.
109 Wheatcroft. 'Famine and factors affecting mortality in the USSR: Appendices', 24–28.
110 Wheatcroft, 'Famine and factors affecting mortality in the USSR', 25.
111 Carr and Davies, *Foundations of a planned economy Volume 1*, 740–741.
112 A. I. Shtreis, 'Osnovye etapy', 1927, 114. As a result of this work, the proportion of rejected food samples fell from 13% in 1925 to 6.4% in 1926; bad bread fell from 96% in 1922 to 50% by 1926 and poor-quality milk from 63% to 20% over the same period (A. I. Shtreis, 'Osnovye etapy', 114). These efforts continued in 1927, with attempts being made to improve the quality of stolovaia food and dairy products (see 'Bor'ba za zdorovoe pitanie', *Krasnaia Gazeta* 23 February 1927, No.51, 3 and 'Maslo, syr, moloko – pod kontrolia', *Krasnaia gazeta*, 5 April 1927, 90, 3).
113 The following discussion is based on Ye D Gribanov, *Vserossiikie s"ezdy zdravotedelov i ikh znachenie dlia praktiki sovetskogo zdravookhraneniia* (Moscow 1956), 73–74.
114 Jack Minkoff, 'The Soviet social insurance system since 1921', PhD Dissertation, Faculty of Political Science, Columbia University, 1960, 261. I am grateful to Dr Christopher Davis (Nuffield College Oxford) for drawing my attention to this source.
115 Gribanov, *Vserossiikie s"ezdy zdravotedelov*, 68.
116 Ivanov argues infant care was locally funded (P. V. Ivanov, 'Organizatsiia lechebno-profilaktiocheskoi pomoshchi detiam rannego vozrasta v Leningrade v pervoe desiatiletle sovetskoi vlasti (1917–1928gg), Avtoreferat candidate degree medical science, Leningradskii pediatricheskii medltsinskii Institut, 1955, 16).
117 Gribanov, *Vserossiikie s"ezdy zdravotedelov*, 69.
118 Ibid., 70.
119 Ibid., 75.
120 Ibid., 76.
121 C. Davis, 'Economic problems of the RSFSR Health system, 1921–30', CREES, University of Birmingham, SIPS Discussion paper No. 19, 1978, 7.
122 According to Ball, private trade in medicines was legalized (subject to special permission) and private clinics were allowed to open in early 1922 (A. M. Ball, *Russia's last Capitalist: The Nepmen, 1921–29* (University of California Press, Berkeley and Los Angeles 1987), 211.
123 While Urals oblast was spending 26.3r and Moscow 21.7r per person on health care, Petrograd/Leningrad was only spending 10.3r. Only the South Eastern region had a lower expenditure level, with 6.3r per head on average being spent on health in the budget year, 1922–23 (M. Ginzberg, 'Mestnyi buidzhet i zdravookhranenie', *Izvestiia Narkomzdrav* 1924 No. 1, 67).
124 R. W. Davies, *The development of the Soviet budgetary system* (Cambridge University Press, 1958), 55
125 *Biulleten' Leningradskogo gubzdravotedela* June 1924, No. 1, 5.
126 *Biulleten' Leningradskogo gubzdravotedela* June 1924, No. 1, 6.
127 Davis, 'Economic problems', 16–17.
128 Davies, *The development of the Soviet budgetary system*, 88.
129 Ibid., 16–17, 21.
130 M. Ginzberg, 'Voprosy zdravookhranenie v predstoiashchem buidzhete', *Izvestiia Narkomzdrav* 1925, No. 2–3, 16.
131 *Zdravookhranenie v g. Leningrade i gubernii* (Leningrad 1927), 15 and *Otchet Leningradskogo oblastnogo ispolkom Noiabr' 1927g – Aprel' 1929g* (Leningrad 1929), 89, 140.

132 G. Dreisin, 'Narodnoe zdravookhranenie v mestnom biudzhete SSSR na 1925/26gg', *Biulleten' Narkomzdrav* 1926, No.7, 13–15.

133 *Otchet Leningradskogo Soveta I gubispolkom 9 s 1-go ianvaria po 7-oe iiulia 1925g)* (Leningrad 1925), 34.

134 *Zdravookhranie v g. Leningrade gubernii: K dokladu zavediaiushchego Leningradskom gubzdravotdelom na plenume Leningradskogo Soveta 29 iiulia 1927g* (Leningrad 1927), 15 and Otchet Leningradskogo ispolkom Noiabr 1927 – Aprel' 1929g (Leningrad 1929), 89.

135 Carr and Davies, *Foundations of a planned economy, Volume 1*, 358–359.

136 Narkomzdrav Circular No.76, 'O rezhime ekonomii v oblasti zdravookhrane-niia', *Biulleten Narkomzdrav* 1926, No.11, 58–59.

137 N. A. Semashko, 'Rezhim ekonomii v dele zdravookhraneniia', *Biulleten Narkomzdrav* 1926, No.13–14, 3. My italics

138 V. Kul'vanovskii, 'Itogi proizvedeniia rezhima ekonomii v dele zdravookhrane-niia'. *Biulleten Narkomzdrav* 1927. No. 4, 4.

139 Kul'vanovskii, 'Itogi'1927, 4, 6–8.

140 E. K Golubeva, 'Massovaia ekonomrabota lechebnykh uchrezhdeniiakh g. Leningrada', *Leningradskii Meditsinskii Zhurnal*,1927, No.7, 60–62.

141 Golubeva, 'Massovaia', 63.

142 Golubeva, 'Massovaia', 63–64.

143 G. Karanovich, 'Etapy razvitiia mestnykh organov zdravookhraneniia', *Biulleten' Narkomzdrav* 1929, No. 10, 19.

144 At regional level in 1921 these were Administration and cadres; finance; supply; out-patients; secretariat; sanitary-epidemiology; mother and babies; children's and military (Karanovich, 'Etapy', 19).

145 By 1923 at regional level these were Administration, economics, cadres and finance; supply; out-patients; secretariat; sanitary-epidemiology; mother and babies and children's (Karanovich, 'Etapy', 19).

146 By 1924 these were administration and economics; out-patients; legal medical expertise and health education (Karanovich, 'Etapy', 19).

147 At regional level in 1921 these sub-sections were under administration – cadres; under out-patients – legal and medical aid, general and specialised aid and den-tistry; and under sanitary-epidemiology – sanitation, statistics, health education and housing (Karanovich, 'Etapy', 19).

148 By 1923, these sub-sections were under organisation and economics – finance and cadres; under out-patients – dentistry, supplies and legal; under sanitary-epidemiology – sanitation, statistics, social diseases and health education (Karanovich, 'Etapy', 19).

149 By 1924 these were sub-sections under adminstration and economics – finance and general cadres; under health education – statistics, mothers and babies and children's (Karanovich, 'Etapy', 19).

150 *Izvestiia komissariata zdravookhraneniia Soiuza kommuna Severnoi oblasti*, November 1918, 123–125; *Ves Petrograd 1922g* (Petrograd 1923), 237–253, 281–288; *Ves Leningrad i Leningradskaia oblast' na 1926 god* (Petrograd 1929), 177.

151 GARF f. A-482 op. 10 d. 37, list 15; GARF f. A-482 op. 10 d. 1914, list 116; *Statisticheskie materialy po soistoianiiu narodnogo zdraviia i organizatsii med-itsinskoi pomoshchi v SSSR za 1913–1923gg* (Moscow 'NKZ' 1926), 82–83, 86–87; S. Mamushin, 'Obzor deitel'nosti bol'nichnoi i ambulatornoi seti v g. Leningrada', *Voprosy zdravookhraneniia* 1930, No. 1, 63 and *XV let diktatory proletariat* 1932, 69.

152 Minkoff, 'The Soviet social insurance system since 1921', 304, 308.

153 Ibid., 310–311.

154 Ibid., 311.

155 Ibid., 311–312.
156 *Trud* 11 January 1925, 4 and A I Vishnevetskii, *Razvitiia zakondatel'stva o sotsial'nom strakhovaniia v Rossii* (Moscow 1926), 120–124.
157 Minkoff, 'Soviet social Insurance system since 1921', 311–312.
158 Sally E Ewing, 'Social insurance in Russia and the Soviet Union, 1912–33: A study of legal form and administrative practice', unpublished PhD dissertation, Princeton University, June 1984, 175.
159 A. I. Vishnevetskii, *Razvitiia zakondatel'stva o sotsial'nom strakhovaniia v Rossii* (Moscow 1926), 86.
160 On the trade union and NOT see M. Dewar, *Labour policy in the USSR, 1917– 28* (London: Royal Institute of International Affairs, 1950); I. Deutscher, *Soviet trade unions: Their place in Soviet labour policy* (London; Royal Institute of International Affairs, 1950) and Jay Sorenson, *Life and Death of Soviet trade unionism, 1917–28* (Atherton Press, New York 1969). On the productivity question and the Taylorism debate see Z. A. Sochor, 'Soviet taylorism revisited', *soviet Studies* Volume 33, No. 2 April 1981, 246–264 and S. A. Smith, 'Taylorism rules OK? Bolshevism, Taylorism and the Technical intelligentsia in the Soviet Union, 1917–41', *Radical Science Journal* 1983, No. 13.
161 On the various types of benefits available see N. I. Bynovskii, *Chto daet rabo- chemy sotsial'noe strakhovanie* (Moscow 1922) and Minkoff, 'The Soviet social Insurance system since 1921', Chapters 4–9.
162 Quoted in Gribanov, *Vserossiikie s"ezdy zdravotedelov*, 79, 82.
163 Gribanov, *Vserossiikie s"ezdy zdravotedelov*, 82–83.
164 The insured included all wage earners, except seasonal and part time workers (B. G. Danskii, *Sotsial'noe strakhovanie ran'she i teper'* (Moscow 1926), 83–85).
165 Gribanov, *Vserossiikie s"ezdy zdravotedelov*, 84.
166 *Sotsial'noe strakhovanie*, 1 February 1923, No. 6, 12; *Voprosy Truda*, No. 11, November 1924, 141; *Rabota i dostizheniia Leningradskikh profsoiuzov* (Leningrad 1925), 230; *Otchet Leningradskogo soveta i gubispolkom (s 1-ian- varia po 1-oe iiulia 1925g)* (Leningrad 1925), 111; *Statisticheskii sbornik po gor. Leningradu* (Izd. Leningradskogo oblispolkoma 1930), 211; XV let dikta- tory proletariat, 1932, 116–117.
167 *Stanovlenie i razvitie zdravookhraneniia v pervye gody Sovetskoi vlastii 1917– 1924gg: Sbornik dokumentov i materialov* (Moscow 1966), 421.
168 *Biulleten' Leningradskogo gubzdravotedela* June 1924, No.1, 5.
169 Complaints about the poor quality and lack of availability of medical facili- ties for the insured were made emphasising that although average per-capita expenditure by the kassy had increased from 20r in 1923 to 75r by 1925, less of the FMP was being used on the insured. Thus out of the 130 million roubles budget in 1924–25 only 6.5million (or as little as 5%) was spent on insured workers (L. Nemchenko, 'Fund "G" tol'ko dila zastrakhovaniiu' *Vestnik Truda* No. 4 April 1926, 10–13).
170 *Biulleten' Leningradskogo gubzdravotedela* June 1924, No.1, 20.
171 Ibid., 23.
172 B. Beleliubskii, 'Rost' zabolaevaemosti zastrakhovannykh v Leningrade', *Voprosy truda* December 1924, No. 12, 150.
173 B. Beleliubskii, 'Zabolaevaemosti zastrakhovannykh v Leningrade za 1924– 1925 godakh', *Voprosy truda* October 1925, No. 10, 158.
174 *Biulleten' Leningradskogo gubzdravotedela* June 1924, No.1, 21.
175 M. Rubinshtein, 'Medpomoshch' zastrakhovannym v Leningrade', *Voprosy strakhovaniia* No. 8, 25 February 1926, 28–30.
176 R. 'Fond "G" i fakticheskaia medpomoshch' zastrakhovannym (Leningrad)', *Voprosy strakhovaniia* No. 23, 10 June 1926, 16–17.

177 A. Aluf', Meditsinkoi pomshch' i zastrakhavannym', *Vestnik Truda*, April 1923, No. 4, 51.
178 Ibid., 52.
179 Ibid., 53–54.
180 *Rabota i dostizheniia Leningradskikh profsoiuzov* (Leningrad 1925), 236.
181 A. K. 'Ocherednye voprosy sotslal nogo strakhovanila', *Vestnik Truda*, May 1923, No. 5, 32.
182 A. Magaziner, 'Obzor finansovoi deiatel'nosti soiuznykh organizatsii', *Vestnik Truda*, November 1923, No. 9, 146.
183 Dr Abramov, 'Petrograd: organizastsiia medpomoshchi', *Voprosy Strakhovaniia* No. 35, 4 September 1923, 18–19.
184 Yu. S. 'Kratkii obzor deiatel'nosti raistrakhkass g. Leningrada (v 1924–25 oper-atsionnom gody)', *Voprosy truda* No. 12, December 1925, 174.
185 Dr A. la. Katsman, 'Petrograd: Voprosy kontrolia', *Voprosy strakhovaniia* No. 51–52, 15 December 1923, 25–27.
186 Cited in M Golovin, 'Sotsial'noe strakhovanye v Leningrade', *Voprosy strakho-vaniia* No. 4–5; 2 February 1925, 59.
187 V. Pachkin,' Kak rabotaet Leningradskaia gubstrakhkassa', *Voprosy strakhova-niia* No. 44–45, 7 November 1925, 47 Dr Abramov, 'Petrograd: organizastsiia medpomoshchi', *Voprosy strakhovaniia* No. 35, 4 September 1923, 19–20.
188 Abramov, 'Petrograd', 19–20.
189 la. Svetiakov, 'Neschastnye sluchai na Petrogradskikh predpriiatlkh', *Trud* 18 Jan 1922, 3 and *Otchet Leningradskogo Soveta i gubispolkom 9 s 1-go ianvaria po 7-oe iiulia 1925g)* (Leningrad 1925), 209.
190 A. Solov'ev, 'Neschastaye sluchai i bor' ba s nimi' *Trud* 30 June 1925, 23.
191 Ibid.
192 See A, Kats, 'Okhrana truda v period rekonstruktsii khozyiastva',*Voprosy Truda* April 1927, No. 4, 63.
193 L. H. Siegelbaum, 'Okhrana truda: Industrial hygiene, psychotechnics and Industrialisation In the USSR', in Susan Gross Solomon and John F. Hutchinson (ed.), *Health and Society in Revolutionary Russia* (Indiana University Press, Bloomington and Indianapolis, 1990), 230.
194 N. D. Vigdorchik,'Leningradskii institut po izucheniia professlonal'nykh zabole-vanii', *Gigiena i zdorov'e rabochikh sem'i* No. 22, 20 November 1924, 8–9.
195 D. N. Vigdorchik, 'Invalidnost v Petrograde v 1918 1919gg', in *Materialy po statistike Petrograda, Vyp.4* (Petrograd 1921), 311. Payments in the first three categories were as follows:

Invalidity category	Per-capita benefits as of:		
	October 1923	*January 1924*	*April 1925*
I	12r 53k	16r 50k	24r
II	8r 56k	11r	16r
III	6r 26k	8r 25k	12r

(Otchet Leningradskogo Soveta i gubispolkom 9 s 1-go ianvaria po 7-oe iiulia 1925g) (Leningrad 1925), 122 and *Rabota i dostizheniia Leningradskikh profsoiuzov* (Leningrad 1925), 234).

As we can see all benefits had doubled in this period, draining Narkomtrud kassy funds further.

196 D. Gorfin, 'Medpomoshch' zastranovannym i raboche organizatsii, *Voprosy strakhovaniia* No. 22, 15 June 1924, 13–14.

197 On these differences See Davis, 'Economic problems', 41–42.
198 *Otchet Leningradskogo Soveta i gubispolkom 9 s 1-go ianvaria po 7-oe iiulia 1925g)* (Leningrad 1925), 91, 95 and *Zdravookhranenie v g. Leningrade i gubernii* (Leningrad 1927), 17.
199 On these establishments see *Rabota i dostizheniia Leningradskikh profsoiuzov* (Leningrad 1925), 242–248.
200 S. Ryss, 'Zabolevaemost' zastrakhovannykh v Leningrade' *Voprosy strakhovaniia* No. 24, 15 June 1925, 43 and V. Pachkin, ' Kak rabotaet Leningradskaia gubstrakhkassa', *Voprosy strakhovaniia* No. 44–45, 7 November 1925, 47.
201 *XV let diktatory proletariat* 1932, 118–119.
202 My calculations are based upon dividing the FMP by the number of insured, on the one hand, and by dividing the state and local health budgets by the total population minus the insured on the other. No distinctions have been made for dependants. According to Gorfin, there were 2.3 dependants per insured worker by 1927 [D. Gorfin, 'Okhrana zdorov' ia proletariata za '10 let', *Biulleten Narkomzdrav* 1927,No. 20, 31). In that case the revised per-capita health expenditure for Leningrad would be as follows:

Year	Insured workers plus dependants [in roubles]
1923–24	6r 99k
1924–25	14r 87k
1925–26	12r 18k
1926–27	12r 63k

203 A. Vainshtein, 'Skhema raskhodovaniia lechfonda', *Voprosy strakhovaniia* No.27, 7 July 1927, 14.
204 'Uchranit' nedostatki, uvelichit' dostizheniia. K perevybornoi kampanii v Leningrade', *Voprosy Strakhovanie* No.89, 27 September 1928, 10.
205 Vainshtein, 'Skhema raskhodovaniia lechfonda', 14.
206 Ibid., 15.
207 This situation was created by numerous factors – personnel shortages, high turnover of staff, failure to update instructions, excessive pressure etc (see Ewing, 'Social insurance in Russia and the Soviet Union', 1984, 313–332)
208 M.G., 'Leningradskaia volokuta', *Voprosy Strakhovaniia* No.32, 11 Aug 1927, 8.
209 Vainshtein, 'Skhema raskhodovaniia lechfonda', 16.
210 V. Karibskii, 'Moskva i Leningrad (Sravnitel'nyi obzor medpomoshchi zastrakhovannym)', *Voprosy Strakhovaniia* No. 30, 26 July 1926, 13.
211 This was far more than the amounts spent in other cities. For example, the corresponding figures for Perm were: 30k, 1r 56k and 86k respectively. With the exception of a Moscow figure of 2r 97k devoted to hospital beds for the insured, Leningrad was spending more on this than its old rival (Karibskii, 'Moskva i Leningrad', 14–15).
212 Semashko letter dated 23 May 1922 in APRF f. 3. Op. 58 d. 2, ll. 3–4 cited in David R. Shearer and Vladimir Khaustov, *Stalin and the Lubianka: A documentary history of the political police and security organs in the Soviet Union* (Yale University Press, New Haven and London 2015), 28.
213 Semashko letter dated 23 May 1922 in APRF f. 3. Op. 58 d. 2, ll.3–4 cited in Shearer and Khaustov, *Stalin and the Lubianka* 2015, 28–29.
214 APRF f. 3. Op. 58 d. 2, ll.3–4 cited in Shearer and Khaustov, *Stalin and the Lubianka* (2015), 28. The term zemshchina here refers to proponents of zemstvo medicine

215 Ibid., 29.
216 RGASPI f. 17 op. 3, d. 296, ll. 2–3 cited in Shearer and Khaustov, *Stalin and the Lubianka* 2015), 32. The term spetsy refers to specialists and has a pejorative connation implying bourgeois and opposition tendencies.
217 A similar conciliatory policy was adopted towards the technical intelligentsia (Kendall E. Bailes, *technology and Society under Lenin and Stalin: Origins of the Soviet Technical Intelligentsia, 1917–41* (Princeton University Press 1978), 5 and lawyers (Eugene Huskey, *Russian lawyers and the Soviet State: The origins and development of the Soviet Bar, 1917–1939* (Princeton University Press, New Jersey 1926), 54.
218 *Statisticheskii spravochnik 1922* (Petrograd 1922), 117.
219 Konecny, *Builders and Deserters* 1999, 64–65. The grants system was in a state of flux during this period, but despite this, one third (700 out of 2,170) of the students attending the State Institute of Medical Science received government assistance (W. Horsley Gantt, 'A review of education in Soviet Russia', *British Medical Journal* 14 June 1924a, 1058).
220 The Leningrad Medical Institute consisted of 4 basic hygiene departments: general, social, school and labour. For more information see V. M. Merabishvili, 'Iz istorii Leningradskogo sanitarnogo meditsinskogo instututa' *Gigiena i Sanitariia* 1971, No. 4, 52–55; S la Freidlin, '50 let kafedre sostial'noi gigieny i organizatsii zdravookhraneniia I Leningradskogo meditsinskogo instituta im. I. P. Pavlova', *Sovetskoe Zdravookhranenie* 1973, No, 3, 66–69; V. la. Belitskaia and K. I. Zhuravleva, 'K 60 letiiu kafedry sotsial'noi gigieny i organizatsii Leningradskogo sanitarnogo Meditsinskogo meditsinskogo instituta', *Sovetskoe Zdravookhranenie* 1982, No. 7, 61–63; T. G. Iakubovich et al, 'Kafedre gigieny truda Leningradskogo sanitarno-gigienicheskogo meditsinskogo Instituta 60 let', *Gigiena truda i professional'naia zabolevaniia* 1986, No.6, 57–59 and S V Alekseev, 'K 75 letiiu Leningradskogo sanitarno-gigienicheskogo meditsinskogo instituta', *Zdravookhranenie Rossiiskoi Federatsii* 1987, No. 1, 35–39.
221 Ye. V. Poliakov, 'Studenchestvo LMI kak professional'no-bytovaia gruppa', *Sotsial'naia gigiena* No. 2 (1925), 69–77.
222 A. A. Kurepin, 'Ideino-politicheskoe vospitanie studentov Leningradskikh institutov v pervye gody sovetskoi vlasti (1920–1928)', *Sovetskoe Zdravookhranenie* 1979, No. 2, 56–60.
223 Kurepin, 'Ideino-politicheskoe vospitanie studentov', 57.
224 Horsley Gantt, 'A review of education', 1057.
225 There were 57 disputes involving medical workers between January-April 1923 but these were economic in character relating to wages, the violation of labour protection regulations and so forth (*Biulleten' Petrogradskogo biuro statistiki truda* No. 38, June 1923, 19). The number of strikes in Petrograd fell from 66, involving 21,011 persons in 1922 to 26 with 5,388 people by 1923. But no medical workers were involved ('O zabastovkakh v Leningrade za 1922 I 1923gg', *Voprosy truda* No. 4, April 1924, 51–53).
226 Composition of the 11th Leningrad Soviet as stated in *Leningrad i guberniia* (Leningrad 1925), 137.
227 W. Horsley Gantt, 'The medical profession, soviet science and soviet sanitation, Part II', *British Medical Journal* 2 Feb 1927, 245. On the contribution of specific scientists see W. Horsley Gantt, 'Scientific work', *British Medical Journal* 20 September 1924b, 533–536 and 'Work of Pavlov and other scientists', *British Medical Journal* 11 June 1927, 1070–1073 and *British Medical Journal* 22 October 1927, 739–742.
228 See Susan Gross Solomon, 'Soviet social hygiene and Soviet public health, 1921–1930' in Susan Gross Solomon and John F. Hutchinson (eds), *Health and Society in Revolutionary Russia* (Indiana University Press, Bloomington and

Indianapolis, 1990), 175–199 and Susan Gross Solomon, 'David and Goliath in Soviet public health: The rivalry of social hygienists and psychiatrists for authority over the Bytovoi alcoholic' *Soviet Studies* Volume XLI, No. 2, April 1989, 254–278.

229 For background details see *Nauka i nauchnye rabotniki SSSR. Chast' II: Nauchnye uchrezhdenie Leningrada* (Leningrad 1926). It is impossible to go into detail on the role played by the Leningrad Occupational diseases Institute but we shall come across the latter in Chapter 4. On the maternity Research institute see Dr Iu. A. Mendeleva, 'Leningradskii nauchnyi institut okhrany materinstva i mladenchestva' in *Trudy III Vsesoiuznogo s"eda po okrane materinstva i mladenchestva (Moskva 1–7 Dekabria 1925 goda)* (Moscow 1926), 161–164

230 Of course, the transition onto local budget sources in 1922 together with the monetary reform (in force from February 1923 to May 1926) and hyperinflation, all had a negative impact on the operational capabilities of these establishments. For example, by 1923, the Military-Medical Academy had a budget of 24,000 gold roubles and the Leningrad medical institute one of nearly 34,000 gold roubles. These compared with 1915 and 1924 levels of 875,000 and nearly 378,000 gold roubles respectively (W. Horsley Gantt, 'A review of education', 1924a, 1058).

231 *Biulleten' Leningradskogo gubotdela soiuza 'Medsantrud'* No. 1 June 1924, 4 and No. 22, 28 May 1925, 25; *Biulleten' Leningradskii oblastnoi otdel soiuza 'Medsantrud'* No. 1 1928, 7, 16 and *XV let diktatory proletariat* 1932, 96.232

232 *Vseoiuznaia perepis' naseleniia 17 dekabria 1926 goda. Kratkii svodki, Vyp 9: Sotsial'nyi sostav i zaniatiia g. Leningrada* (TsSU Soiuza SSR, Moscow 1928), 66.

4 Health plans, medical disorder and repression: the health of the collective in crisis, 1928–41

This chapter considers developments in the Leningrad health service from 1928, the start of the 'Revolution from above'[1] to the Winter War with Finland and the siege of Leningrad, 1939–41. We analyse the aims and priorities of the Stalinist regime such as rapid industrialisation and forced collectivisation and the implementation of health planning, and the impact all this had on Leningrad – population growth, the influx of workers, shortages of housing, food etc. – and the financial and political constraints on health service development during the purges and preparation for the Great patriotic war. We then examine the response of local and central government and the medical profession to major increases in disease levels from social and infectious diseases and abortion and childhood illnesses and the ability of the health service and its staff to eradicate these problems in view of resource availability and political repression in the 1930s. Health care was still assigned a low priority and despite all the rhetoric, improvements in the health of the collective in Leningrad proved increasingly difficult to achieve as the Stalinist era progressed. The argument advanced is that increased morbidity and mortality were caused by poor diet, inadequate housing, the pressures of industrialisation and collectivisation, and by the failure, due to financial issues and political repression, to satisfy the population of Leningrad's medical needs. All in all, the health service was ill-prepared for the new challenges brought on by Stalinist policies and suffered from the consequences of the new leadership's demands and policies.

Life and death in Leningrad, 1928–40

The population of Leningrad increased from 1.7 million to 2.69 million during the First five-year plan (1928–32) or by around one million. It is noteworthy that by 1931, the size of the Leningrad population had surpassed its pre-war (1913) total. By 1932, the number of production workers had increased to 51.4% (compared to 24.4% in 1926) and the First FYP period and beyond saw an unprecedented rise in Leningrad's industrial base so that the number of industrial workers rose from 197,253 in 1925–26 to 540,000 by 1935.[2] During the Second FYP, 1932–36, the population only rose by another 9% (93,000) and then from 1936 until the 1939 census, the Third FYP, the population of Leningrad increased from 2,728,500 to 3,191,304 or by nearly half a million (462,804). Overall, from 1928 until 1939, the population rose by nearly 1.5 million. Thus the rapid rate of recovery experienced under the NEP was continuing, though growth was uneven throughout the 1930s. The birth rate stood at 22.6 per 1,000 in 1928 but declined to 15.9 by 1934 but then increased to 22.0 by 1940, close to its 1930 level; whilst the death rate increased slightly from 14.4 per 1,000 in 1928 to 17.6 per 1,000 in 1940.[3]

From 1922 to June 1930, the city had six districts (Petrograd side, Vyborg, Vasiloestrovskii, central city (from 1930 renamed October), Moscow-Narva and Volodarskii. In July 1930, Smolnyi was added and Moscow-Narva was split into two separate districts. From 1934, Narva was called Kirov. Leningrad oblast was created in 1927.[4] Throughout the 1930s, the number of districts increased. For instance, the central district was created from Smolnyi. In April 1936, the number of districts increased to 15 including Red Guards (*Krasnogvardeiskii*) from Vyborg; maritime (*Primorskii*) from Petrograd side; Lenin from Kirov; Sverdlov from Vasiloestrovskii and Dzerzhinskii, Kiubyshev and Frunze districts from central (suburb). In August 1936, Prigodskii was abolished and then three more new districts were added: Kolpin, Detskoesel'skii (from 1937 renamed Pushkin) and Peterhof.[5]

These territorial changes complicated the residential mixing issue as well as the workings of the health service. Medical professionals now had to deal with a wider geographical area and a more highly dispersed population.

The 1939 All-Union census is acknowledged to have been distorted and only covers 19 districts of Leningrad and its gubernia – 15 urban districts and four towns (Kolpino, Kronstadt, Puskin and Peterhof), which affects the availability of data and its accuracy[6] but archival and other sources have been used to fill some of the gaps.

There are a number of factors which affected demographic patterns. Leningrad was undergoing tremendous change from 1928 onwards in terms of its economy, job opportunities etc. and so recovery was rapid. New migrants entered the city in search of jobs in heavy industry, metallurgy and allied trades, as well as in construction, transport and the civil service.[7] Some of these groups responded to priority areas in local government policy. Unfortunately, health was assigned a low priority alongside social services and education, making it difficult for the health system to cope with the growing demand for medical care by the expanding industrial working class and incoming peasantry. Growth was particularly acute in 1929–30 and 1931–32, and so strains on the city's health service were especially high in these years. According to one source, in-migration accounted for nearly 80% of the increase in the Leningrad population between 1928–31.[8] Clearly expectations regarding the possibility of employment were high given the ongoing industrialisation drive. The additional population changes between

1932–36 were partly the result of the 1932–33 famine and the adverse effects of collectivisation which led to the arrival of peasants from the countryside and to a low level of out-migration. In the rest of the 1930s, in- and out-migration figures changed. Thus in 1935–38, in-migration was 479,300 whereas out-migration was greater at 456,200.[9] We can speculate that this was due to peasants returning to the post-famine countryside or certain sections of the population trying to avoid Stalin's great and mass terrors from 1934–37 as Leningrad was deemed a Terrorist centre. 1939 marked the start of mobilisation and preparation for a possible war. Leningrad was in a vulnerable military and strategic position and close to the frontier. Population levels were influenced by Soviet-Finnish War of 1939–40 because 147,000 reservists and new recruits were drafted into the Army, Navy and NKVD units. As a result, out-migration exceeded in-migration by 101,054 in 1939; although there was greater in-migration by 51,021 in 1940 according to Cherepenina's calculations.[10] The departure of able bodied men into the Army, and the mobilisation of women into industry, meant fewer births compounded by increases in illegal abortions and the infant mortality rate. Finally, the demography of Leningrad was affected by a shifting pattern of illness, with the death rate reaching 17.6 per 1,000 population by 1940.[11] We shall now turn to analyse the underlying reasons for this situation.

The health of the collective in danger

One 1939 document for the Leningrad council elections argued that life expectancy in the city had improved by 12 years in comparison to the pre-revolutionary era and concluded that this was a clear sign of the elimination of exploitation of workers and poor peasants and evidence that there had been an improvement in the living standards of workers, a key part of the Stalinist collective.[12] This chapter challenges the accuracy of this overall official verdict that the quality of health conditions improved in the Stalin era and argues instead that in the period 1928–40 morbidity and mortality trends fluctuated and in many cases increased which had an adverse impact on the workers and peasants lives in Leningrad.

In Leningrad in 1928–29 illness and death rate levels were initially down on the NEP period. This was of course prior to full blown rapid industrialisation and forced collectivisation. Once the latter got underway and other changes occurred, the situation was reversed and the sanitary infrastructure was made worse by Stalinism and its policies. There were problems obtaining clean, uncontaminated water to wash in or drink; sewage polluted places where Leningraders lived and worked and the quality of water meant that the population were unable to maintain the basic levels of personal and domestic hygiene necessary to prevent sickness and disease. This led to dysentery and gastrointestinal problems and infections. The water supply was controlled by the Leningrad Soviet and industrial enterprises but unfortunately the latter polluted the local rivers (Neva) due to location of paper, chemical, metallurgical, textile, leather tanning and food industry in the city. The lack of legislation and the demands of the five-year plans (FYPs) failed to prevent hazardous discharges into Leningrad's water supply. Thus, ironically meeting Stalin's FYP targets was done at the expense of workers and peasants, the core of the collective, and also influenced the lives of the non-insured in Leningrad. As we shall see later, the local Party and government expanded the provision of water and tried to create a more comprehensive sewerage network but due to shortages of funds and building materials, it failed to achieve this goal. A lack of housing, poor standards of health and safety at home and in the factory and the ever-increasing speed and irregular nature of work, as the city's workers dealt with high FYP targets, overbearing managers, Party and state, made workers' lives harder leading to absenteeism, high labour turnover and illness.

Certain infectious diseases, which were the most widespread cause of death in nineteenth and early twentieth century St. Petersburg/Petrograd, were no longer a major challenge to the city's medical profession in the late 1920s. For instance, morbidity levels from typhoid in 1928 were just over a tenth of their 1913 level or comparable with 1917 levels. Typhus, which was transmitted by lice, like typhoid, was comparable in 1928 with 1926, below its 1913 total and only a mere fraction of the peak year of 1919. Morbidity from relapsing fever was negligible at this time. Typhoid, typhus, scarlet fever and diphtheria all declined between 1933, amidst famine, and 1940, after the end of the Soviet-Finnish war. The use of health inspectors of various kinds in factories, on trains and water transport (boats), disinfection stations and staff to check for lice and any contaminated clothing, the availability of reasonably good urban bath houses and other bathing facilities in Leningrad, and factory-based health points, undoubtedly helped the situation.

However, this was not the case with all diseases due to overcrowded housing, workers living in dormitories or barracks, warm summers and cold winters, and mass population movement (with the homeless children, industrial workers, peasants and 'alien elements' on the move). Table 4.1 shows the threat posed by infectious diseases.

According to Catriona Kelly '[t]he Soviet state placed children's affairs at the heart of its political legitimacy, emphasizing that children were treated with greater care than they were anywhere in the world'.[13] However, health conditions in Leningrad were most unfavourable for children and teenagers. While morbidity from smallpox was continuing to fall, much as it had done since the mid-1920s, scarlet fever and measles were now on the increase between 1928–31. For example, there were 11,198 cases of measles in 1928, as against only 1,638 in 1921, but this was still much lower than in 1913 levels. Scarlet fever had surpassed its 1920 and 1927 levels by 1932, and was just below the pre-revolutionary 1913 total, at 8,064 in 1932 as against 8,442 in 1913.[14] By 1936, scarlet fever had reached 17,301 (double its tsarist level), declining thereafter (Table 4.1). This impacted upon the health of children and adults.

Illness rates for diphtheria, a serious bacterial infection, show that during the first half of the First FYP period, 1928–30, the basic upward trend experienced during the late 1920s continued. As a result, by 1930, this disease was

Table 4.1 Incidence of infectious diseases in Leningrad, 1928–40 (absolute numbers)

Type of disease	1928	1929	1930	1931	1932	1933
Typhoid	1,424a	2,5081	-	-	-	7,971
Typhus	116b	240	-	-	-	6,483
Measles	11,148	8,232	10,198	-	-	11,223
Scarlet fever	10,261	10,478	16,905	11,585	8,064	5,722
Diphtheria	1,841	2,959	4,149	4,391	-	3,525
Dysentery	82b	36	-	-	-	4,131
Malaria	-	-	-	-	-	5,347

Type of disease	1934	1935	1936	1937	1938	1939	1940
Typhoid	3,938	2,576	2,400	-	1,534	624	1,951
Typhus	1,415	733	785	-	309	253	143
Measles	12,877	24,680	18,777	-	31,760	21,123	14,321
Scarlet fever	5,196	8,413	17,301	-	9,840	8,196	2,946
Diphtheria	3,099	2,743	2,308	-	-	-	1,855
Dysentery	12,491	9,287	20,696	-	14,621	15,781	40,731
Whooping cough	2,407	5,900	8,263	-	-	-	18,107
Malaria	7,876	11,155	8,497	6,595	-	-	4,577
Influenza	-	169,829	474,870	599,876	926,687	681,198	-

Source: GARF f. A-482, op 10, d. 2448, list 1, 1ob, 1ob ob; 4, 4ob, 4ob ob, 10, 10ob, 10 ob ob, 13, 13ob, 13ob ob, 16, 16ob, 16ob ob, 19, 19ob, 19ob ob, 22, 22ob, 22ob ob, 25, 25ob, 25ob ob, 28, 28ob, 28ob ob, 32, 32ob, 32ob ob; GARF f. A-482, op 10, d. 1914, list 112; GARF f. A-482, op 47, d. 2424, list 10; GARF f. R-3009, op. 3, d. 214, list 83, 90, 107, 109; GARF f. R-3009, op. 3, d. 70, lists 1–7; GARF f. A-482, op. 47, d. 5045, list 242ob; GARF f. A-482, op. 47, d. 6164, lists 75–77,102,127; GARF f. R-3009, op. 3, d. 74, lists 81; GARF f. R-3009, op. 3, d. 214, lists 5, 107, 109; *Statisticheskii sbornik Leningradskogo oblastnogo otdela zdravookhraneniia za 1928 god* (Leningrad 1929), 30

three times more common than in 1927 (4,149 cases as against 1,477) but still less prevalent than in 1913 (6,249 cases).[15] By 1936, there were 20,696 cases. In the period 1934–39, the goal was to increase the proportion of the population inoculated against diphtheria.[16] There was concern that the number of cases of diphtheria among children which rose from 65,000 in 1931 to 133,000 by 1937.[17] Between 1934–39, 500,000 schoolchildren in Leningrad were vaccinated against diphtheria and 75% of 1–14-year-olds were vaccinated from 1937–40.[18] The Pasteur Institute in Leningrad, liaising with the Zhakty, children's establishments and staff at vaccination points, played a key role in anti-diphtheria inoculations using 50,000 medical detachments in the city to carry out this mass inoculation campaign. Nevertheless, although diphtheria levels fell for the rest of the 1930s, by 1940, disease levels had doubled again to 40,731 cases. This was over six times its pre-revolutionary level (see Table 4.1). This increase, would have probably been higher if left untreated and if vaccines or inoculations and revaccinations had taken place up to 1940.

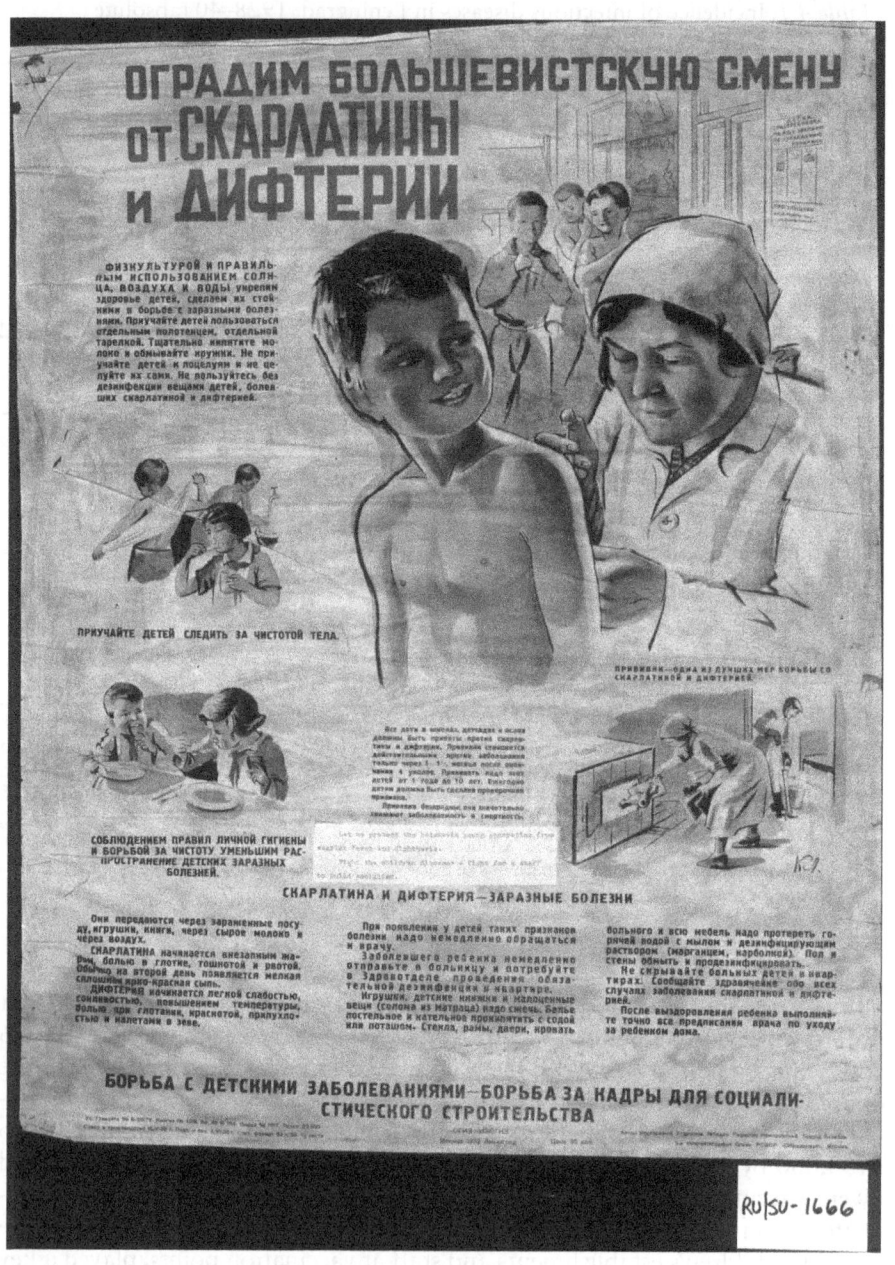

Poster 13 Combating scarlet fever and diphtheria among children

Source: 'We protect the Bolshevik guard from scarlet fever and diphtheria.... Fight against children's diseases, fight for the cadres of socialist construction' 1932 poster. Artist Lebedev. Poster collection, Poster ID # RU/SU 1666, Hoover Institution Archives.

Public health campaigns of the time, as shown in Poster 13, highlighted the need to fight diphtheria and scarlet fever among children through immunization achieved through visits to medical personnel, better hygiene and proper diet and food. This poster consists of four reinforcing images: the main one focusing on a caring doctor treating a smiling child (top right) observed by others in the background; children bathing (top left) or eating a healthy meal (bottom left) and staff cleaning and keeping the environment hygienic (bottom right). The poster includes various messages about clean environments and personal hygiene in order to defeat these children's diseases.

Dysentery, which is an intestinal inflammation that can lead to severe diarrhoea, is caused by poor hygiene and sanitation, and had declined to negligible levels by 1929 (32 cases in first six months of the year), which was a marked improvement on developments during the NEP and in relation to tsarist St. Petersburg.[16] Unfortunately between 1933–40, dysentery became a serious challenge rising almost 10-fold from 4,131 cases in 1933 to 40,731 cases by 1940 (see Table 4.1).

Whooping cough, which is a respiratory disease also spread via the coughs or sneezes of an infected person, affects all ages and can be deadly for infants and young children. Cases of whooping cough increased from nearly 2,500 in 1934 to over 18,000 by 1940 (see Table 4.1). The use of antibiotics was seen as the best treatment in these cases, but they were not available until the 1950s. Although, as Table 4.1 shows malaria reappeared in the 1930s, reaching a peak of 11,155 in 1935, it was on the decline in Leningrad by 1940.

By far the biggest threat of all to Leningraders was influenza, which spread across the city in very large numbers affecting nearly 170,000 people in 1935 peaking at nearly 930,000 cases by 1938, before falling again to over 68,000 cases by 1939 (Table 4.1).

In view of the trends in Table 4.1 the Soviet government sought to produce vaccines and serums. Archival data for 1936–38, which is detailed in Table 4.2, demonstrates that the local government and the medical profession were making concerted efforts to produce numerous vaccines and serums to combat a wide range of key infectious diseases such diphtheria, dysentery as well as social diseases such as TB.

Table 4.2 Production of serums and vaccines in Leningrad to combat infectious diseases, 1936–1938

Serums and vaccines	1936	1937	1938
Stolbiianch serum (dozens)	150,700	169,352	189,000
Gangrene serum (litres)	592.8	398	898
Stolb. antitoxin (litres)	-	1,189.4	7,500
Meningitis serum (litres)	383.5	308.9	394.0
Pneumonia serum	61.5	153.7	297.0
Streptococcus serum (litres)	333.3	254	197
staphylococcus anti-virus (litres)	321.9	344.1	150
Dysentery tablet (000s)	6,135	9,141	7,000

(continued)

Table 4.2 Production of serums and vaccines in Leningrad to combat infectious diseases, 1936–1938 (*continued*)

Serums and vaccines	1936	1937	1938
Dysentery serum (000s)	352,000	237,933	442,000
Diphtheria serum (000s)	468,000	342,500	806,000
Diphtheria antitoxin (litres)	1,878.3	2,768.3	3,000
Scarlet fever serum (litres)	-	497.9	1,153.0
Scarlet fever toxin (litres)	-	1,381.7	1,200.0
TB serum (litres)	-	88.6	150.0
Staphylococcus vaccine (000s)	-		4

Sources: GARF f. R-3009, op. 3, d. 34, lists 1,11; GARF f. R-3009, op. 3, d. 74, lists 1,11

Health conditions clearly dramatically declined during the 1930s for adults, children and babies under Stalin as Table 4.1 shows. As a consequence, the Party, medical professionals and the press increased its interest in all health aspects of the domestic and factory sphere. Numerous health issues – abortion, alcoholism, children's lives, infectious diseases, TB – were all viewed as potential or real health hazards. Health education efforts targeted women, men, children in clinics, industrial enterprises, workers' dormitories and clubs, schools and abortion clinics and a variety of settings including public venues. The posters and health dialogues discussed in this chapter and throughout this book underscored the health risks facing different parts of the collective and so there were various anti-alcohol, anti-abortion and anti-industrial accidents campaigns, with some lifestyles being deemed 'improper', and this was contrasted with pro-women, pro-family, pro-crèches and pro health and safety factory campaigns, with the latter indicating the Stalinist regime's view of what constituted a 'proper' lifestyle as recommended by the one Party state and medical professionals. This created as we shall see a tension between various emancipatory and traditional stances on women and related issues, such as abortion.

Having shown that at the start of this chapter that everyone's health was in danger due to prevalence of infectious diseases, we can now consider how other diseases hit different parts of the population of Leningrad in the Stalin era.

The adjusted Infant Mortality Rate (MR) stood at 17.2 in 1927 and had fallen to 15.3 by 1929. Leningrad still had the highest IMR in this year followed by Moscow, Paris, London, New York and Amsterdam. By 1930 the IMR had only fallen slightly to 15.2 but a year later it had risen to 18.0. By 1940, the IMR was 17.9, so just below its 1931 level.[19] During the 1920s, it was believed that the main cause of high infant and child mortality was illiteracy and ignorance of the population and so Soviet enlightenment campaigns sought to plug the gap in knowledge by providing advice about hygiene, prophylaxis and the upbringing of children.[20] Elizabeth Waters argues that throughout the Soviet period, including the Stalinist era, there was an attempt made to modernise motherhood by the state and the medical profession. The idea in health posters and sanitary enlightenment campaigns, as we have seen in the previous two chapters, was to ensure that mothers met their responsibilities to their children by guaranteeing they were brought up in healthy environments and it was the role of medical professionals to ensure that any mother's ignorance was eradicated.[21] In the process, as Waters points out control passed 'from women to men – from female healers, friends, relatives, neighbours and from mothers themselves, to male doctors; everywhere decision making passed from individuals and their communities to the experts'.[22]

The causes of rising infant mortality are widely acknowledged to be poverty, poor sanitation, limited access to clean water, overcrowded housing and a basic understanding of personal and public hygiene. As we saw above, the rise in certain infectious diseases (influenza, diphtheria) should have increased the IMR, but the lack of IMR data for 1932–39 does not allow us to assess how these diseases impacted upon the IMR. The goal of the Stalinist State was to protect the health of women and infants. Sustained anti-alcohol campaigns launched during the First FYP period might have reduced the drinking levels of women in the city (see below) and some mothers' willingness to breastfeed their children, providing them with breast milk and all its nutrients, probably improved the health of their children. However, we must set this against a series of other factors. First, poorer diet (detailed below though stopping short of malnutrition) especially among low income and less privileged social groups, and second, the fertility of economically active women, which was generally lower than that of dependent women.[23] In the case of Leningrad, a higher female participation rate in the labour force was evident in the late 1920s and into the 1930s. According to Lebina, the proportion of women working in Leningrad's industry rose from 37% in 1928 to 45.7% by 1934 increasing again to 49.8% by 1937.[24] This meant that more women were now having to juggle being wives, workers and mothers (which impacted upon family life) and women were also working in arduous and dangerous occupations, such as construction, and for longer hours.[25] This labour participation rate affected the birth rate and the IMR.

The number of marriages increased from 27,972 (or 16.45 per 1,000 population) in 1928 to 34,456 in 1931 (a lower rate of 14.12 per 1,000 population)[26] and the divorce rate rose from 19,509 in 1928 (or 114.8 per 1,000 marriages) to 20,733 (a lower level of 113.4 per 1,000 marriages) by 1929.[27] ZAGS data for Leningrad in 1928 indicate that in 70% of cases (based on an analysis of 500 Leningrad institute for the protection of women and infants questionnaires), divorce was initiated by males, in no more than 20% of cases by parents, in 7.5% of cases by both partners and in 2% by women. The reasons cited for divorce were incompatibility, differences over starting a family, money worries, arguments, drinking and religious differences.[28] By 1929, 77.5% of male and 68% of female teenagers, had intimate relations with two to three partners, which indicates issues of commitment to lasting relationships in the early Stalin era.[29] Of the 17% of young people getting married by 1929, 10% ended up in divorce.[30] This influenced family size due to an indirect relationship between family stability and the average number of children per marriage and the IMR.[31]

The total fertility rate (TFR) continued its downward trend dating from 1926, reaching 2.26 in 1928 and 3.08 in 1932.[32] This TFR was however just high enough to guarantee possible population replacement. It was changes in the age composition of females within the child bearing age range, which above all had an adverse impact on fertility. In this case, the proportion of females in Leningrad aged 19–24 years, the prime reproductive group, had recovered by 1926, in comparison to 1910–23, but then fell back again by 1932.[33] This trend was contributing to a declining TFR. Family size in Leningrad during the First FYP period and later, was therefore influenced by the IMR, inadequate housing, falling fertility and a high level of abortions.

As we saw in Chapter 2, a 1920 decree decriminalised abortion and give women a personal choice as to whether or not to keep their child. Accounts by Western visitors to the Soviet Union in the late 1920s–early 1930s – such as those of Fannina Hall, Alice Withrow Field and Dr Arthur Hewsholme and John Kingsbury – suggest first that contraceptives were in short supply and second that this sector of the health service was underdeveloped at this time.[34] The decline in the birth rate from 22.6 per 1,000 population in 1928 to 20.9 by 1931 was due to many factors including a change in the age composition of the female population of Leningrad and the tendency among some women to have repeated abortions. Furthermore, more peasants tended to reside in the city of Leningrad by the early 1930s and they gradually acquired the low fertility behaviour of the indigenous urban population. These factors affected fertility and abortion trends.

Under Stalinism from 1928–36 abortion remained the main method of birth control. The upward trend in the number of legal (i.e. hospital-based) abortions continued, with totals reaching 53,562 in 1928 and 67,000 in 1929. The number then fell to nearly 40,000 in 1931. Despite a gap in the data for some years, Ministry of Public Health, RSFSR archival sources show that the number of abortions had reached over 106,000 by 1935 (see Table 4.3). They declined thereafter for reasons explored below.

Table 4.4 demonstrates in 1931, towards the end of the First FYP, that the majority of those having abortions in Leningrad were workers, followed by white collar workers and then students and craftspeople. The age range of those having abortions before the new 1936 law was introduced, varied according to social group, with the majority of those seeking abortions being workers, white collar workers and craftspeople aged between 20–39 years (93.7%, 94.4% and 91.1% respectively) whereas amongst students, the largest group were 20–29-year-olds (83%).[35] Of the 39,636 having abortions, 32,138 were married and 12,314 had one child, 5,607 two children, 2,148 three children and 1,155 four children.[36]

Ministry of Health declassified materials show that poverty/money worries (46.9%) ranked the highest followed by other motives, including

Table 4.3 Abortion in Leningrad, 1928–40

Year	Number of abortions a	b	Overall total	Legal abortions d	Illegal abortions d
1928	53,562	-	53,562c	-	-
1929	67,000	-	67,000c	-	-
1930	-	-	-	33.7	-
1931	39,636	-	39,636c	36.3	-
1932	-	-	-	32.0	-
1933	-	-	-	39.4	4.0
1934	-	-	-	43.4	5.0
1935	89,361	17,181	106,542	-	-
1936	38,768	21,411	60,179	-	-
1937	1,991	22,468	24,459	-	-
1938	4,177	30,116	34,293	-	-
1939	6,946	35,542	42,488	-	-
1940	8,459	29,421	37,880	-	-

Notes: n.a. no data available [a]in hospital [b]outside hospital
[c]excludes illegal abortions [d]rates per 1,000 population
Sources: GARF f. A-482 op 24, d. 13, lists 2–3; GARF f. A-482 op 29, d. 18, lists 7–8;
TsGANTD SPb. f. 24, op. 2v, d. 5324, list 2; 'Aborty v Leningrade', *Gigiena i zdorov'e rabochei
sem'i* No. 23, December 1930, 16 and Sarah Davies, 'A Mother's Cares': Women Workers and
Popular Opinion in Stalin's Russia, 1934–41' in Melanie Ilic (ed.), *Women in the Stalin Era*
(Palgrave, Houndsmills 2001), 101, 106

Table 4.4 Abortions by economic situation/social class in Leningrad, 1931

Socio-economic category	Number of abortions
Worker	18,470
White-collar worker	14,795
Handicrafts	874
Students	2,177
Other	3,320
Total	39,636

Source: GARF f. A-482, op. 24, d. 13, list 2

still nursing; large family and not wanting any children or another child.
These factors influenced Leningrad women's decisions to have an abortion
towards the end of the First FYP.[37]

Excess demand for abortions in Leningrad was initially dealt with on
a 'social need' basis – unemployed single women first, followed by single
mothers with many children, all remaining categories of the insured and,
finally, all other citizens. The introduction of a fee for performing abortions in April 1927 was gradually followed by the introduction of a 'class
line' as in other spheres.[38] Because of excess demand, negative labelling of
those having abortions and concern about the birth rate, many women were
turned away by the abortion commissions and some women ended up as the
customers of the babki.

There was also a cost factor. By late 1930, the Leningrad health service was spending 1.2 million roubles performing abortions.[39] For women, abortions involved a cost. Lebina points out that according to two public health department orders (No. 80 and No. 144) approved in 1933, three years before the new anti-abortion law, the scale of cost of abortions, depending upon wage, was set, as detailed in Table 4.5.

Women in Leningrad now faced a vicious circle, poverty led to a desire on the part of women to have an abortion, on the one hand, and the new fees introduced in 1933 now put a further monetary restriction on Leningrad women's ability to make their own choice, on the other. Although some allowance was made for income, with the lowest abortion cost of 25r applying to the lowest paid wage earner on a 31–40r salary, whilst if the wage earners salary was more than 500r, then the cost of an abortion in Leningrad was at its highest at 300r. The intention was to prevent women seeking abortions as the lowest cost abortion was 62.5–80.6% of a woman's wage or 60% for those on higher wages. The risk of introducing such fees was that this might backfire by forcing women into the hands of the babki, if their costs were lower, and if women were not granted permission by the abortion commissions. At the same time this fee was introduced, a survey was carried out of 33 abortion cases in Kiubyshev hospital in Leningrad. Of this sample, the age range of the women was 23–30 years, of which eight had already had previous abortions (from as low as one to as high as eight), several were newly married or married to military personnel away serving their country, some women seeking abortions were ill (with TB) and two of the 33 women had alcoholic husbands, so did not want any more children.[40]

In public debates on abortion on 28 May 1936 before the new abortion law was introduced, *Pravda* argued that under the NEP there were too many survivals of bourgeois attitudes towards marriage, women and children, which encouraged sexual debauchery and non-progressive attitudes in the 1920s. Such views were said to be incompatible with socialist principles,

Table 4.5 Abortion fees in Leningrad in 1933

Family member wage	Cost of abortion
31–40r	25r
41–60r	35r
61–80r	55r
81–100r	75r
101–125r	95r
126–200r	120r
201–500r	175r
More than 500r	300r

Source: TsGASPb f. 7384 op. 2, d. 52, lists 27–28 cited in N. B. Lebina, '"V obstanovke sovetskikh bolnits" (Novye dokumenty o sovetskoi abortnoi politike pervoi poloviny 1930-kh-gg)', *Noveishnaia istoriia* No. 2, 2014, 170.

ethics and the expected conduct of the new Soviet citizen. *Pravda* argued in 1936 that certain bourgeois enemies within society had promoted the wrong values and tried to undermine the foundations of the Soviet family and marriage.

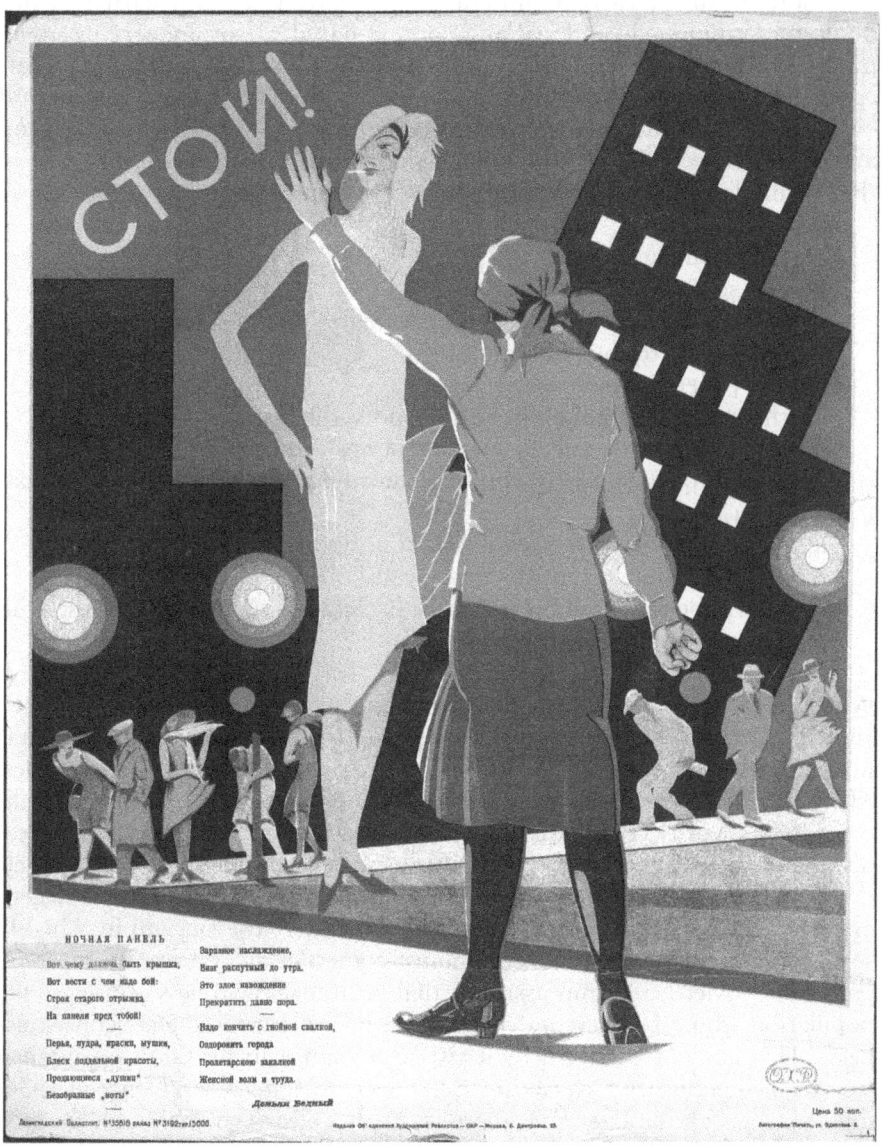

Poster 14 Eradicating prostitution under Stalin

Source: 'Stop' (*Stoi!*) poster 1930. Courtesy of Soviet Poster Collection, Swarthmore College Peace Collection

Prostitutes were also deemed to be a danger to the fabric of Stalinist society. It is in this context that we must view the 1930 anti-prostitution poster 'Stop'. Poster 14 with the warning 'Stop' includes poetry from the proletarian poet, Dem'ian Bednyi, and is meant to increase its popular appeal. The poster promotes a proletarian, communist ideal of femininity and morality in the early Stalin era. It was part, as we saw earlier in this book, of a continued gendered and context-based use of imagery in Soviet public health posters which drew subtle distinctions between different categories of women. This poster compares two women of the Soviet period – the enlightened and class-conscious comrade in red head band, orange top and purple skirt, and the contagious female prostitute in white. The text in the bottom left states:

Night Pavement
Here is something that must be ended.
Here is something that needs to be fought:
A throw-back to the old regime
On the pavement before you!
Feathers, powder, make-up, beauty spots, the luster of false beauty,
'Little Darlings' for sale, disgusting 'pimps', contagious delights,
the squeal of debauchery until the morning, this evil frenzy of sexual passion;
it should have been stopped a long time ago;
this festering dump, must be destroyed.
Cities will be rendered healthy with proletarian tempering and the will and labour of women.

Poster 14, which urges communist women to persuade other women not to engage in prostitution, asks them to once and for all eradicate female exploitation and rid Soviet society of prostitution. It implicitly criticises NEP attitudes. There is a clear message that prostitutes pose a danger to society as indicated by the words 'contagious delights' (suggesting that they spread venereal diseases) and negative stereotyping of prostitutes who are criticised for their decadent characters ('feathers, powder, make-up, beauty stops') and degenerative ways. They are portrayed as inappropriately dressing up in a highly sexual manner to tempt male communist comrades away from the 'correct' path. The Soviet leadership assumed that such 'backwardness' amongst the population would be overcome by enlightenment (increased class consciousness). This has not occurred by 1930 so a change in direction on women was deemed necessary to eradicate such bourgeois tendencies. Hence in 1930, midway through the First FYP, there was still a clear fear that some women were undermining morale, loosening Stalinist morals and their vice posed a danger to the family the birth rate and the health of the collective.

It was concluded that the time was right for Soviet women to fulfil their duty 'as a citizen and as a mother responsible for the birth and early upbringing of her children'.[41] Prostitutes were clearly bad role models. *Pravda* concluded that 1936 was the moment to complete the final emancipation and equality of women and eliminating prostitution was part of this too.[42]

The Stalinist government was therefore extremely concerned about certain types of women – prostitutes – and in the same context about other women given the abortion levels shown in Table 4.3.

This change in government attitudes culminated on 27 June 1936 in the introduction of a new abortion law that prohibited abortions. This was justified by the harm caused by abortions. A ban was placed on all abortions whether or not they are performed in hospitals, at doctor's homes or where the pregnant women lived. Abortion was now only permissible on medical grounds, namely if a continued pregnancy threatened the health of the baby or mother. In cases were permission was granted, abortions could only be performed in a hospital or maternity home. Abortions performed outside of these venues were punishable by one to two years in jail and if abortions were performed in unsanitary conditions by people without the necessary medical training (an implicit reference to babki) then it was a crime that led to three years' imprisonment. Anyone found forcing a woman to undergo an abortion received a two-year fixed sentence. Moreover, any pregnant women who herself violated the law would be reprimanded in the first instance, and fined 300r for any repeat abortions.[43]

From the mid-1930s, there was a shift in Soviet family policy from emancipatory to traditionalist stances on abortion. This was a sign of pronatalism and a move to more traditional and conservative stance on social and family issues. Thus, divorce was made more difficult and abortion was re-criminalised to reverse the decline in the birth rate, stabilize the Stalinist family and ensure that women could contribute to the Stalinist economy.

This new 1936 law contributed to an almost three-fold decline in the overall number of abortions in Leningrad. The proportion of abortions performed in hospitals declined 10 times from nearly 90,000 in 1935 to nearly 8,500 by 1940. However, this fall in officially sanctioned abortions was partly offset by a rise in the number of abortions performed outside the hospital sector, which rose from 17,181 in 1935 to a peak of 35,542 in 1939 before falling to 29,421 in 1940 (see Table 4.3).

As Sarah Davies notes:

> Soviet propaganda stressed the fact that women who resorted to back-street abortions were reverting to the mores of a pre-socialist and pre-modern Russia. As these were performed principally by old women lacking scientific skill and knowledge, it was inconceivable that the modern Soviet women would patronise such butchers.[44]

Women's protests against the new law and the fact that abortion infringed their free will were ignored by the Stalinist state. Furthermore, the new law also failed to address the irresponsible sexual behaviour of males. The fate of women wanting abortions was now in the hands of the abortion commissions. By 1938, there was one central abortion commission in Leningrad, with the President being Savelova, deputy head of the city public health department, plus three other members with different specialities, and 15 district abortion commissions in Leningrad.[45] These commissions decided who was granted an abortion. Not everyone was successful and granted permission for an abortion, so they resorted to other means.

According to Lebina, archival documents reveal that in 1935 of those performing criminal abortions prior to the new 1936 law, 23% were doctors and nurses; 21% workers; 16% white collar workers and housewives and 24% people from other social groups.[46] One person who performed illegal abortions after the new 1936 law, was 35-year-old Maria Morozova from Miginsk district of Leningrad, who was found guilty of performing an illegal abortion on 17 April 1941. From 1938–41, Maria had apparently performed 17 criminal abortions on numerous foreign trade employees in unhygienic conditions.[47] Out of fear of being persecuted under the 1936 law, some pregnant women unfortunately performed abortions on themselves, which put their health and lives at risk.[48]

The 1936 law led to incentives for women having children by providing allowances for new mothers, bonuses for women with seven and more children, and promises were made to increase the number of maternity clinics, day-care institutions and other services for mothers and children. In relation to the new abortion decree, the aim was to significantly improve the number of maternity facilities. One 1938 Narkomzdrav document compared the tsarist era with the Stalin one pointing out that only 10% of the population had access to stationary maternity aid before 1917 forcing them to rely upon babki. Under the Soviet regime, the number of maternity beds during the Second FYP increased in the RSFSR up to 40,000 by 1937 and there were also plans to build new collective farm (*kolkhoz*) maternity homes with 11,000 beds by 1937 and to increase the number of midwives. By the end of the Third FYP the goal was to have 54,000 maternity beds in villages and 56,000 in kolkhozy. It was also pointed out that in tsarist times there were the equivalent of nine women's consultation clinics, but by the end of the Second FYP there were 2,751 women's consultation clinics in cities and 1,611 in villages of the RSFSR. This provision was aimed at protecting the health of women and children in general and during industrialization and collectivization in particular.[49]

Both the demands for more female workers and the new abortion law led to calls for an expansion in the number of crèches (*iasli*) in the USSR. By 1937, there was an extensive crèche network serving six million children in seasonal rural facilities with 777,100 permanent beds. As a sign of the government's commitment 12 million roubles was spend on crèches during the Second FYP, increasing their number to 105,000 places in RSFSR. During the Third FYP, the aim was a 2.5-fold increase in crèches to one million crèche places, of which 500,000 were to be located in rural areas.[50] However in the Second FYP, there was a serious shortfall in meeting the target for crèches (138,600) in the RSFSR, as a figure of only 39,700 was achieved.[51] In Leningrad too, the protection of mothers and infants became a priority. In the period 1928–35 there was an increase in the number of crèches and places in them due both to the construction of new buildings and to a more intensive usage of the existing ones during the First FYP (see Table 4.6).

Specialists in Leningrad research Institutes aided these developments by devising model plans for the structure and development of crèche and nursery school buildings in the city. They determined the optimal number of children in a crèche should be no more than 150, with an ideal children-staff ratio of 12 to15 children for every two staff members.[52] To make arrangements more efficient and economic, in 1937, eight crèches were closed with 522 beds and 454 places but they were replaced by a new crèche with 4,989 beds and 5,360 places.[53]

In line with the medicalisation of motherhood discussed earlier, the medical profession in Leningrad also sought to medicalise other areas, including crèches and nurseries. According to Chernyaeva, hygienic standards in crèches were in fact modelled on a hospital regime segregating children of different ages to prevent the spreading of disease with staff wearing white coats (see Poster 15) to convey the idea of medical knowledge and reassurance.[54] Between 1932–34, during the First and second FYPs, public health services for children were reorganized and the division between well-baby clinics (*detskiie polikliniki*), monitoring child development in year one, and children's outpatient hospitals or consultancies (*detskie konsultatsii*) who treated sick children, was abolished, and both institutions were merged. Narkomzdrav also required children's polyclinics to keep records of all children up to the age of four and to make home visits at least twice a year.

Table 4.6 Creches network in Leningrad, 1928–40

Year	Number of crèches	Number of children
1927–28	99	5,848
1928–29	106	6,661
1929–30	119	7,867
1930–31	154	11,714
1931–32	338	25,370
1934	247	13,500
1935	157	20,434
1936	-	22,574
1937	-	18,614
1938	250	18,645
1939	-	21,129
1940	-	23,106

Sources: GARF f. A-482, op. 10, d. 2523, list 3; GARF f. A-482, op. 10, d. 2683, list 41ob, 42; GARF f. A-482, op. 10, d. 2972, list 7; GARF f. A-482, op. 47, d. 5655, list 5; *XV let diktatory proletariata: Ekonomiko-statisticheskii sbornik po gor. Leningradu i Leningradskoi oblasti* (Leningrad 1932), 158 and *Otchet Leningradskogo soveta XIII sozyva 1931–34* (Izd. Leningradskogo oblispolkoma i soveta 1934), 115.

Finally, children's clinics now operated on a strict territorial principle. The clinic's patient base was now split into smaller districts (*uchastki*), each run by a doctor and a nurse, and parents were no longer permitted to choose their own family paediatrician, instead they had to utilize the one operating in their district.[55] Thus parent choice and what was best for their children was now being decided by the Stalinist state.

Soviet posters of the period depict a happy life for children. Poster 15 is typical of the official viewpoint and shows children in a non-life threatening green garden setting, safely protected by the state (represented by crèche employees). It seeks to depict a model Soviet day care institution to show the best side of the Soviet experience and to demonstrate how caring the Soviet state is towards its children. The crèche children are probably from factory worker families (their workplace is shown in the background, with smoke rising from its red brick chimney). Children are shown playing in a pleasant clean, sunny outdoor setting and doing a range of approved activities – playing a game in a circle in the top left and/or playing together in a sand pit in the bottom left. The setting looks extremely hygienic, with children well looked after by staff. Thus Poster 15 is showing how the state enables women to help build socialism by providing crèches. In this connection at the bottom of Poster 15 is a lengthy quote from Lenin demonstrating his support for establishing communal nurseries and women's liberation.

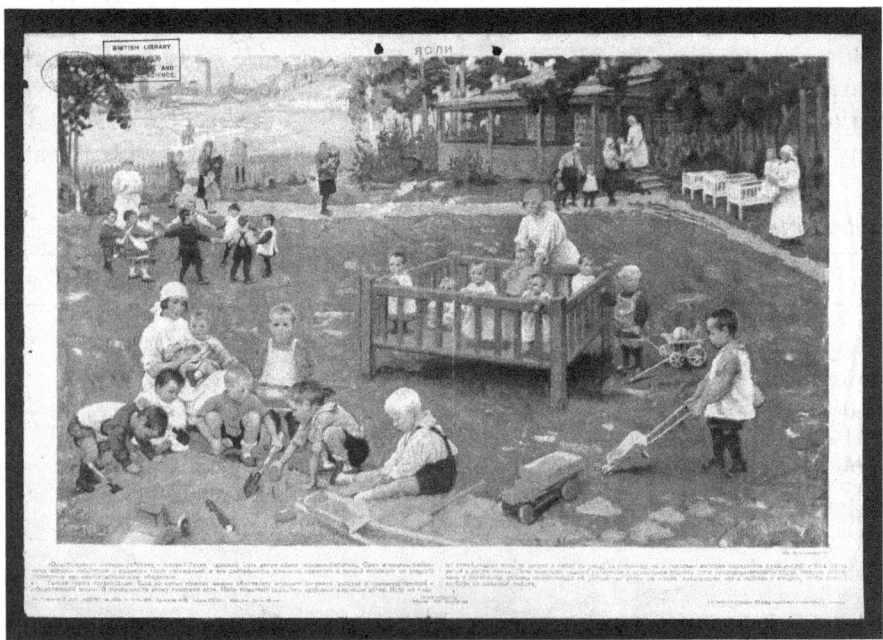

Poster 15 Crèche is best

Source: 'Creche', published by Ogiz-Izogiz, Krasnyi proletariat (Red proletariat) printers, Moscow/Leningrad 1931. This image is courtesy of and from the London School of Economics Library's collections, COLL MISC 0719/8

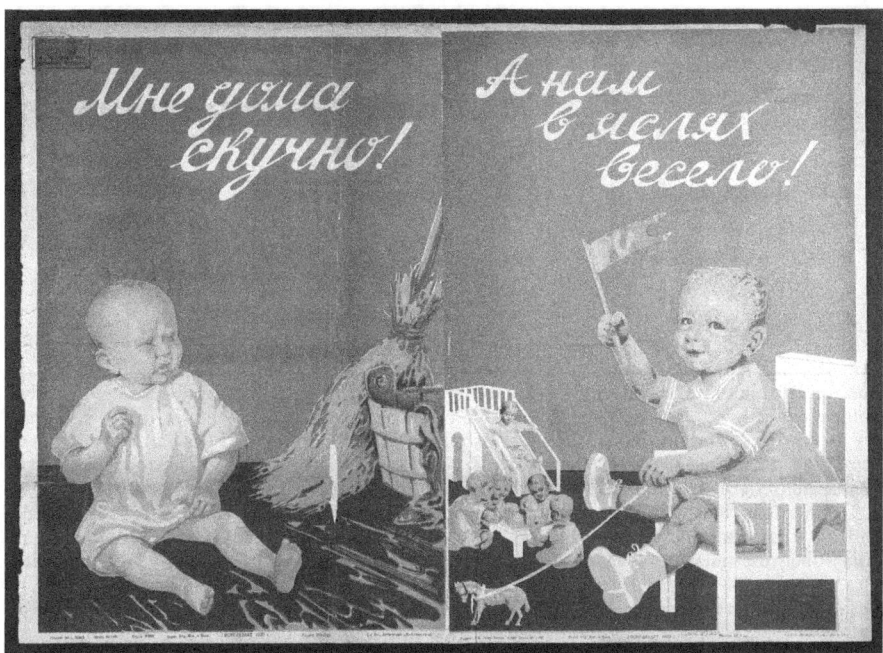

Мне дома скучно!

А нам в яслях весело!

Poster 16 Home or crèche?

Source: 'I am bored at home, but I am happy in the crèche'. Publisher: Gosmedizdat, Mospoligraf printer, Moscow 1931. This image is courtesy of and from the London School of Economics Library's collections, COLL MISC 0719/16.

Poster 16, by contrast, deploys the standard 'before' (on the left side) and 'after' (on the right) approach in Soviet health education propaganda comparing a sad unhappy, bare footed crying baby in a dirty, wooden floored room, symbolised by the broom and bucket (on the left), with a happier baby, who is well clothed, and sitting on a chair in a well decorated, clean room with toys to play with and accompanied by other children in the background (on the right). Poster 16 also depicts a positive shift from the traditional to the modern and legitimises implicitly the legacy of the October Revolution and Stalinism which allegedly allowed such progress to take place. So in this representation a crèche is seen as preferable to a home where the child might be neglected. Unfortunately, the reality contradicted such health propaganda.

We will now discuss social diseases in Leningrad between 1928–41.

One of the major social diseases threatening the collective in Leningrad was tuberculosis (TB). TB trends from 1928, at the start of the First FYP, until 1937 at the start of the Third FYP are detailed in Table 4.7. The death rate from TB started at 23.7 per 1,000 population in 1928 and then declined to 21.7 per 1,000 by 1931, but increased by 1932, the end of the First FYP to 33.6 per 1,000, or by nearly 55%. Thereafter TB deaths in Leningrad

Table 4.7 The TB crisis in Leningrad, 1928–1937

Year	Death rate from TB per 10,000 population	Number of TB dispensaries	TB dispensary patients
1928	23.7	17	576,449
1929	23.5	18	659,587
1930	21.7	20	560,042
1931	21.7	20	627,328
1932	33.6	20	737,946
1933	40.8	20	821,839
1934	47.5	20	1,466,036
1935	55.0	20	1,105,232
1936	62.7	20	1,126,354
1937	63.7	20	1,063,991

Sources: 'Kon'iunkturnye obory epidezabolevanii po gorodam Kyubyshevu, Leningrady, Molotovy, Moskve za 1947g' (1947) in GARF f. A-482, op. 47, d. 6164, list 163; *XV let diktatory proletariata: Ekonomiko-statisticheskii sbornik po gor. Leningradu i Leningradskoi oblasti* (Leningrad 1932), 144; Ye. E. Ben et al, *Trudy Leningradskogo tuberkuleznogo nauchno-issledovatel'skogo instututa (Iubileinyi sbornik)* (Izd. Lentubinstituta, Leningrad 1933), 14; M. L. Goldfarb, 'K istorii bor'by s tuberkulezom v Peterburge-Leningrade' in Ye. E. Ben et al, *Voprosy sotsial'noi gigieny tuberkuleza* (Izd. Kargosizdata Leningrad 1939), 34; Ye. E. Ben et al, 'Tuberkuleznaia zabolevaemost' i smernost' sredi batsilliarnykh kontaktov v Leningrade' in Ye. E. Ben et al, *Voprosy sotsial'noi gigieny tuberkuleza* (Izd. Kargosizdata Leningrad 1939), 88; G. E. Al', 'Osvedomlennost' o sluchaikh letal'nogo tuberkuleza v Leningrade' in Ye. E. Ben et al, *Voprosy sotsial'noi gigieny tuberkuleza* (Izd. Kargosizdata Leningrad 1939), 118

went on rising throughout the 1930s, reaching 40.8 by 1933; 55.0 in 1935 and 63.7 per 1,00 by 1937 or by 2.7 times since 1928.

To combat TB, the number of dispensaries in Leningrad increased from 17 to 20, but they remained fixed after 1930, while death rates from TB significantly increased. These TB dispensaries were in heavy demand, with the number of TB patient levels increasing from over 576,000 in 1928 to nearly 738,000 by 1932, then increasing further to 1,466,036 in 1934 before falling to 1,063,991 by 1937, still double the 1928 level (Table 4.9). The TB dispensaries studied and treated the roots of TB. Staff carried out health and hygienic work among TB sufferers' families. Health visitors and district nurses visited homes and a study was made of the patients working and living conditions and their way of life. TB was linked in Soviet medical and social hygiene thinking above all to poverty, urban overcrowding and malnutrition.[56] After the relevant information had been collected then appropriate health measures were taken, such as isolation, use of the BCG vaccination (approved from December 1927 after trials in Leningrad),[57] improved housing (with the assistance of the local housing administration), a recommendation of special diets and/or advising a trip to a health resorts or sanatoria for recuperation.[58] The difficulty was that workers did not always receive the health passes necessary to go to the TB and other sanatoria when recommended by medical staff. On 28 September 1929, the Party criticised the situation as only 70% of passes were given to workers. In subsequent Party debates, it was argued that the proletariat must be given preferential treatment in terms of access to medical aid (sanatoria, health resorts, rest homes) because of their importance and the role industrial enterprises played in meeting FYP targets and Party objectives. The target for the number of workers (*rabochie*) going to these facilities was set at 80%.[59] Towards the end of the First FYP (1931) it was recommended that 85–90% of the sanatoria, health resorts, rest home passes go to workers[60] and by 1932, this target had almost been reached, as 84% of workers were actually sent for such treatment or vacations at sanatoria, health resorts and rest homes.[61]

Treatment at these facilities was free, as were health passes and up to 1936 travel to these establishments was also paid by the state. After 1936, however, part of the travel costs was now met by the sick individuals with contributions depending upon earnings.[62] Thus if a TB patients' salary was 600r, they paid all their travel to health resorts; but if wages were less than 250r a 50% contribution towards travel to health resorts was made by TB patients. By 1940, everyone paid for their own travel to sanatoria, health resorts and rest homes.[63] The policy on this, which affected TB and other patients in Leningrad, was constantly changing, and the social insurance system was trying to help members of the collective recover from illness. Later on, as more policy shifts took place, not just skilled but shock workers were prioritised. It will not be until 1936 that any distinction between worker and white-collar worker was dropped with regards to paying for their travel to receive insurance medicine.[64]

TB patients received Bacillus Calmette-Gurein (BCG) vaccinations and the BCG was supposed to be manufactured locally and distributed via TB dispensaries. However, Michael David argues that this drug was underfunded between 1930–34[65] at a time when TB was on the rise in Leningrad. A 1934 decree called for improvements in TB control and this led to increased funding and so the BCG programme was expanded and introduced in 18 cities, including Leningrad, which already possessed a bacteriology institute. Vaccinations were given by nurses and the programme was monitored by TB dispensaries.[66] By 1938, the percentage of eligible infants vaccinated against TB in Leningrad maternity homes had reached 53%.[67]

Based on data from 3,131 TB cases in six districts of Leningrad (Volodarskii, Vyborg, Moscow, Narva, October and Smolnyi) in 1931, the age range of TB patients in Leningrad was as follows: 148 were aged under a year, 374 were one to four years old, 179 were aged 5–14 years and the largest number of cases (2,430) were among those 15 years and above.[68] There were more female than male cases – 20.8 per 10,000 for males compared to 357.3 per 10,000 for females.[69] Even bearing in mind the boundary changes mentioned above, the spread of TB of all forms and TB of the lungs varied according to district of the city in 1931, as Table 4.8 indicates. The districts with the highest level of cases include Vyborg, first in all forms and second for TB of the lungs, whilst October district was bottom in all forms of TB and second from bottom for TB of the lungs. In 1927, 2,665 BCG vaccinations were given but by 1931, the figure had risen to 6,809 BCG vaccinations in these six districts, of which 39 were administered to children and 6,770 to adults.[70] Despite these efforts, 3,131 Leningraders died from TB in 1931, 1,221 at home and a further 1,910 in hospital.[71]

Table 4.8 TB in Leningrad in 1931 according to district

District	TB of all forms	TB of lungs	BCG vaccinations
Vyborg	454	182	936
Narva	414	264	683
Volodarskii	333	154	832
Smolnyi	306	136	1,832
Moscow	304	90	323
October	176	113	419
Average of all districts	312	150	1,832

Source: Ye. E. Ben et al, 'Tuberkuleznaia zabolevaemost' i smernost' sredi batsilliarnykh kontaktov v Leningrade' in Ye. E. Ben et al, *Voprosy sotsial'noi gigieny tuberkuleza* (Izd. Kargosizdata Leningrad 1939), 27–28

Table 4.9 TB in Leningrad in 1931 according to industrial sector (rates per 10,000 workers)

Sector of industry	TB of all forms	TB of lungs	BCG vaccinations
All workers, of which:	436.7	254.7	31.8
Metalworking	494.9	283.1	38.0
Machine building	472.5	270.4	35.9
Coal	707.2	405.0	59.3
Textiles	696.3	422.9	26.9
Chemicals	615.0	372.0	32.0
Printing	678.4	433.9	60.4
Woodworking	515.6	293.8	41.6
Leather and tanning	617.9	367.6	34.9

Source: Ye. E. Ben et al, 'Tuberkuleznaia zabolevaemost' i smernost' sredi batsilliarnykh kontaktov v Leningrade' in Ye. E. Ben et al, *Voprosy sotsial'noi gigieny tuberkuleza* (Izd. Kargosizdata Leningrad 1939), 38

TB levels also varied according to sector of industry in Leningrad, as Table 4.9 demonstrates. With regard to TB of all forms, first place was occupied by workers in the coal industry followed by textiles and lowest levels were among those in machine building; whereas for TB of lungs, it was printing workers in first place followed by textiles and once again lowest levels were in machine building. Ben's research shows regarding TB of all forms that first place was occupied by males in the printing industry (436 per 10,000) and women in textiles (432 per 10,000); whereas for TB of lungs it was women in chemical industry (411 per 10,000).[72]

Poster 17, though it dates from the late NEP period, is a drawing of several workers at their factory work stations. It focuses on the role of the foreman in black shirt, blue apron and cap. Its message is that it is his responsibility to ensure that work stations are clean and spacious. This is portrayed as the key to preventing TB among the industrial proletariat. The foreman (*mastera*) was responsible for running the workshop, maintaining labour discipline, the allocation of work, meeting output targets, preventing conflict and in this case keeping a careful eye on the health of the workforce. The way in which the foreman is depicted here is with respect due to his conscientious attitude towards his work. However, worker-foreman relations and the authority they actually exercised varied from factory to factory and, in some instances, he might be seen by workmates in a positive way, but in other instances, especially as the rate of industrialisation intensified and the five-year plans got underway, as demanding, bureaucratic etc. It is possible that some Leningrad workers viewed their factory foremen as either siding with them against enterprise management or the Stakhanovites[73] or acting as agents of the Stalinist state.[74]

If there were good relations on the shop floor, it might have been possible to protect workers' health; if not and conflict and discontent were high, due to the demands of FYP targets, heavy workloads, overtime, coping with new recruits, food shortages, falling working and living standards and the pressures exerted by the purges, on veteran foreman and other factory workers, then the ideal situation portrayed in Poster 17 would have been more difficult to achieve after 1928. Stephen Kotkin highlights cases in relation to Magnitogorsk were alleged negligence (high temperatures, dust, the lack of ventilation and periodic gas poisonings) were blamed on the foreman though the situation was not their fault and beyond their control.[75] Poster 17 suggests that the factory foreman cooperate with the state and the medical profession to prevent TB among factory workers.

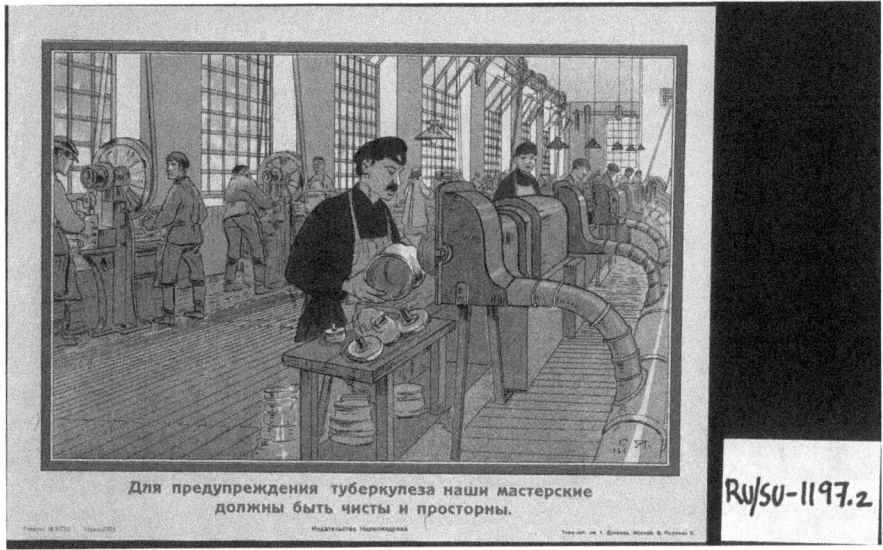

Poster 17 TB prevention in factories

Source: 'For the prevention of tuberculosis, our factory shops should be clean and spacious'. Poster c. 1926. Artist S. Ia. Poster collection, Poster ID # RU/SU 1197.2, Hoover Institution Archives.

During the NEP, there was a rather liberal approach to alcohol that allowed the sale of 14° wine (from August 1921), beer (from February 1922) and the reintroduction of 40° vodka (in October 1925). At the same time, moonshine (*samogon*) production was common as agricultural producers used excess grain to produce alcohol and this contributed towards the grain crisis of 1927.[76]

In this context, Poster 18, produced in the Stalin era, is a drawing divided into two sections by bags of grain. On the left-hand side, peasant children are depicted eating at a table, with well-built accommodation with heating shown at the top. Agricultural supplies are being loaded on wagons and agricultural machinery and tractors are located nearby (bottom right) signifying modernisation and progress. This is contrasted on the right side, with a family shown suffering in a room, as a man and wife selfishly drink moonshine produced using a primitive still (shown at the bottom). On the top right, grain is being sold to a kulak. This poster successfully connects one danger to the collective (moonshine and distilling) to new class enemies such as grain hoarding kulaks. It also presents the possible benefits of collectivisation, as symbolised by the better more prosperous peasant lives shown on the left.

Alcoholism was a major issue at this point. The number of litres of spirits in the USSR, according to Deichman, increased from 48 million litres in 1924/25 to 480 million litres by 1927/28, and the revenues raised by the start of the First FYP from alcohol reached 1,200 million roubles.[77] In Soviet

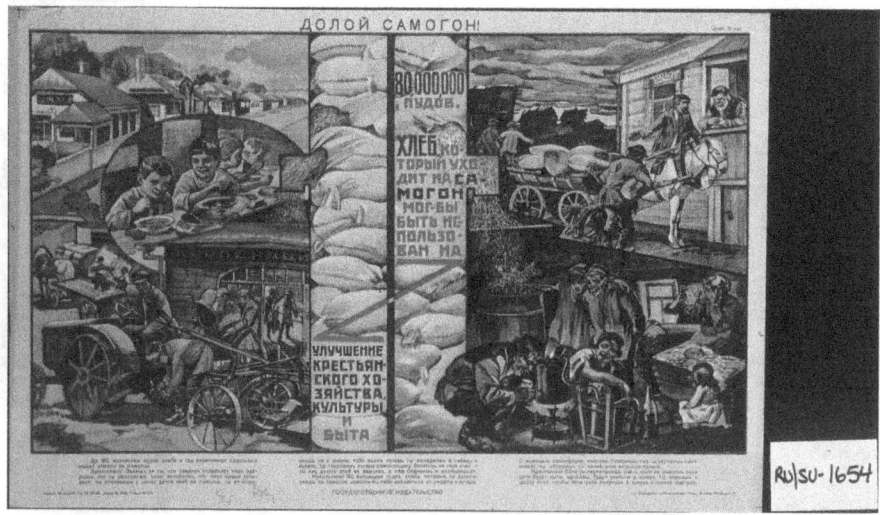

Poster 18 Moonshine and the kulaks – two dangers to the collective

Source: 'Down with moonshine! ... 80,000 poods (4,884kg) of bread are used to produce moonshine. This could be used to improve the peasant economy, culture and way of life'. Produced c. 1930–40. Poster collection, Poster ID # RU/SU 1654, Hoover Institution Archives.

minds, alcohol consumption was linked with the spreading of VD (as an estimated 75% of VD cases were contracted during alcohol intoxication),[78] the break-up of families and with declining production. The products of particular Party and medical professional concern were vodka and especially moonshine, and campaigns were launched against producers of the latter given the health consequences, the 1927 war scare and the grain crisis which led to the introduction of forced collectivisation.

A new law on alcohol was passed on 14 February 1929 prohibiting trade in alcoholic beverages and the anti-alcohol campaign got underway in earnest. Phillips argues that, by 1929, Leningrad became virtually a 'non moonshine region'.[79] By 8 August 1932, Leningrad had 190 bars, 51 restaurants, 142 buffet and snack bars, 277 stores and 265 other trading organisations selling alcohol.[80] Stricter controls were put in place on the distribution and consumption of spirits such as vodka which led to the closure of alcohol sales outlets reducing the number to only 881 by 1929 (compared to 3,386 in 1913).[81] The production of non-alcoholic drinks (fruit juice) was also stepped up. Thus by 1928–29, 5.4 million non-alcohol beverages had been produced in Leningrad (up from 2.5 million in 1926–27).[82]

Poster 19, produced in 1930, was aimed at encouraging the population to either drink non-alcoholic beverages or to avail themselves of more cultural pursuits by going to the cinema (*kino*), (depicted below the main title), clubs (on the left) or to tea shops (in the background) rather than drink alcohol. This was part of the Stalinist temperance drive.

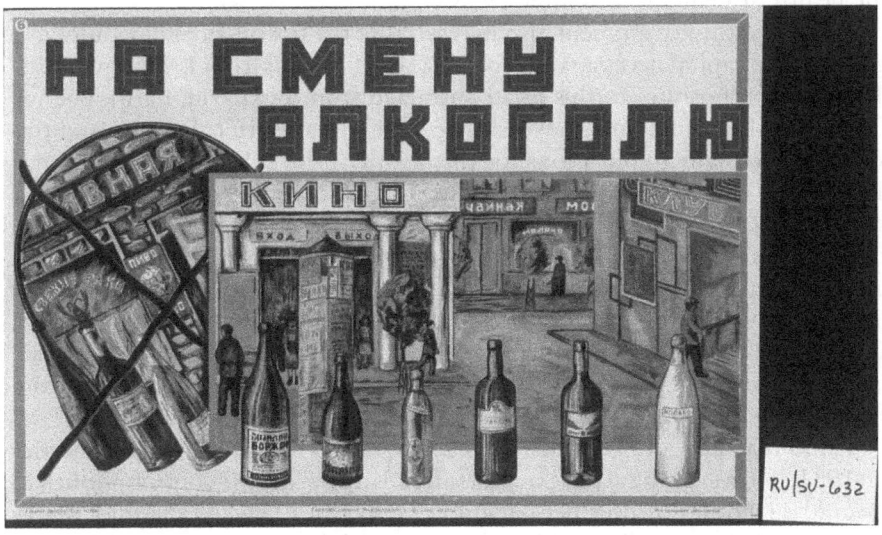

Poster 19 Tea and culture as alternatives to alcohol

Source: 'To replace alcohol …'. 1930 poster. Poster collection, Poster ID # RU/SU 632, Hoover Institution Archives.

The administrative strategy used under the NEP continued into the 1930s, so many police arrests were made, with the number of alcoholics detained totalling 135,000 in 1928 and a further 127,000 were arrested in 1929.[83] The Stalinist leadership was well aware of the way in which alcoholism was a threat to health and everyday life and that it occasionally led to hooliganism (drunk and disorderly issues).[84] In the 1930s, there was also a debate on selling alcohol to under age children and about the location of alcohol sales outlets too near to factories and schools, out of a fear of encouraging children to drink.[85]

As in earlier Russian and Soviet periods, fiscal considerations influenced government action on alcohol from 1928 onwards. Stalinist debates on drink centred on the impact of drinking on economic growth through reduced productivity, absenteeism[86] and industrial accidents. Health education efforts therefore targeted industrial enterprises and the industrial working class. In December 1928 anti-alcohol cells were established in local factories, probably to improve labour productivity and prevent injuries at work.[87]

Poster 20 explores the link between drink, employment and industrial safety hinting at the fact, which shall be explored later, of the problem of industrial injuries in the Stalin era. This 1931 poster states that 'it is not true that alcohol nourishes' and argues instead that 'alcohol consumption causes industrial accidents' and that alcohol is the 'enemy of healthy labour'. Thus Stalinist health propaganda depicted drunken workers as endangering their own lives and potentially those of their factory workmates by drinking at work. This poster overlooks the role played by breakneck industrialisation, ignorance of machinery, the factory setting and the threat which this put on the health of Leningraders after 1928.

Stalin and the government also realised that the tax on alcohol would help generate the capital necessary for socialist development from 1928 onwards.[88] There was opposition to this fiscal approach from Bukharin, Larin, Bednyi, Deichman, Budennyi and Podvoiskii because of its unethical nature and this strategy had many implications for the health of the collection and nation.[89] Table 4.10 details how per capita worker consumption of vodka doubled between 1927/28 and 1939. Vodka consumption initially declined during the First FYP falling from 6.47 litres per person in 1927/28 to 4.39 litres in 1931 but then increased to 10 litres per person by 1935, rising by one litre per person each year until 1938 rising to 12.7 litres per capita by 1938, though vodka consumption declined by 0.7 litres by 1939 over the previous year. Similarly, per capita worker consumption of beer initially fell from 18.33 bottles in 1927/28 to almost 15 bottles (14.81) at the start of the First FYP and reaching a third of its 1928/29 level by 1931 at nearly four bottles in 1931. However, by 1935, a year after Kirov's death, consumption had risen to 21 bottles of beer per person in Leningrad. Thus by the mid-1930s, members of Leningrad's working class were drinking on average 10 litres of vodka and 21 bottles of beer per person. These consumption levels, which damaged people's health, generated nearly 430 million roubles for the state.

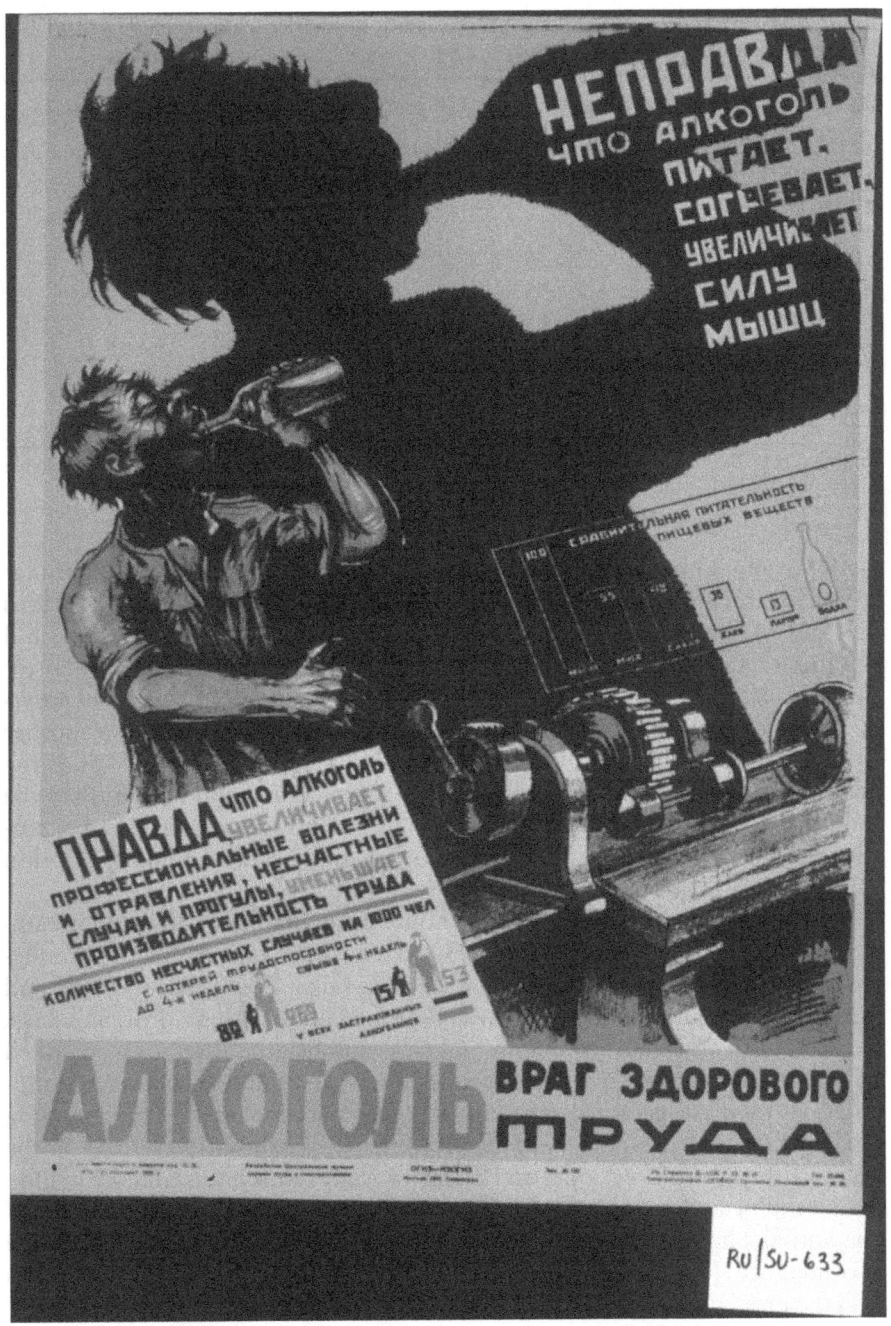

Poster 20 Drink and industrial accidents

Source: 'It is not true that alcohol nourishes, warms and increases the strength of the muscles, it is true that alcohol increases occupational diseases. Alcohol is the enemy of healthy work/labour'. 1931. Poster collection, Poster ID # RU/SU 633, Hoover Institution Archives.

Table 4.10 Per capita alcohol consumption among workers above 16 years old and
state revenues from alcohol sales, Leningrad, 1927/28–1939

Year	Vodka (litres)	Beer (bottles)	Income from sales (million)
1927–28	6.47	18.33	-
1928–29	5.94	13.81	-
1929–30	3.81	5.76	-
1931	4.39	3.97	-
1934	-	-	428.6
1935	10.0	21.0	429.4
1936	-	-	435.8
1937	11.1	-	-
1938	12.7	-	-
1939	12.0	-	-

Source: Ye. D. Tverdikova, " 'O pivnom uklone i torgashchevskikh izrashcheniiakh': torgovliia
alkogolem v Leningrade 1930-kh-gg ", *Noveishaia istoriia Rossii* No.2, 2012, 95–96.

A Society to combat alcoholism was set up in Leningrad in February
1928. It targeted drink and drinkers in order to protect the lives of various
sections of the collective. A priority was the industrial working class and
another section were children and the family. For instance, one 1930 poster
'Who causes children to drink alcohol' (*Kto prichaet detei k spiritnym napitkam* …) shows three images: a father giving alcohol to his son, a mother
giving alcohol to her daughter and schoolboys sharing alcohol.[90] Thus the
overall message is that alcohol is a danger to the family and the future of the
collective – fathers and mothers must be fit parents, not set up a bad example, by encouraging their children to drink and hence alcohol prevention
within the family and at work is essential.

The government advocated temperance in its Stalinist anti-alcohol campaign of the late 1920s and early 1930s. Campaigns pushed for the production of non-alcoholic beverages, not serving vodka after 6pm, and beer and
wine after 8pm, and a campaign was launched on drinking during holidays,
jubilees, festivals etc. Trade unions and other public organisations were asked
to be particularly vigilant in these periods.[91] Twenty million roubles were allocated to food cooperatives for setting up temperance organisations among
the workers and peasants. Anti-alcohol films and exhibits were held in the
cultural theatres of key industrial enterprises and in schools and 15 million
roubles allocated for this health education programme.[92] The first stage of
the anti-alcohol campaign started in Leningrad on 25 December 1928 with
a conference. It was agreed that a key target would be industrial enterprises
and the message would be 'It is possible and necessary to live without alcohol'
and to do this the Stalinist regime needed to generate greater awareness and
a new byt so that Leningraders became 'new persons who were healthy and
abstained from drink'. This necessitated a 'cultural revolution' in citizen's way

of behaving and thinking.[93] Health officials advocated the closure of beer and wine stores, cultural programmes in factories with more than 2,000 workers and debates on alcohol took place in groups of 50 chaired by a group of three activists. Themes for discussion included 'Alcoholic fathers' and 'Drinking amongst Komsomol and youth'.[94] Canteens were also encouraged to hold non-alcohol based celebrations, including the use of tea.[95] These efforts had some positive results as the number of deaths from alcoholic poisoning fell in Leningrad's case from 440 in 1928 to 189 by October 1929 or from 18.0 to 12.7 per 100,000 population in Leningrad between 1928–29.[96]

The difficulty was that the Societies for the struggle against alcoholism and the All-union Society for the struggle against alcoholism did not always enjoy universal support and, unfortunately, they were associated, in official circles, with the Right Opposition to Stalin in Leningrad. Thus, in early 1930 they were censored and 'for all practical purposes, institutions concerned with the issue of drunkenness ceased active work, and discussions of alcohol largely disappeared from the press'.[97] By 1932, the Societies for struggle against alcoholism were merged into the new 'Healthy life Society' and alcoholism started to be played down though alcohol was still a threat to the collective and viewed as uncultured and backward. The dilemma was that alcohol was also a source of state revenue. Laura Phillips believes that the reduced attention on drink was also due to the fact that alcohol was associated with comradeship, friendship, part of the rites of passage in factory life, and working-class cohesion as a group.[98] Thus by the start of the Second FYP there was perhaps an acknowledgement that the early Stalinist regime hard-line on alcohol was negatively impacting on its relationship with workers so the regime backed off.

Thus, combating alcoholism was far more complicated than it looked and 'excesses' (arbitrary closures, summary arrests of alcoholics, seizure of stills) potentially jeopardised the regime's relationship with the working class and peasantry. The Soviet regime made the mistake of assuming that it if attacked the alcohol outlets or drinkers politically, economically and in organisational terms, everyone would abstain from drinking alcohol, but this did not prove to be the case. Furthermore, eradicating any 'backwardness' amongst the population, through anti-alcohol enlightenment using the types of posters displayed and discussed in this chapter, which was supposed to lead to increased class consciousness, through schools, trade unions, the Komsomol, Party, factory managers did not work either. Thus, as Table 4.10 demonstrates, citizens of Leningrad continued to drink beer, vodka and other spirits and budget surveys of workers in the city show that from 1930–39 families spent at least 2–3% of their budgets on alcohol.[99]

Lenin and Stalin were faced, as already explained, with a legacy of alcoholism from the Tsarist era, and the transition to Socialism promised the population a better quality of life. This drive was headed up by social hygienists who in the new socialist utopia sought to influence lifestyles for the better. One of the main health policies pursued was geared toward drink. We saw that the Soviet state sponsored institutions and launched numerous anti-alcohol campaigns and posters 'trumpeted a clean, ordered life',[100] but this was not always the case in Leningrad after 1928. Regime success must mainly be gauged by the extent to which the anti-alcohol propaganda actually changed people's beliefs, attitudes, and behaviour. Despite the stress on hygiene, purity, and a healthy life and body since the 1920s, and on the fact that alcohol destroyed the body, mind, and Soviet society, the aforementioned propaganda was only partly effective. Part of the reason for this lies in the fact that alcoholics were portrayed by the Soviet state and medical and related professions as 'bad role models'. The idea was to re-educate them because the Soviet regime believed 'drink endangered workers and society'.[101] The aim of reforming people's views in Leningrad and improving their health failed. This meant, in Stark's view that

> [t]he messages of decades of propaganda on hygiene and rational living had not achieved its intended outcome. The body Soviet was neither healthier, nor stronger, nor more physically fit than any other nation on the globe. Nor had the surveillance, propaganda, and hygiene programs created the anticipated changes in lifestyle, the body, and the mind.[102]

On top of TB and excessive drinking, shortages of housing and food supply difficulties also impacted upon health conditions and status, as we shall now see.

The increases in the size of Leningrad's urban population, the failure to achieve the projected rise in labour productivity, losses in agriculture and wastage in industry and the major housing problems now detailed led to a declining standard of living among the city's industrial workers between 1928–1941.

A new law of 1 January 1928 'On housing policy' recognised that there was a need to accelerate housing construction and expand dwelling space. In 1929, restrictions were placed on the leasing of municipal housing to private individuals, in particular 'non the working elements' (the children of clergy, former merchants, landlords, kulaks, or other 'alien' groups).[103] Per capita housing space[104] in Leningrad declined from 8.70m² in 1926 to 8.50m² in 1928, before falling to a meagre 5.6m² by 1932.[105] Dwelling space was also much smaller in the traditionally working-class areas of the city, such as Vyborg, Moscow and Narva districts, than in the former upper-class city centre parts of the old capital.[106]

As the population expanded, overcrowding became a major problem. The local municipal authorities launched housing programmes to rectify this, but for a variety of reasons their solutions failed. Because of breakdowns in the supply system, which resulted in severe shortages of workers or building materials,[107] new housing construction failed to keep pace with demand and existing housing was left to rot. Problems with plan fulfilment,[108] an issue to which we shall return again later, merely exacerbated these difficulties.

Although under the NEP, changes in housing policy had had a positive effect on health conditions, Stalinist industrialisation impeded developments in the housing sector. In this context, Block argues that building resources were diverted from public housing to factory building in order to attract key skilled and semi-skilled workers into Leningrad industry[109] or to provide demobilised Army personnel with housing.[110] In the Stalin era, different parts of the collective were prioritised at different times and this generated a housing crisis in Leningrad.

Many communities and parts of the city lacked adequate water supplies. The sewage network had expanded from 539km in 1914 to 880km by the end of 1931, but 403km of this network was unsanitary and still made of wood.[111] Drainage had always been a problem ever since pre-revolutionary times. Such a system had yet to be systematically installed, and sewage by the late 1920s, was still not channelled in such a way as to prevent seepage into the surface or ground water used for drinking and washing.[112] After 1928, the local council discussed the need for improvements. Due to financial constraints, new water supply and sewage systems took longer to complete and older ones longer to repair. Moreover inefficient, old and out-dated filter systems were still in place, offering no real guarantees against water pollution. Nevertheless, the water supply network was gradually expanded and additional filtration systems installed, but projects were hampered by shortages of experienced staff and a lack of suitable equipment. For instance, the 'Red Chemical' plant failed to meet its production target for alumina and so purification of the Neva was behind schedule.[113]

Housing finance difficulties also played their part too. Although capital investment in housing increased from 24 million roubles in 1928 to 120 million by 1932, this was insufficient to meet local needs.[114] For example, at a plenum meeting of the Leningrad Soviet, held in January 1928, 55 million roubles was needed to resolve the housing crisis but only 20–21 million had actually been allocated.[115] As a result, housing repairs lagged behind and new buildings were started before adequate plans had been drawn up. Leaking roofs, cracked floors and low ceilings were, therefore, extremely common.[116] Basic amenities were also rare in Leningrad. Zelson, President of the health department's Sanitary Commission, found in early 1928 that 12% of the city's houses were without water; 14% without a sewage system and an additional 40% lacked adequate washing facilities due to shortages of finance.[117]

A decree of 14 May 1928 formally introduced a 'class line' in the housing sphere whereby former landowners, kulaks and other so-called 'alien elements' were evicted from their homes. This was to create more living space and to eliminate the kulaks as a class as they opposed government policy. This law was supposed to take effect on 1 June 1928 but in Leningrad's case it was not actually implemented until 1929–30. Occupants officially defined as kulaks were gradually evicted from 266 rooms in February and 250 in March 1930.[118] But this exclusion of kulaks did not eradicate the housing crisis because its origins lay in excessive pressure applied by the FYP targets and Stalinist low priority policies regarding welfare policy. Other problems, such as red tape, meaning that houses were left unoccupied[119] or the failure to utilise resources efficiently[120] compounded matters. The housing council in Leningrad was reorganised but this had little impact.[121]

For example, the Leningrad housing trust only fulfilled its 1931 plan target by just under half (44.8%) and so by June 1932, housing was still in short supply and of extremely poor quality.[122] The level of repairs carried out was also low. In the first half of 1932, for instance, only 36% of the city's housing repairs had been carried out. The severity of the situation varied according to district, but was found to be at its worse in Smol'nyi (22.5% repairs) and Volodarskii (21.5% repairs).[123] Not everyone was this bad off. Olga Filipova, a student at the Leningrad Medical Institute, lived in a communal apartment with 18–20 others and had a good-sized room, a big kitchen and good neighbours.[124]

In overall terms, then, by the end of the First FYP period, housing in Leningrad was in a deplorable state. Demand exceeded supply, and families, as a direct consequence of rapid population growth, were left with less living space per capita. Forced to live in close proximity with one another and to share the same basic amenities, when they were available, disease spread quickly. This situation undoubtedly contributed to declining health conditions in Leningrad in the First FYP and beyond. An illustrative example is TB. Soviet hygienists and medical professionals believed that TB was a 'housing related disease'. In 1932 Al' from the Leningrad TB Institute carried out an analysis of the housing conditions of 5,906 TB patients given BCGs. Regarding workers with TB, 3% had up to $2m^2$ dwelling space, 26.1% between $2–4m^2$ dwelling space, 35.9% $4–6m^2$ dwelling space, 19.9% $6–8m^2$ dwelling space and 15.1% more than $8m^2$ of dwelling space.[125] The government housing norm was officially $8.25m^2$ and Leningrad's norm was set higher at $9m^2$, but around 85% of Leningrad's TB sufferers did not reach this ideal housing level. Instead, on average, almost a third (29.1%) of workers with TB had half this norm and 29.6% of single workers in hostels and 42.3% of working class families with a member with TB had less than the USSR norm.[126] We saw above in our discussion of TB that the district with the highest level of TB cases was Vyborg and whilst October district was bottom in terms of TB levels. With regards to living space in 1932, Vyborg had an average of $3.9m^2$ and October $5.3m^2$, but residents of October district were top in terms of BCG vaccinations whilst Vyborg residents were fifth. Overcrowding was one aspect allegedly contributing to the spread of TB among workers, but TB experts found some residents were living in dark, dimly lit residences (7.9% of this group) damp conditions (among 31.5% of sample) and in Leningrad houses in a bad state of repair. Thus, in Vyborg district with the highest level of TB cases, 17.6% of houses required repairs whilst in the October district of Leningrad which was bottom in terms of TB levels, 17.1% of apartments required repairs. Of this group of TB patients, 81% lived in communal housing. Among Vyborg district TB sufferers, 27.1% lived alone, 24% shared communal housing with one family, 21% with two families and 27% with more than two families. The comparable figures for October district TB sufferers, were that 23% lived alone, 11.9% shared communal housing with one family, 18.1% with two families and 47% with more than two families.[127] The Stalinist state might have wanted its children to have their own bed but given housing crisis in the 1930s, workers and their families in Leningrad had to share rooms and so there with no possibility of separate beds for babies or young family members. Thus of the aforementioned TB sufferers in 1932, 24% had children under 16 years old and 2.2% children under one year old, sharing the same accommodation.[128] Hence the risk was that parents would infect their children with TB due to close proximity.

Sosnovy argues that the Second FYP for housing only fulfilled 41.9% of its target in terms of providing more dwelling space[129] and the collective in Leningrad still often occupied housing before essential plumbing, electricity and other key facilities were in place after 1932 as well.[130] The lack of plumbing encouraged dysentery. By 1936 of working class families in Leningrad, 10.8% occupied the entire or several rooms of an old apartment; 46.5% one room and 25.6% part of a room; 5.2% had a kitchen and 11.9% lived in a communal dwelling; whereas of working class families in Leningrad living in new apartments, 16.2% occupied the entire apartment or several rooms, 69.5% one room and 14.3% part of a room.[131] Others were more fortunate. Lilian Issakian, who was born in Tiflis, but moved to Leningrad in 1936 to become a third-year student at the Institute of experimental Medicine in Leningrad, was fortunate enough to be able to share a communal 15–16m^2 space with her mother, who worked as a gynaecologist/feldsher at the Leningrad Otton Institute, and her communal apartment was located near the Philharmonic, RNB and Hermitage, and included officers and trade officials as residents.[132]

From 1937–41 housing construction was no longer financed through the social insurance budget which meant that money for housing had to be found elsewhere and this increased the pressure on the Leningrad authorities.[133] Nevertheless expenditure on housing in Leningrad increased from 87 million roubles in 1936, to 94.8 million roubles in 1937, 123.8 million roubles in 1938 before reaching 144.7 million roubles in 1939. In difficult times the Leningrad authorities were spending more and more on housing. The aim was to build 2,370m^2 more new houses, to expand the canal network to 1,059km and to increase the size of the sewerage system to 1,137km by 1939.[134] During the Third FYP, the goal was to improve the water supply, the quality of water pipes, to launch a chlorination programme and reduce the level of raw sewage. To achieve this, a law of 14 May 1932 gave inspectors greater power over the water supply network and in January 1937, a new drinking water facility was built with 300cm^2 of new water pipes.[135] In the Third FYP for public health, nearly 3.6 million was set aside to improve the quality of Leningrad's water supply.[136]

The housing situation steadily declined until the late 1930s and the Party and the medical profession realised that providing better quality housing and cleaner water and better sewerage systems was required to improve health and eliminate infectious and social diseases, like TB. By 1939, the plan was to increase the number of new houses from 170,000–190,000m^2 in 1939 to 255,000m^2 in 1941 and to complete the water supply station on the Southern side of Leningrad as well as improve the gas supply and sewage systems.[137] To this end, the housing construction budget was substantial and Leningrad's council allocated 37.9 million roubles for house building, 154.5 million roubles for repairs, 96 million roubles for communal dwellings, 29 million roubles for plumbing, 15.1 million roubles for sewerage systems, 2.8 million roubles for cleansing, three million roubles for public baths and 8.2 million roubles for gas supply improvements.[138] An extra 3.2 million roubles was allocated to plumbing in relation to the completion of the water supply station on the southern side of Leningrad. To improve plumbing in Kolpino in Leningrad oblast, 770,000r was allocated from the Leningrad Party housing budget.[139] The problem achieving these ambitious goals and housing improvements was the shortage of construction workers and materials, and in this respect little had changed since the start of the First FYP.[140] So on the eve of the war with Finland, Leningrad's housing was receiving more funding but meeting the demand and ensuring its quality was still a problem which threatened people's health.

Like housing, food supply difficulties also contributed to the hardship's facing the Leningrad population. Here we will consider food availability, consumption and the influence of diet on health status.

Poster 21 'Build a new way of life – Healthy eating' contrasts the old backward ways of preparing food (on the left side) with the new healthier post-revolutionary way (on the right-hand side). This provides an example of the advice that the Soviet regime was giving to Leningraders about a healthy diet at this time. We will now explore how easy it was to put this official viewpoint into practice.

Diets had improved under the NEP as we saw in Chapter 3. Under Stalinist industrialisation, the food situation declined. Statisticians were placed under pressure to provide favourable impressions of food trends, plan fulfilment etc.,[141] but it is now acknowledged that during the period 1928–34, per capita consumption declined.[142] Moshe Lewin concludes that 'the process of industrialisation as carried out by the Soviet authorities entailed an enormous wastage of human and material resources. This inevitably led to a fall in living standards and further strained an already critical situation'.[143] Erlich points out that

> sweeping collectivisation with its shattering impact on living standards, centralisation pushed to the extreme and attempts to impose on the economy a rate of growth defying human and technological constraints ... was not a very efficient way to increase the productive potential of the economy.[144]

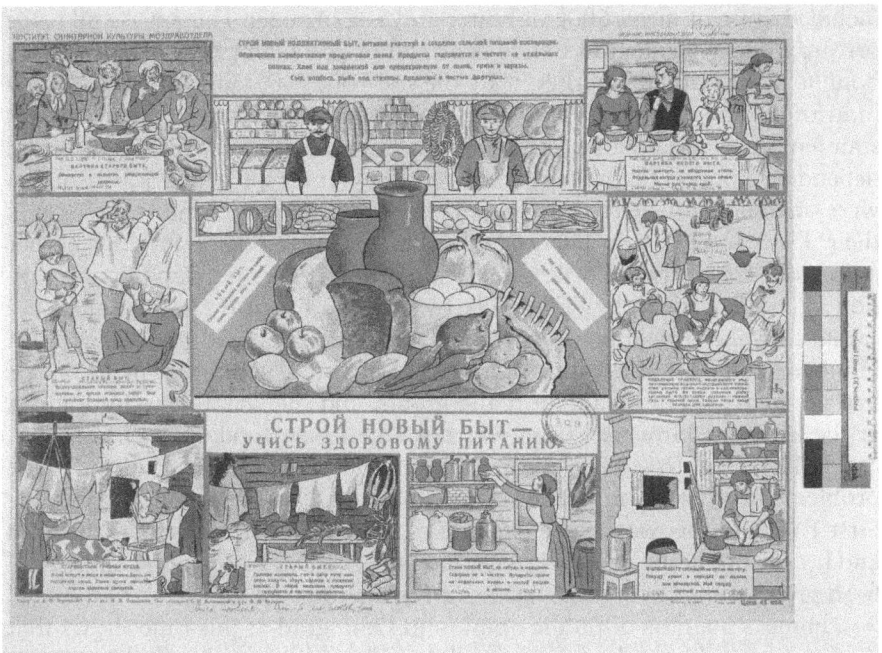

Poster 21 Promoting healthy eating

Source: 'Stroi novyi byt – uchil' zdorovomu pitaniiu' (Build a new way of life – Healthy eating'), Soviet poster courtesy of Woodburn Collection, Reproduced by permission of the National Library of Scotland.

The burden of industrialisation weighed heavily on the USSR population, affecting different social classes in various ways.[145] John Barber's work shows that the standard of living of the Soviet industrial working-class declined throughout the 1930s, though there were improvements between 1934–37.[146] Workers' food consumption compared favourably with other sections of the population, and workers ate more rye, bread, potatoes and fish than others but less meat, eggs, butter, milk and sugar in 1929–30 as compared to 1927–28. Wheatcroft concludes that daily calorie intake levels in the USSR fell from 2705kcal in 1928 to 2,425kcal by 1932, which was lower than 1920 (2,469kcal), after the civil war, and 1921 (2,441kcal), early NEP levels. Daily protein also decreased from 101.13g to 94.53g between 1928–32, as did animal protein availability from 34.33g to 20.85g per capita over the same period.[147]

Food rationing was introduced in Leningrad in November 1928. Fortunately, Leningrad was better supplied that other cities because it had 'regime' status and Kirov fought hard to minimise the impact of rationing.[148] The Stalinist state controlled wholesale and retail prices and suppressed inflation but there were still an increased number of goods in short supply.[149] In 1929, according to Barber, workers' rations were set at around 800g and included 200g of meat, 600g of butter and 50g of sugar. There was still some private trade in Leningrad but citizens had to pay high prices for any goods bought in the kolkhoz market.[150] By the start of 1930, most foods and many industrial goods were rationed and goods in Leningrad were distributed to state employees via a fixed ration system, with a person's allocated ration depending upon their branch of the economy and type of work.[151] Rations were often not sufficient, and as retail prices by 1932 were almost three times their 1928 level, it was increasingly difficult to purchase food.[152] Barber points out that between 1928–32, Leningrad workers per capita consumption of meat declined by 77%, milk by 64% and fruit by 63% though per capita consumption of potatoes rose by 11% and rye bread by 39%.[153] Olga Filipova, a student at a Leningrad medical Institute, noted that in 1931, she had no potatoes but bread, meat and groats, and she was able to have lunch at the Institute. However, Olga was not able to get food at the Institute in 1933–34, so had to sell her library books to buy bread, meat and fish.[154] The problem was that Stalin's government sought to build heavy industry in the First FYP and this was at the expense of the consumer. Consequently, food and bread supplies were inadequate and in Sarah Davies opinion commercial food prices were 'beyond the means of the majority' of workers.[155]

Rimmel's analysis of public opinion in Leningrad at this time shows that women worried how they would feed their families; some Leningraders criticised the government for taking grain from peasants and selling it at high prices, which they saw as effectively robbing peasants and the general population and finally, Rimmel cites Korodev, a worker at the Red Putilov factory who argued that the price increases would not impact on those earning 500–600r a month but would hit those on 100–150r very hard. It appeared as if the government did not care.[156]

To ease the pressure, in March 1932 the rationing of eggs, milk, cheese and fish was abolished, but flour, bread, groats, meat and herring as well as vegetable oil, butter and sugar were all still rationed.[157] Unfortunately in 1932–33 there was a food crisis and famine, and retail prices rose once again. This affected all population groups especially the most vulnerable, such as those under one year (linked to the IMR) and younger children. The population of Leningrad was better off than elsewhere because it was among the 'special' list of towns. In June 1934, the price of rationed rye breads increased from 25k to 50k per kilogram.[158] On 16 December 1934, the Party in Leningrad passed a resolution urging everyone to ensure that the bread supply would be adequate by taking action to remove deficiencies in the retail trade network and checking that bread quality was high.[152] This clearly indicates the Party's concerns about supply bottlenecks and its impact on population morale. In 1934–35 food supplies and workers' diets improved but bread rationing was not abolished until 1 January 1935, when the price of bread reached 1r per kilogram.[159] Rationing on all remaining food goods was not removed until 1 October 1935.[153] At this point the situation was extremely tense. Kirov had been murdered in December 1934, instigating the start of Stalin's Terror, there were insufficient bread supplies and a typhus epidemic was raging.

Medical workers in Vinnitsa district had reached crisis point and threatened to leave if no more flour was available.[160] On 25 September 1935, rationing on meat, fish, sugar, fats and potatoes was abolished and the price of rye bread fell to 85k a kilo.[161] Rationing on all industrial consumer goods was removed on 1 January 1936. Khlevniuk and Davies argue that following the abolition of rationing, prices increased due to excess demand. Nevertheless, basic foods were available in majority of Leningrad shops by 1936.[162] There was a famine in the countryside in the Winter of 1936–37 and this caused an influx of peasants into the city searching for bread. This put pressure on the retail system and shortages became more widespread.[163] Food consumption was also reduced in 1937 due to the economic disruption caused by the height of Stalin's purges. By 1937, according to Barber, workers in Leningrad were consuming less meat and dairy products than they did in 1929.[164]

Food supplies and nutrition is important to health as they determine calorie and protein intake in Leningrad. One way of gauging how these trends affected Leningrad is to examine Soviet budget surveys. These were carried out since the 1920s and are based upon average wage and the primary wage earner. Table 4.11 examines a series of such surveys compiled for Leningrad between 1922–39. The 1922–25 NEP surveys are included, for the sake of comparison. Because the absolute amount spent on each category varied with income, and inflation distorted wages and costs, the table lists only percentages, so as to allow comparisons. The figures shown are average wages, so excludes those on higher wages and more importantly those on less than the average in Leningrad who might be poorer.

It is evident that Leningrad workers spent nearly 43–46% of their income on food by 1929–31. Sarah Davies argues that by 1934, expenditure had reached 55.9%, increasing to 58% by 1935, falling to c. 55% by 1936–38,[165] but increasing, as Table 4.11 shows, to over three quarters of the family budget (87.2%) by December 1939. Archival material shows that: the average monthly consumption in Leningrad of meat fell from 4.2kg in 1930 to 1.7kg in 1932; animal protein increased from 0.14kg to 0.18kg by 1931; milk and vegetable consumption fell from 0.47kg in 1930 to 0.35kg by 1932; bread consumption fell from 1.3kg in 1930 to 1.2kg in 1932; and margarine consumption remained the same at 0.12kg between 1928–32.[166] The most remarkable thing to note in Table 4.11 is that, by the early 1930s, nothing much had changed since early NEP. By the late 1930s, following the Great and mass terrors, the greatest family expenditure was on food and most of other categories had declined in importance. The Third FYP ran from 1938 until the outbreak of war. Investment in defence occurred at the expense of food and consumer goods, so queues and shortages occurred from 1939 onwards and by that time, prices had doubled. Once the Winter War with Finland broke out, the Soviet government prohibited the sale of flour and bread in the countryside and although there was no official rationing, food prices started rising in April 1940 and continued going up in July and October that year.[167] Maria Kunkite's analysis shows that average wages stood at 439r in September–October 1939, but by 1940 had increased to 459r[168] and

Table 4.11 Budget surveys of Leningrad, 1929–39 in comparison to 1922–25 (expenditure as percentage of income)

Expenditures	NEP period			First five-year plan			Third five-year plan
	June 1922	Apr–June 1925	Jan–June 1929	Jan–June 1930	Jan–June 1931	Oct–Dec 1939
Food	62.3	50.4	44.4	43.1	46.4	78.2
Rent	2.8	6.1	6.5	6.4	5.1	8.8
Fuel, electricity	6.8	4.4	4.2	3.2	2.8	0.2
Household items	3.5	1.9	-	-	-	-
Clothing	10.5	18.3	14.4	15.2	14.4	6.4
Alcohol, tobacco	2.0	4.9	5.1	4.4	6.1	2.2
Health, hygiene	1.1	0.3				0.7
Entertainment, culture	1.8	3.6	2.7	2.8	2.9	0.3
Trade Unions	2.7	3.9	3.2	3.0	3.8	-
Family aid	0.3	6.1*	1.9	1.5	1.7	-
Other	5.0	-	4.7	5.0	5.0	0.7
Total	99.8		87.1	84.6	88.2	97.5

Note: *both family assistance and miscellaneous items combined
Sources: 1922–25: S. Prokopovich, 'Buidzhety rabochikh i krest'ian posle revoliutsii', *Russkii ekonomicheskii sbornik* VI (Prague 1926), 173; 1929–31: *Ekonomiko-statisticheskii spravochnik Leningradskoi oblast'* (Izd. Oblispolkom i Lensoveta 1932), 452–453; 1939: TsGAIPD f. 25, op 2v, d. 4282, lists 127–128

new work norms were introduced in May 1940.[169] At the time of the Soviet-Finnish war of 1939–40, rent cost 349r for the average family rising to 389r in Leningrad by 1940.[170] Thus rent cost a high proportion of a wage earners income, squeezing family finances further. Kunkite argues by October 1940 in comparison to the same time the year before, meat, fish, milk, eggs, sugar, tea and pasta products existed in sufficient quantities, though meat consumption fell whilst fish consumption rose.[171]

In overall terms, despite the fact that after 1926, the real wages of Leningrad workers exceeded those of 1913, most of the city's proletariat remained relatively poor and rising prices neutralised any increases in nominal wages. Few general members of the population possessed luxury items and most of their income was devoted to basic necessities, such as food, shelter and clothing. Collectivisation had caused a severe deterioration in diets, and even though the social security and health care systems provided them with a measure of security unknown before the October Revolution, the quality and accessibility of housing and basic amenities, still left much to be desired. All these difficulties when combined, led to increasing sickness at different stages in the period 1928–39. The lack of general infrastructural improvements (especially in urban sanitation and housing), falling standards of public hygiene and inadequate nutrition, together with heavily polluted washing and drinking water, posed a considerable threat to health. However,

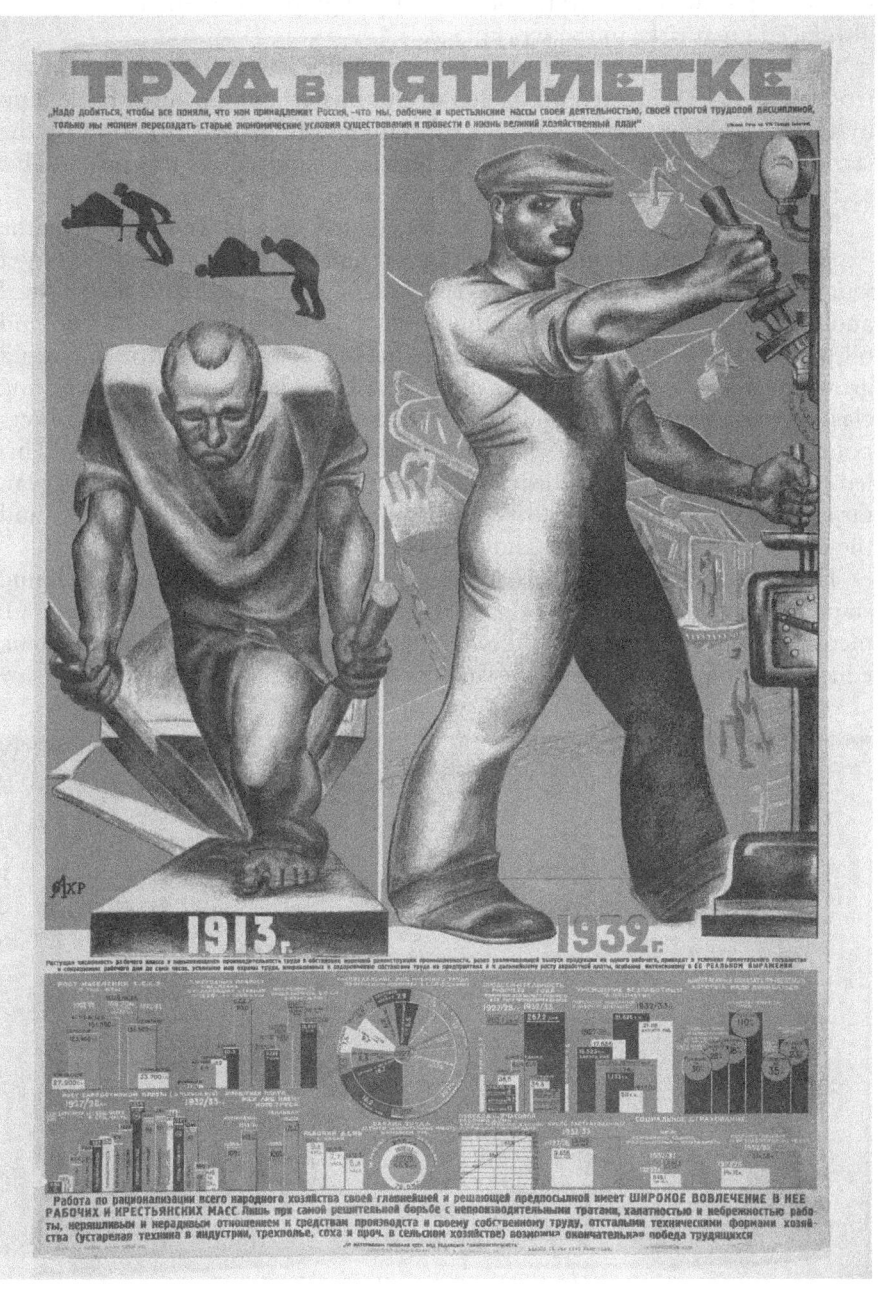

Poster 22 Labour in 1932 as compared to 1913

Source: 'Labour in the First Five Year plan', Soviet poster courtesy of Woodburn Collection, Reproduced by permission of the National Library of Scotland

it was not just at home that the health of Leningraders was endangered, they also faced great risks in the workplace.

Poster 22 suggests that workers' lives in Russia went from being down-trodden in 1913 (depicted on the left of this poster) and certainly backed up by the material in Chapter 1, to a substantially improved situation by the start of the First FYP, as illustrated by the right-hand side of this poster. This section of the final chapter challenges this assumption.

Rapid industrialisation, which was depicted as a class war, led to the expectation that the economy would grow quickly and that the FYP target would be achieved in four not five years. Between 1928–40, Soviet steel and coal output increased more than four-fold, machine tools 21-fold and oil production three-fold and this breakneck development led to the rapid growth of industrial labour force in the USSR.[172] The size of Soviet working class as a whole grew and millions of unskilled peasants and new workers poured into the towns as large-scale industrial projects got underway.[173] This led to an ever-changing industrial landscape, the setting of unrealistic plan targets, the emergence of priority sectors – heavy industry and defence – and the use of role models (Stakhanovites)[174] to increase labour productivity.

This policy shift led to a reduction in worker's real wages, a declining standard of living among workers (with food consumption deteriorating), increased pressure on towns like Leningrad (in terms of its health system, education, transport) and there was overcrowding and disease, as we saw

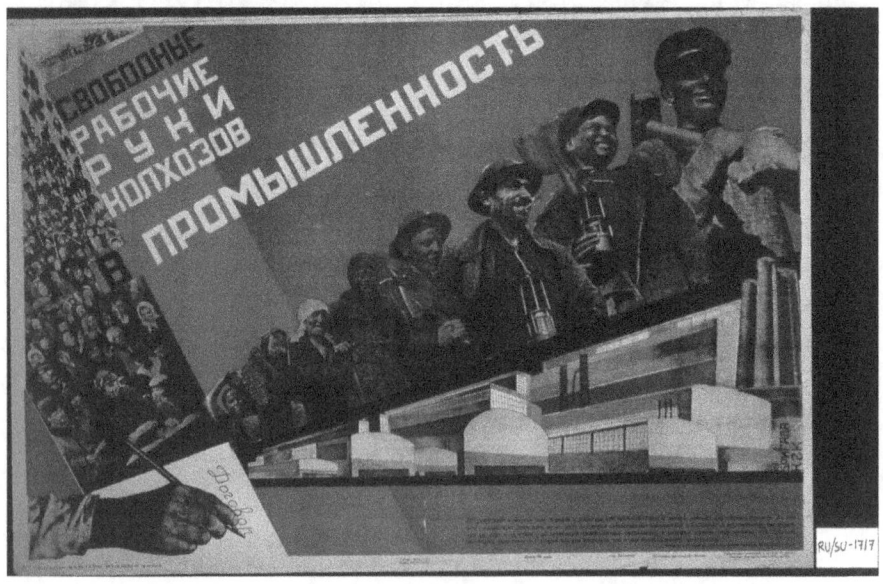

Poster 23 Generating support for the industrial and agricultural goals of the
            Stalinist era

Source: 'The free labour of collective farms in industry'. 1931. Poster collection, Poster ID # RU/SU 1717, Hoover Institution Archives

earlier. In factories, the low level of labour discipline (alcoholism, conflict on shop floor) as well as socialist competition between factories to meet targets increased the demands on factory managers and the workforce.[175]

Poster 23, from 1931, towards the end of the First FYP, was meant to mobilise the population. It is a montage of two photographs and depicts farm workers (crucial for collectivisation) and the industrial working class (crucial for industrialisation) smiling, looking joyful and determined, carrying the tools necessary to complete the goals of the FYP. An example of their achievements is the large factory complex shown in the bottom right. A hand with the word 'agreement' (*dogovor*) in the bottom left of the poster implies to the viewer that the narod agreed with the economic policy of the Stalinist regime, and that they supported the economic transformation envisaged by the Soviet government in the early 1930s.

Leningrad too was impacted by these changes. The workforce of the giant Red Triangle Rubber plant, for instance, quadrupled, but many were 'raw' recruits, often peasants. According to Donald Filtzer, during the NEP industrial workers had a high degree of control over the intensity and organisation of their work, but Stalinist industrialisation took this away. It removed workers' control over their tasks, as inexperienced peasants needed time to 'master more complex organisations'.[176] The new factory entrants were allegedly undisciplined and had difficulties operating machinery, often damaging it and causing accidents.[177] This situation arose out of the need to meet labour shortages and fulfil targets as well as due to the fact that unskilled newcomers in Leningrad had insufficient technical training and little time to adapt to the new factory context and the machinery therein. Newcomers in Leningrad's industry were also discriminated against, harassed and treated as 'outsiders' by the more experienced 'older' workers. They were sometimes disliked because of their higher work ethic, and older workers and managers saw newcomers as challenging the old work norms and as an obstacle to achieving FYP targets. Furthermore, norms (quotas) increased over time whilst wages dropped so workers had 'to produce significantly more merely to keep their earnings stable'.[178] This led to strikes over wage reductions[179] and contributed to labour turnover. These workforce and work culture tensions and the tempo of industrialisation, posed challenges for the Stalinist regime and in particular the Ministries of Labour and Health which dealt with different aspects of labour and its protection.

The 1922 Labour Code and later amendments set the number of working hours (eight hours per day, but six in hazardous trades and seven for night work), overtime levels (four hours in any two consecutive days), breaks (30 minutes to one hour) for meals and other adjustments (times for nursing mothers), whilst other Labour laws stipulated that new machinery needed inspecting and safeguarding and all industrial enterprises were required to provide protective clothing and devices or products (masks, soap, antidotes to poisons) for employees. It was the role of various inspectors (under the auspices of the Ministry of Labour) to investigate conditions in industry, mines, transport (rivers, rail, harbours), forestry and in prisons.[180] There were three types of inspectors: first, labour inspectors dealt with different branches of industry, mills, railroads, rivers, forestry and construction and they determined hours, overtime, lunch breaks, identified defects in ventilation and lighting and ensured clothing and baths were provided; second, technical inspectors, normally engineers, addressed the safety of boilers for example, light and electrics and were concerned with accident prevention; and third, sanitary or medical inspectors (under the auspices of the Ministry of Health), were each responsible for 9–10,000 workers, the hygiene and sanitation in factories and they investigated industrial hygiene in relation to specific occupations and trades and were responsible for preventing epidemic and contagious disease outbreaks and combating TB and other diseases among the factory workforce.[181]

The aim was to classify any injury, its frequency and register the disease. These records were normally compiled by a range of agencies including first aid points at enterprise level; patients seeking medical treatment, the insurance funds and by labour protection organs, all responsible for ensuring that enterprises complied with the law.

The level of occupational diseases in Leningrad as elsewhere was linked to the conditions of labour, the nature of the labour process, the dangers posed by a particular occupational setting or job and by the level of industrial hygiene prevailing. The role of the Ministries of Labour and Health inspectors was to analyse the relationship between pathology and hygiene and to advise the appropriate therapy and to recommend that a worker was 'fit for work' or classified as an 'invalid', either temporarily or on a more permanent basis.[182]

A range of factors influenced the level of industrial accidents, poisoning and injuries including the level of experience, length of service, age, gender[183] the skills of new workers, factory manager's adherence to Labour Code regulations and doctors and others knowledge of occupational pathologies and hygiene. The reporting of accidents was chaotic during the late 1920s and 1930s hindered by the large influx of seasonal workers, phenomenal turnover rates, changes in factory conditions and the political arena within which industrial accident statistics were collected and reported. Under reporting of accidents was common and workers, fearful of losing their jobs, often failed to report to the medical stations at enterprise level.[184]

Friedlin's data in Table 4.12 assesses the overall fluctuation in the number of industrial accidents in over 150 enterprises in Leningrad employing just over 330,000 workers by 1933, and the resulting number of deaths in this period from their injuries. Despite a rising number of workers (up 138,143) in more enterprises (increased by 38) between 1928–33 as well as the pressure of higher targets, the number of accidents reportedly fell from 75.5 per 1,000 in 1928 to 69.4 per 1,000 by 1933, though the number of deaths from these injuries rose from 27 to 37 in this five-year period, after reaching a peak of 45 in 1932.

Table 4.13 provides a breakdown of the number of industrial accidents per 1,000 workers according to branch of industry in Leningrad between 1928–33 and shows that at the start of the First FYP in 1928, the highest rates were in forestry (135.2) and metallurgy (124.4) and the lowest level of accidents was in printing (28.4) and tobacco (30.5). By 1933, the start of the Second FYP, industrial accidents in all branches had fallen and now metallurgy (89.5) had the highest accident rate whilst sewing (15.8) had the lowest.

Given changes to workers control over the intensity and organisation of their work between 1928–40, the pressures of industrialisation, the rapid tempo of work, the increased expectations from workers in terms of meeting rising norms and workers' desires to preserve their income, one would expect the level of industrial accidents to substantially increase but this is not the case according to Table 4.12 or 4.13.

Table 4.12: Industrial accidents and deaths per 1,000 workers in Leningrad, 1928–1933

Year	Number of enterprises	Average number of workers	Industrial accidents	Number of deaths		Changes over previous year	
				Absolute	Rate per 1,000	Injuries	Deaths
1928	118	199,959	75.5	27	0.135	-	-
1929	126	216,347	73.3	42	0.148	–3.0	+9.6
1930	130	283,391	85.1	41	0.144	+16.1	–2.8
1931	130	346,188	75.7	44	0.127	–11.1	–11.9
1932	139	360,177	65.7	45	0.124	–14.6	–2.4
1933	156	338,102	69.4	37	0.096	–9.6	–22.6

Source: S. Ia. Friedlin, 'Proizvodstvennyi travmatizm v Leningrade i opyt organizatsii traumo-logicheskoi pomoshchi', *Sovetskaia Vrachebnaia Gazeta* 31 August 1934, 1203, 1205

Table 4.13: Industrial accidents by sector of the Leningrad economy, 1928–33 (per 1,000 workers)

Branch of industry	Rate per 1,000 workers	
	1928	1933
Metallurgy	124.4	89.5
Sewing	43.1	15.8
Chemicals	57.5	44.0
Minerals	79.1	56.1
Food	76.5	59.5
Tobacco	30.5	20.8
Leather and tanning	75.1	40.2
Forestry	135.2	86.6
Printing	28.4	22.2
Hydro electric power	79.0	67.7
Total	75.5	59.4

Source: S. Ia. Friedlin, 'Proizvodstvennyi travmatizm v Leningrade i opyt organizatsii traumo-logicheskoi pomoshchi', *Sovetskaia Vrachebnaia Gazeta* 31 August 1934, 1204

There are numerous possible explanations for these trends. First, factory management provided sufficient rest, breaks and other forms of support; second, workers, as Filtzer's research shows, tried to control the situation themselves by moving to other jobs[185] and factories, when things became too unbearable as there were only mild restrictions on their movement before 1940 or else they left work early or turned up for work late;[186] third, absenteeism and circumvention by workers, managers and doctors of the these and other laws (by losing work books, not dismissing workers and forging sick notes)[187]; and, fourth, these trends were the product of the chaotic nature of production cycle in Leningrad. Managers, trade unions, the Party and inspectors of various kinds did their best to protect workers in Leningrad under Stalin, but labour protection was still not enough to prevent diseases and death.

Moving on to consider the case of industrial poisonings, Table 4.14 shows a similar trend with the number of poisonings from lead, carbon dioxide, benzine, chlorine and other substances in Leningrad industry as a whole[188] as well as in two key sectors, namely metallurgy and chemicals. Thus although the number of workers in industry almost doubled between 1927/28 and 1935, the number of poisonings in industry as a whole declined from 498 to 309, with the coefficient of frequency falling from 1.97 to 0.57 cases per 1,000 workers. Industrial poisonings in the Metallurgy sector follows this general pattern, but poisonings in the chemical industry in the city, with a more than doubling of the workforce, saw a greater fall in the number of industrial poisoning cases from 246 to 140 or from 10.9 to 2.9 cases per 1,000 workers. Archival data shows that this downward trend continued in the late 1930s. Thus, the number of industrial poisonings in Second and into Third FYP stood at: 292 in 1937; 201 in 1938 and 152 in 1939, with the number of victims falling from 929 in

Table 4.14: Industrial poisonings by branch of industry in Leningrad, 1927–1935

Year	Metallurgy			Chemicals			All industries		
	a	b	c	a	b	c	a	b	c
1927–28	89,074	155	1.8	22,609	246	10.9	254,458	498	1.97
1928–29	98,337	138	1.4	24,795	225	9.9	267,292	473	1.77
1929–30	173,919	252	1.4	33,822	160	4.7	396,848	487	1.23
1930	-	78	-	-	34	-	-	140	-
1931	244,849	185	0.8	53,582	154	2.9	532,137	392	0.7
1932	239,367	146	0.6	43,989	331	7.5	485,544	505	1.04
1933	229,125	220	0.9	39,523	176	4.4	482,385	418	0.86
1934	236,218	110	0.46	44,361	201	4.5	512,993	363	0.7
1935	256,713	114	0.44	47,672	140	2.9	539,999	309	0.57
Total number of poisonings		1,979			1,944			4,558	

Notes: [a]Number of workers [b]Number of occupational poisonings [c]Rate per 1,000 workers
Source: V. V. Stroganov, 'Desiat' let bor'by s professional'nymi otravleniiami v Leningradskoi promyshlennosti (1925–1935)', *Gigiena truda i tekhnika bezopasnosti* 1936, No. 6, 6–7

1937 to 436 by 1938. There were only 226 victims by 1939, or a two third fall since 1937.[189] Stroganov's figures as well as the St. Petersburg archive of Historical and Political documents unfortunately tell us nothing of the severity of the accidents or the disabilities which resulted from them.

Regarding the causes, Lewis Siegelbaum concludes that

> hygienists isolated several factors unrelated to work. Poor living conditions, alcoholism and family problems – the latter often the result of the first two – were frequently cited. But overwhelmingly, it was the conditions in the factories that bore the brunt of criticism.[190]

We saw above that diet was poor and that housing provisions failed to keep pace with the development of the economy at a time of rapid population growth. Vol'fson's investigations of 30% of cases at Krasnyi Putilovets (the former Putilov factory) engineering factory, shows that of workers visiting dispensaries in Leningrad in early 1928-mid 1929, 85% of the sample lived in accommodation below the sanitary norm of 10m² and a further 25% in housing four times below this standard. The food that they ate was also of poor quality and most consumed alcohol excessively and smoked heavily. Workers' level of personal hygiene was also low. For example, 32% bathed two to three times a month, 52% once a week and only 16% more frequently than that. 43.5% failed to brush their teeth.[191]

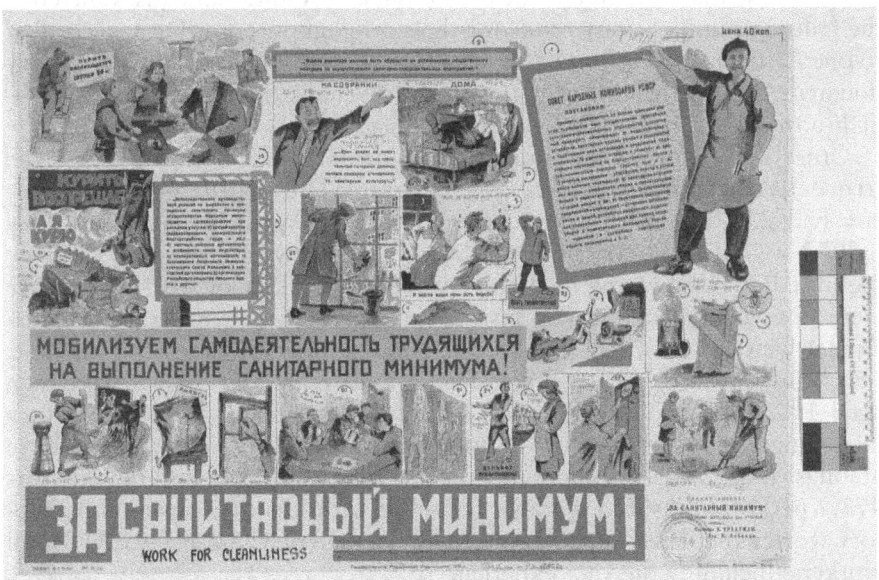

Poster 24 Achieving minimum factory cleanliness

Source: 'Za sanitarnyi minimum' (Mobilising workers to achieve minimum cleanliness in a range of settings)', Soviet poster courtesy of Woodburn Collection, Reproduced by permission of the National Library of Scotland.

Poster 24 tried to encourage the factory labour force under Stalin to keep their place of work as clean as possible, and to achieve 'sanitary minimum' standards; but for reasons set out below this was goal not achieved. Accidents at work, and the particular conditions and strains associated with the workplace – noise, dirt, cold, damp and dust and speed – all prematurely impaired workers' health. This, together with poor levels of diet, public hygiene and sanitation, as well as overcrowded housing, led to a declining standard of living among those living and working in Leningrad.

Numerous studies carried out from the late 1920s onwards highlight fatigue before and during work, insufficient rest periods, socialist competition, unhygienic conditions within the factories (inadequate lighting, excess temperatures, humidity, dust, obsolete equipment, too many workers and machines in a cramped space) and violations of safety regulations and labour rules as the main reasons for industrial accidents and poisonings of the collective in Leningrad. Thus, in one 1929 study, the factory Administration failed to adhere to Article 72 of the Labour Code of 29 August 1928.[192] Two five-year plans later, little had changed. In the period 1937–39, the causes of industrial poisonings in Leningrad were still the incorrect organisation of labour (at the Zhdanov factory and Oktenskii chemical combine), the failure to observe safety measures and poor ventilation (at the Krasnyi Vyborzhets and the Listokratnyi factory), the failure to supply or utilise gas masks (at the Nevskii chemical combine and Lenin mill) and breaches of technical processes (at the Nevskii chemical combine).[193] Additional causes included the failure to utilise safety funds for their original purpose. Thus, according to one *Leningradskaia Pravda* article of 25 March 1931, the Putilov factory donated 690,000r to improve safety in Narvskii district but the district public health department squandered the money.[194]

Other reasons cited for industrial accidents in Leningrad included the frequently changing workforce and its nature. Thus in 1928–32 alone, the city had 250,000 workers, and the number was growing on average by 8,800 between 1928–31 and by 8,700 per year between 1931–34.[195] Newly mobilised arrivals, young men and women with a lack of work experience were amongst the victims of industrial accidents. Of the workers in 'Znamia Truda' factory No. 1 in 1930 who had suffered eye injuries, for example, 79.1% of the cases were women aged 14–30 years and 67.6% were men aged 19–30 years old.[196] Another study, a year later of the same factory in Leningrad, found that of 3,660 industrial accident cases, 2,886 were amongst those with less than one year's factory experience and the rate was 477.9 per 1,000 insured workers for those with less than six months' factory work experience as compared to an average of 177.2 per 1,000 for all workers (including the very experienced).[197]

Shmerling's data in Table 4.15 suggests that there was a strong correlation between the branch of industry and the severity and-frequency of accidents. Thus, metalworkers in Leningrad required 10.9 days to recuperate in 1929 but 11.6 days by 1933; chemical workers 14.1 days in 1933

Table 4.15 Average duration of temporary incapacity due to Industrial accidents in various branches of industry in Leningrad, 1929–1933 (in calendar days)

Branch of industry	Year					Difference between 1929–33
	1929	*1930*	*1931*	*1932*	*1933*	*(%)*
Metalworking	10.9	11.8	11.8	11.6	11.6	+6.4
Timber	11.9	12.7	13.1	13.1	13.2	+10.9
Food	10.7	11.5	11.9	11.8	11.9	+11.2
Paper	11.6	14.4	13.3	12.9	15.1	+30.2
Garments	5.7	7.6	9.0	8.3	9.5	+66.7
Leather and tanning	10.7	10.8	12.6	12.0	12.2	+14.0
Chemicals	9.9	11.7	13.1	14.0	14.1	+42.5
Textiles	11.5	12.2	13.0	12.0	12.5	+8.7
Printing	10.5	11.8	13.0	14.1	13.7	+30.5
Tobacco	14.1	12.5	13.1	13.4	11.5	-18.5
All sectors of industry	10.8	11.7	12.0	11.9	12.0	+11.1

Source: S. G. Shmerling, 'Promyshlennyi travmatizm v Leningradskoi oblast ii puti ego likvidatsii' *Gigiena, bezopasnost' i patologiia truda* 1935, No. 1, 49

compared to 9.1 days in 1929; printing workers 13.7 instead of 10.5 days and those in the garment industry, the worst offenders, 9.5 days by 1933 instead of 5.7 days in 1929 to recover from accidents. This research contradicts Stroganov's data in the sense that workers from all branches of the city's industry required longer periods to recover from accidents in the early 1930s than in the late 1920s, with the exception of the tobacco industry. Labour productivity drives, launched on top of the earlier 'regime of economy' and rationalisation initiatives, were therefore damaging workers' health.

Victims of industrial accidents and poisonings in Leningrad industry needed more time to recuperate and lost working days were extremely costly in terms of lost production and social benefits. For instance, social insurance agencies in Leningrad paid out 37 million roubles in 1930–31 to workers temporarily incapacitated, and the value of lost production, over the same period as a result of this, was 268 million roubles.[198]

Unfortunately, expenditure on safety and labour protection measures decreased dramatically in comparison to previous years. Hence actual expenditure on these measures in Leningrad oblast' initially increased from 2.7 million roubles in 1926/27 to seven million by 1928/29, but already by 1931 expenditure was down to 5.7 million and in the first half of 1932 it fell sharply again to only 1.6 million roubles.[199] In order to try and reduce the level of industrial accidents, a Ministry of Health RSFSR resolution of 28 May 1931 sought to improve the level of medico-sanitary facilities for workers in industrial districts, such as Leningrad.[200] Labour protection organs and medical service staff were required from 27 May 1925 to record all accidents and poisonings and to offer medical-prophylactic care and treatment.[201] Despite factory managers diverting health and safety monies into other areas, the labour protection organs and medical service staff did their best but criticisms were still made of the care offered to factory workers. The treatment of I. V. Zhukov of the 'Znamia Truda' factory is a case in point. He was admitted to the Nechaev' hospital suffering from typhus in early November 1928 and upon being sent to the third floor, he was left unattended for 20 minutes and died 15 minutes later. Lack of funds had led to staff shortages, leaving only one senior nurse and two junior ones on duty at the time.[202]

Factory medical staff were not to blame. They had a very heavy workload and had to deal with all sorts of illnesses among the factory workforce – influenza, TB, gastro-intestinal diseases, VD alongside industrial injuries. In another factory survey of the 'Company Front' in the Smolyni district in 1937, where the workforce consisted of 82% females, factory doctors and Polyclinic No. 38 staff, dealt with the aftermath of abortions among workers.[203] Thus industrial accidents, poisonings and injuries were just one of the many demands placed upon overworked factory medical point personnel.

This situation relates to the bigger issue of invalidity among the Leningrad workforce under Stalinism. Here the work of the medical labour expert commissions (VTEK) staff came into play. They had to evaluate any patient referrals and make an expert judgement on whether or not those injured, poisoned or ill were fit to return to work or required invalidity status and support. According to Vigdorchik's data, the number of patient evaluations made by VTEK staff in Leningrad increased from 36,912 in 1930 to 54,833 by 1932 rising further to 76,740 in 1936 before finally reaching 85,778 by 1939 or by over 2.3 times.[204] The outcome was that of the cases reviewed between 1930–39, the number declared fit to return to work increased from 13.2% in 1930 to 20.8% by 1939; the number temporarily incapacitated rose from 0.9% to 6.0% and those declared category I to III invalids fell from 85.9% in 1930 to 63.4% by 1939.[205]

Table 4.16 provides an indication of the reasons for incapacity in Leningrad which shows that the large majority of workers were incapacitated as a result of heart disease, which prevailed in nearly a quarter of the sample. Next came TB, closely followed by diseases of the nervous system. Industrial accidents (5–6%) are low down the list. The gender breakdown was largely the same for males and females.[206] Workers, provided they could prove they were not malingerers or wreckers, went to rest homes, sanatoria or health resorts to recuperate. With regards to industrial related problems – accidents and poisonings – factory medical point staff, the Leningrad Institute of Labour hygiene and occupational diseases, the city and district medical inspectors and emergency aid staff might have been successful in combating industrial intoxifications, poisonings, air pollution by offering medical treatment as quickly as possible and to the highest standard possible

Table 4.16 Causes of incapacity among Leningrad workers, 1937–39

Type of disease	1937	1938	1939
Heart	25.2	24.8	24.1
TB of lungs	17.0	16.7	16.5
Diseases of the central nervous system	11.6	11.8	11.0
Breathing	7.7	7.8	7.9
Other nervous diseases	4.6	5.7	6.0
Psychiatric	6.0	5.5	5.2
Industrial accidents	6.0	5.5	5.2
Digestive organs	3.3	3.4	3.5
Malignant disorders	3.4	3.2	3.4
Gynaecological	1.3	1.6	2.3
Eye diseases	2.5	2.2	2.1

Source: N. A. Vigdorchik, *Statisticheskii analiz dannykh o rabote Leningradskikh VTEK-ov na poslednie gody* (Leningrad 1941), 22

under the circumstances. Thus, although the number of workers rose by 195% between 1925–37, as did the tempo of production, the level of industrial poisonings during the same period declined by 70% for the reasons highlighted earlier as well as due to all of the hard work and cooperation between these labour protection and medical organs.[207]

Ambitious health plans for the RSFSR under Stalin

The question we must now consider is whether or not central planning was part of the problem, but before doing so a few comments are in order. What distinguishes Soviet industrialisation and the modernisation of agriculture and industry from other countries was the use of central planning. It was used to apply pressure, mobilise resources and establish priority sectors in line with Stalinist policy. The following sections analyse the impact of central planning on health care – political interference in medical affairs and economic irrationality – and the consequences in trying to address the threats to the health of the collective in Leningrad from 1928 until 1941.

Central planning had three functions: first, it applied pressure via the way resources were allocated and so everyone in the health service had to meet FYP targets and as we saw above the breakneck speed of Stalin's policies had consequences for the health of the population. Second, planning was used to mobilise resources via a reward-penalty system and was based on plan fulfilment or non-fulfilment. Thus, factory manager's resources and bonuses were tied to meeting FYP targets and this had consequences for workers health. Finally, Soviet central planning established priority sectors, such as heavy industry and defence, which developed at the expense of health, not just in relation to housing, food and other areas as detailed above.

Health planning as such did not fully emerge in the health field until after the first Narkomzdrav (NKZ) planning conference was held in April 1928. At this time an initial draft of the five-year financial plan for public health (1927/28–1931/32) was published. It contained control figures for 1927–28 and three variants of projected expenditures from the major sources up to 1931–32. These were used as a means of framing public health policy. On 26 April 1928, the First FYP period was changed to 1928/29–1932/33 and public health departments were asked to submit by 1 June, complete statistical reports on finance and on the state of their health systems in the years 1925–28. NKZ promised to publish the final figures on 15 September 1928.[208] Christopher Davis' analysis of 'Theses concerning the five-year perspective plan of the RSFSR health service' shows that only modest increases in RSFSR health service indicators were forecast.[209] Semashko, the RSFSR Health Minister, declared that these 'plan targets were too low to radically alter the situation by 1932/33 given the tight financial constraints hindering health service development'.[210] The biggest problem areas, according to Davis, were capital investment, the supply of medical manpower and inadequate finance.[211] NKZ called in May 1929 for 'significant correctives and supplements in all plans'.[212] At the Third Planning Conference held in September 1929, the health targets set were much more ambitious, unrealistic levels. Although local public health authorities were asked for amended targets by 1 December 1929, the long awaited second variant of the RSFSR First FYP for health was not completed until August 1930.[213] Davis concludes that second variant fulfilled the demand of the party that the rate of development of the health service be more in line with that of the rest of the economy.[214]

These ambitious targets could not be attained. Davis argues that this applied to the number of doctors and hospital beds and if any quantitative advances were achieved, it was at the expense of the quality of inputs, for example, accelerated medical training.[215] It was political aspiration rather than realism that dominated Stalinist health planning. Such a situation did not ensure an appropriate allocation of resources. Problems with resource availability and the inefficient use of meagre resources meant that the medical system was unable to cope with adverse changes in health conditions under Stalinism.

According to the first variant of the financial plan for the RSFSR's Second FYP for public health, which was planned to run from 1933–37, the general budget was to rise eight times reaching a planned projected total of 24,591.1 million roubles by 1937. All the main areas of public health expenditure were to be allocated more of the budget than in 1932: capital investment up seven times; crèche aid up 24 times; the expansion of the number of public health points was planned to increase 10 times; investment in hospitals was up by 4.5 times and non-hospital aid was planned to rise five times. Expenditure on mothers and babies was also forecasted to increase seven times.[216]

The biggest focus during the Second FYP was the fight against epidemics. In the First and Second FYPs smallpox immunisation programmes focused upon those under one year old, 10–11 and 20–21-year-olds and then due to further outbreak of smallpox in 1934–35, the age group shifted to 4–5 and 7–8-year-olds and those above thirty as well as the migrant population.[217] Whilst smallpox was under control by 1937, typhus broke out in 1933, with incidence levels three times higher in towns than in rural areas. By 1936–37, typhus cases had also broken out in schools. These policies were needed as infectious diseases were also prominent in Leningrad in the 1930s (see Table 4.1). Such infectious disease outbreaks were due to the mass movement of the population in 1932–36 from villages to towns and to newly constructed areas and this needed to be budgeted for.[218] The challenge was not just a shortage of disinfection equipment, infectious diseases staff in rural areas, poor population awareness of how working and living conditions can spread typhus and the lack of leadership in anti-typhus campaigns but health workers also faced disorganised, chaotic population movements, including politically suspect populations (homeless children, criminals, kulaks, speculators etc.) which enabled typhus to spread easily, which no amount of health planning could easily address.[219] It was this failure to combat the medical disorder that largely caused the medical profession to be a victim of Stalin's terror.

Unsatisfactory hygienic conditions – problems with the sewage network, inadequate cleanliness, unclean water supplies, the tendency to use wells and open water pipes, flies – also caused intestinal and infectious diseases which were often diagnosed late.[220] The number of dysentery cases was initially low but increased from 1936 onwards, and the plan tried to allow for this but due to the failure to isolate the sick, wrong diagnoses, the poor network of bacteriology laboratories (despite production of serums and vaccines) and the failure to prevent a large number of flies, dysentery hit young and school age children the hardest. This situation was caused by the health conditions of the general population, poor quality food and public hygiene and the ineffective work of some health inspectors. Plans to create more bacteriology laboratories, especially in rural areas and to locate them in rural hospitals failed, for reasons beyond the control of the medical profession and health service, and not enough staff had been trained to deal with this health challenge.[221]

Some successes occurred with diphtheria in comparison to the NEP period for reasons discussed at the start of the chapter, but scarlet fever was on the rise at the end of the Second FYP period, which had first spread in key towns, reaching levels of 81.0 per 10,000 population by 1936 in the city of Leningrad.[222] Similarly, measles was initially high in 1930, then fell between 1932–34 but increased from 1935 onwards, reaching a level of 26.8 per 10,000 in towns and 35.2 per 10,000 in villages of Leningrad oblast by 1936. The problem with children's diseases was attributed to a failure to plan effectively, so there was a shortage of paediatricians and insufficient hospital facilities (especially beds) to treat the sick. As a result, those with measles were diagnosed late and this spread the disease in residences and barracks, and only then were the sick hospitalised.[223] One of the biggest challenges was influenza epidemics with around 13 million cases in the RSFSR between 1931–March 1936.[224]

A 1937 report argued that these epidemics occurred because of an inadequate number of anti-epidemic centres especially in rural areas and a shortage of staff. The report highlighted that an extra 1,625 doctors, 1,700 feldshers and nurses, 100 laboratory staff, 1,601 disinfection personnel instructors and 1,307 inoculation and vaccination staff were needed in the RSFSR to combat epidemics. However, these extra staff and shortages were not fulfilled, as there were only 436 trained doctors available in 1937.[225]

The Third FYP for public health in the RSFSR, covering the period 1938–42, had two variants with different targets and different projected expenditure levels. Archival materials reveal that the difference between the two variants was first, extremely large at times (with regard to city hospitals 17,506 higher or children's hospitals by 6,184 more in the first variant); second, large in certain instances (a difference of 499 in terms of the number of feldsher points between the two variants); third, there were minor differences (20 more sanitary-epidemiological establishments in first than second variant) and finally, non-existent differences between the two sets of goals (for example in the number of trauma and emergency aid points, psychiatric hospitals).[226]

In broad terms, the Third FYP envisaged creating 20,000 more maternity beds, 20 more clinical hospitals, a TB hospital with 10,000 beds, 50 more emergency aid stations, a 10,000 bed sanatoria, a new medical institute, a medical hall of residence for 200 students, feldsher and nursing schools, pharmacies, a hostel for junior city hospital personnel and it sought to provide more housing for city and district medical workers.[227] The plan was premised on improvements made during the Second FYP which health officials argued had resulted in a fall in the death rate, the IMR (which had fallen three times in urban and 2–2.5 times in rural areas) and VD (which had declined three-fold since 1936) but the plan acknowledged rising death rates from TB (so the aim of Third FYP was to combat it). It envisaged an increase in the number of crèche and beds which at RSFSR level had reached 240,000 in 1932 but fallen to 95,000 by 1936–37, before increasing again to 145,000 by 1938. A further aim was to build more medical institutions and training facilities (feldsher and midwife and nursing schools) and to improve the quality of student halls of residence.[228]

An assessment was made of the level of progress towards Third FYP targets at RSFSR level in 1939, and it was discovered that 1938 plan targets for several areas had not been achieved. For example, the overall number of hospitals (shortfall of 153), hospital beds (down 6,948), maternity homes (down 5,300), disinfection stations (10 below target) and disinfection points (19 shortfall), and the number of smallpox vaccination staff (by 170), were highlighted. Despite these failures, the 1939 plan targets were set at even higher levels than those for 1938. But in other cases, some progress had been made. Some targets had been achieved (children's hospitals, psychiatric hospitals, out-patient establishments, polyclinics, TB and VD dispensaries) and others exceeded (TB beds by 400, emergency aid stations by 56, industrial health points by 50, the number of food and factory inspectors by 20 and housing inspectors by 10).[229]

We saw above that at Russian Republic level health plan objectives from the First through to the Third FYP varied as did the level of success in meeting objectives. This section examines how this impacted upon the situation in Leningrad. The evidence suggests that the main problem was lack of sufficient resources to deal with the scale of the health problems outlined above. This stemmed from a lack of capital investment, manpower and finance compounded by inefficiency and political repression (see later). The relative importance of each of these variables will be assessed in turn.

Health care planning in Leningrad – a 'regime' city

For Gosplan, health officials, such as Donskoi, the health plans for Leningrad must correspond to the needs of the economy. He wrote, '[t]he tempo of public health development must be in line with the rate of economic and cultural development'.[230] Against this background, the aim of the First FYP was to provide adequate prophylactic medical services, to curtail epidemics, to improve medical provisions in the towns and countryside, to significantly increase the level of facilities for the insured, and finally, to increase the quantity, while at the same time improving the quality, of health care.[231]

The RSFSR health plan envisaged a rapid expansion in many areas including Leningrad.

According to Smirnov, the local head of the health service, the aim of health planning in Leningrad was 'to improve labour conditions and way of life as well as to reduce ill-health among the local population'.[232] More specifically, at a time of socialist reconstruction, the desire was to improve the level of medical provision for the industrial proletariat, factory workers and those in key industries. The broad strategy that was to be employed in Leningrad involved the following:

> the introduction of a dispensarization programme in industry; improving the water supply, sewage system and housing; development of the medical infrastructure; improving health facilities for women and children, industrial workers, the insured, and other key occupational groups, by embarking upon a new construction and capital repairs programme; expansion of the ongoing health education programme; unification of all medico-sanitary establishments on a territorial or district basis, and finally, averting the current staffing crisis by raising the wages and improving the living standards of medical personnel thereby increasing the availability of specialised and secondary medical cadres.[233]

There were two variants of the health FYP for Leningrad, each of which generated fierce debates. The first variant was regarded as too modest, as its targets were set too low and with the projected increases in finance viewed as woefully inadequate. The main problems areas were a low level of capital investment, a lack of medical staff, poor transport links, inefficient management as a result of red tape and inertia, excessive central control and too great a desire to link the pace of public health development to that of the local economy as a whole. As criticism of this variant increased, a second one was devised. It was far more ambitious and premised on the expectation of a significant, though not specified, rise in population in Leningrad.

The aim of the First FYP was to eradicate infectious disease epidemics which had hit the city and especially the region of Leningrad. A malaria station was set up and attached to the Pasteur Bacteriological institute to fight malaria in the city, oblast and surrounding okrug. This kept the level of malaria among workers relatively low at 220 in 1928 falling to 210 in 1929 in Leningrad oblast.[234] The health service was required to carry out disinfection work in public baths, vaccination programmes and to ensure that 'sanitary minimums' were maintained in factory dining rooms and canteens (*stoloviya*) and that food quality levels in buffets and in residences and barracks in key industrial centres were monitored as they were a source of dysentery and typhoid fever.[235] In addition, the goal was to improve housing conditions, the food supply, labour productivity, health care in industrial enterprises, to reduce industrial accidents and to improve health culture.[236] To this end, the number of enterprise public health points increased from 380 in 1930 to 500 by 1932, with the number of doctors serving Leningrad machine building workers, for instance, rising from 132 in 1930 to 35 by 1932 whilst those doctors serving Leningrad textile workers increased from 119 in 1930 to 180 by 1932.[237] Medical facilities for Leningrad machine building workers reached 200 hospital beds, 21 doctor visits, three industrial health points, 100 crèche beds, three sanitary-epidemiologists, one disinfection point, four women and children's doctors, 25 sanatoria for young workers and 25 summer camps for young Pioneer children of workers by 1932, the end of the First FYP.[238]

A discussion of these two variants reveals that targets were not realised. Table 4.17 shows that the number of doctors did not kept pace with the rise in population. Thus, while the population increased by 43.5%, the number of doctors rose by 42%. However, the number of secondary medical personnel increased by 57.2%, much higher than overall population growth. Other targets were not attained. Thus, Ivanov notes, for instance, that the target for psychiatric beds for 1931 was 3,840 and for 1932 was 4,140, but the actual figures achieved were 3,415 and 4,116 respectively, slightly below target. In the First FYP, the number of midwives declined from 5.9 to 2.6 and hospital beds from 8.10 to 7.40 per 1,000 population, respectively between 1927/28–1932/33.[239] The scheduled number of public health points, usually in factories in Leningrad but also in schools, was set, according to Ivanov, at 380 in 1931 and 519 in 1932, but actual levels reached were only 326 and 400,

Table 4.17 The number of medical personnel in the city of Leningrad, 1928–40

Year	Doctors	Dentists	Dental doctors	Pharmacists	Secondary medical personnel
1928	4,267	614		1,568	5,837a
1929	4,068	-	712	2,721	4,790
1930	5,448	-	521	215	1,099a
1931	9,778	653	1,267	21	618b
1932	5,296	-	-	-	-
1933	2,639	-	686	-	-
1934	6,331	-	784	186	-
1935	2,714	-	695	-	-
1936	-	-	-	-	-
1937	20,563	-	753	51	9,224
1938	23,232	661	967	54	9,565
1939	4,612	-	-	-	13,526
1940	9,222	23,245	-	-	-

Notes: ᵃ all categories – feldshers, midwives etc ᵇ nurses, orderlies, technicians
Source: GARF f. A-482, op 10, d. 1689, lists 40–41; GARF f. A-482, op 10, d. 2523, lists 4, 4ob; GARF f. A-482, op 10, d. 2839, lists 99, 99ob; GARF f. A-482, op 10, d. 2972, lists 2ob, 9ob, 10; GARF f. A-482, op 24, d. 1317, list 7; GARF f. A-482, op 24, d. 350, list 130; GARF f. A-482, op 47, d. 5655, lists 7, 60, 62

a considerable shortfall.[240] The main reasons given for non-fulfilment were a failure to submit accurate documents, an inadequate number of staff to over-see the planning process, a lack of finance, poor management and a failure to mobilise the local population.[241] The outcome, according to one 1933 planning document was that

> [b]oth the quality and the quantity of medical care in Leningrad was woefully inadequate – staff were in short supply, hospitals were closed, provisions were highly unsatisfactory, new construction was not forth-coming and capital investment during the First five-year plan was virtu-ally non-existent.[242]

There were also shortages in the number of hospitals. Table 4.18 using declas-sified archival material shows that the number of hospitals in Leningrad declined from 71 in 1928 to 61 by 1932 or by 14.1%, far less than the population increase over the same period. This probably occurred as a result of amalgamations. Attempts were made to avert this crisis by expanding the number of beds from 16,161 to 21,687 (a rise of 34.2%) but this still failed to keep pace with the rise in population so the city of Leningrad's hospitals were becoming more and more overcrowded during the First FYP period. Some recovery was made in 1936 when the number of hospitals reached 83 but a year later in 1937 (at the height of Stalin's purges) the number of

Table 4.18 The number of hospitals and beds in Leningrad, 1928–40

Year	Number of hospitals	Number of hospital beds
1928	71	16,161
1929	61	16,341
1930	56	18,405
1931	61	19,277
1932	61	17,500
1933	-	19,153
1934	-	19,675
1935	-	20,356
1936	83	-
1937	53	22,304
1938	-	23,390
1939	-	25,853
1940	92	20,794

Source: GARF f. A-482, op 10, d. 1914, list 116; GARF f. A-482, op 10, d. 1689, lists 16; GARF f. A-482, op 10, d. 1915, lists 19; GARF f. A-482, op 10, d. 1702, list 19; GARF f. A-482, op 10, d. 2523, list 2; GARF f. A-482, op 10, d. 2839, list 79ob; GARF f. A-482, op 24, d. 266, list 19; GARF f. A-482, op 26, d. 39, list 14; GARF f. A-482, op 47, d. 5655, lists 2, 7, 60, 62; GARF f. A-482, op 47, d. 8887, list 162

hospitals fell again to 53, 25% below the 1928 level. The demand for beds was constantly rising and the FYPs set targets to cope with this. Thus, the number of beds rose from 16,161 in 1928 to 17,500 in 1932 (by 8.2%), then increased again to 20,356 in 1935 (a further 19.1% rise) before the number of beds reached their peak at 25,853 in 1939, some 9,692 hospital beds higher than in 1928 (or 60% in real terms). By 1940, the number of beds in the city of Leningrad hospitals fell back again to 20,794 on the eve of the siege, but this was still an increase of over a quarter (28.7%) since 1928. There were 92 hospitals at this point, 21 more than in 1928. In the hospital sector, as elsewhere, these fluctuations were a result of poor investment in the medical infrastructure which meant that new hospitals and other facilities were not always being built or completed.

During the Third FYP hospital construction was a priority in Leningrad given the decline by 30 hospitals between 1936 and 1937. This was due to a failure to prioritise this issue and shortages of construction workers to build hospitals.[243] The goal was to expand the hospital stock by building a hospital on the right bank on the Neva, the Nechaev hospital, treatment facilities in Kronstadt and more beds at the Obukhov hospital and a third-floor addition at the children's hospital within the Botkin hospital. In addition, the goal was to build two polyclinics.[244] This clearly had an impact as the number of hospitals had increased to 92 by 1940, though beds within them had declined by nearly 5,000 since 1928. One 1938 report pointed out that there was a shortage of trauma, oncology, TB and ontological beds, as well as insufficient junior hospital staff. There was a 50% shortage in secondary medical personnel as well as a shortage of leading staff to run children's hospitals.[245] Additional problems highlighted included a lack of leadership in scientific research institutes, weak coordination between NKZ and the scientific research institutes and poor centre-regional relations and so a recommendation was made that the management of scientific research institutes be reorganised.[246]

However, in recognition of the hard work of medical staff, their wages were forecast to double: the planned increase in doctors' wages was from 196r in 1932 to 450r by 1937; secondary medical personnel from 77r to 200r and junior medical staff wages from 46r to 100r during the Second FYP period. These pay rises were to vary according to grade and experience and the goal was to spread the costs across the duration of the Second FYP as detailed in Table 4.19. Sarah Davies highlights an example of a letter written by a group of low-paid domestics who argued that they earned about 125 roubles for 14 hours' work; whereas their bosses (doctors) received a lot more and also had access to free cars, holidays and luxury flats.[247] Thus, the general public were not always happy about such wage increases and some people seem to have resented doctors and their living conditions. During the Terror these differences came to the fore and were part of the denunciations made.

A comparison of the city of Leningrad's medical establishments at different stages in all three five-year plans – the First (1930), Second (1934) and in the Third (1937) FYP is shown in Table 4.20. This table, based upon declassified Ministry of Public health data, shows staffing levels in the various years by speciality, which departments they worked in, which diseases were viewed as crucial (infectious, social) and the expectation that medical personnel will deal with hygiene at home, carry out food and factory inspections, and these trends indicate which groups are a priority – the insured as a whole, as well as children, mothers as well as those with specific diseases such as TB, VD and epidemics. We can see that the Stalinist health system in Leningrad in the 1930s included the normal health service organisations (hospitals) as well as factory-based facilities, day and night sanatoria and specialised sanatoria facilities for industrial workers' children and aspiring Party members (Pioneers).

Table 4.19 Forecasted pay increase of different categories of medical personnel during the second FYP for public health

Category	Projected pay increases (in roubles)						
	1932	*1933*	*1934*	*1935*	*1936*	*1937*	*1937 as % of 1932*
Doctors	196	250	300	350	400	450	229.6
Medical point doctors	230	300	375	450	525	600	260.9
Leading doctors	240	350	450	550	650	720	300
Surgeons	200	300	375	450	550	600	300
Sanitary doctors	210	300	375	450	550	600	300

(*continued*)

Table 4.19: Forecasted pay increase of different categories of medical personnel during the second FYP for public health (*continued*)

Category	Projected pay increases (in roubles)						
	1932	1933	1934	1935	1936	1937	1937 as % of 1932
Doctors employed in:							
Epidemiological work	220	300	375	450	550	600	272.7
Food	220	300	375	450	500	550	250.3
Disinfection work	220	275	340	410	450	500	227.3
Infectious diseases doctors	200	275	325	400	400	450	243.2
X-ray doctors	175	250	300	340	380	425	242.9
Secondary medical personnel, of which:							
Senior							
rank 1	85	120	155	195	230	265	311.8
rank 2	70	88	110	155	150	185	230.0
rank 3	65	76	90	105	125	140	223.1
rank 4	122	160	195	235	280	310	254.1
Junior:							
rank 1	55	70	85	100	115	135	245.5
rank 2	45	50	60	75	87	100	222.2
rank 3	30	40	48	56	64	72	240.0
rank 4	60	90	110	125	140	155	258.3

Source: *Finansovoi plan organov zdravookhraneniia na 2-e piatiletie (1-i tur) 1933–37gg tom. 1* in GARF f. A-482 op 26, d. 26, list 80).

Table 4.20: City of Leningrad health networks in 1930, 1934 and 1937

Type of health provision	1930 (absolute number)	1934 (absolute number)	1937 (absolute number)
Number of health workers, of which: sanitary-epidemiological department	58	-	180
Housing inspectors	42	55	60
Food inspectors	25	60	52
Bacteriologists	14	109	164
Epidemiologists	23	76	92
Dealing with social diseases:			
TB	128	207	222
VD	171	190	265
Children and teenagers doctors, of which:	360	-	-
Pediatricians	142	787	1,383
Mothers and baby specialist doctors	328	833	437
Legal medical experts	6	17	21
Dental doctors	521	784	753
Pharmacists	215	186	51

(*continued*)

Table 4.20: City of Leningrad health networks in 1930, 1934 and 1937
(*continued*)

Type of health provision	1930 (absolute number)	1934 (absolute number)	1937 (absolute number)
Midwives	415	999	780
Number of out-patient points, of which:	93	-	256
Industrial enterprise based	26	110	-
Emergency aid stations	6	6 (with 79 vehicles)	8
Number of hospitals, of which with:	56	32	53
1–19 beds	2	-	-
20–49 beds	6	-	-
50–99 beds	10	-	-
100+ beds	38	-	-
Number of permanent crèches, of which:	79	157	239
Total number of children	13,778	-	24,244
Factory-based crèches	24	1,979	106
Malaria stations	1	1	5
Disinfection stations, of which:	1	2	-
Number of disinfectionists	-	8	155

Source: GARF f. A-482, op 10, d. 1915 lists 13–14, 19, 22, 24, 26, 28, 30, 32, 34, 36–37, 40;
GARF f. A-482, op 10, d. 2523 lists 1, 1ob, 2, 2ob, 3, 3ob, 4, 4ob; GARF f. A-482, op 10, d.
2839 lists 97, 97ob, 98, 98ob, 99, 99ob, 100

Financial constraints on health service developments in Leningrad

The financial problems which prevailed under the NEP remained in the Stalin era, if anything they got worse. The four sources of finance – state and local budget, insurance funds (FMP) and special means – were still being used as well as additional sources of income. In Table 4.21 information on public health expenditure in the city of Leningrad from 1927/28 until the mid-1930s is given. A number of points can be made. First, direct State funding to enable the Leningrad health system to meet the local population's needs dropped by nine-fold, constituting only 0.3% of the overall total. At regional level, NKZ revenues doubled between 1927/28 and 1935, although as a percentage of the overall budget, this made up only 2% of public health revenue by the mid-1930s. Second, contributions coming from the local budget rose more than six-fold with the total spent on public health in the city rising from 14.4 million roubles 1927/28 to 99.5 million roubles by 1935. Revenues from local budget sources were higher than those coming from the insurance funds in 1928/29 but for the remaining years, the FMP was greater and constituted 20.2% of the overall contribution by 1935. Given the importance of the insured in Leningrad, other insurance funds contributed nearly 215.5 million to the city's health budget or 55.4%, recognising that doctors, nurses and other personnel were needed to provide the highest quality of care to these key components of the collective.

Table 4.21 Source of public health funding in Leningrad, 1927–1935

Source of budget expenditure	1927–28	1928–29	1929–30	1934	1935
State budget	1,225,200	1,290,000	900,000	359,600	111,500
Local budget	15,365,730	19,059,700	22,645,600	65,111,000	99,481,000
FMP	17,913,300	17,203,800	20,630,764	60,146,700	81,500,000
Republican fund	151,600	2,059,000	2,702,700	1,504,000	7,047,400
Insurance funds	-	-	-	-	13,668,400
Other insurance funds[a]	-	-	-	751,000	201,808,300
Industrial cooperatives	-	-	-	2,600,800	-
Special means	3,008,800	2,375,700	2,541,253	1,248,800	-
Total	37,664,630	41,998,200	48,521,217	131,721,900	403,616,600

Note: [a] From various Ministries

Source: GARF f. A-482 op. 10 d. 2523, list 5; GARF f. A-482 op. 15 d. 403, list 5; GARF f. A-482 op. 15 d. 388, list 23, 44; *Zdravookhranie v g. Leningrade za 1928–1929 i na 1929–30 biudzhety god* (Leningrad 1930), 3

Any decline in the FMP, and for that matter other sources of revenue, reflected changes in government policy, inflation, problems with local taxation and/or voluntary rate-paying (*samooblozhenie*) to finance social and cultural measures (public health, education, housing etc) in Leningrad after the late 1920s.[248] In the case of the FMP, attempts were made to try and offset deficits by using fund 'G', but this did not have the desired effect. As a result, priority groups in Leningrad's health policy, such as the insured, were badly affected. Thus Donskoi points out that

> [a]s a consequence of withdrawals from the FMP, it was necessary for Leningrad to close down in 1928/29, 1,250 beds of which 750 will remain inactive in 1929/30. This occurs at a time of rapid growth in the number of industrial cadres.[249]

Medical care for the insured continued to operate much as it had done under the NEP, that is, it was paid for by the bosses, with no contribution directly forthcoming from the workers themselves.[250] Medical treatment was provided free of charge out of social insurance funds and administered by local public health departments.[251] The proportion of the population of the city of Leningrad covered by the insurance medicine system increased from 560,545 in January 1928 to 1,206,824 in July 1932.[252] However, per capita public health expenditure on the insured actually fell by 48% from

31r 29k in 1927/28 to 13r 43k in the first half of 1932.[253] Thus the burden of any cutbacks in health services, as under the NEP, still fell largely on the non-insured sections of the Leningrad population. As Donskoi notes: 'In the current year (1929) assistance to the non-insured population will be severely cut in order to prevent health care for the insured population from diminishing'.[254]

Under Stalinism, as under the NEP, each Republic of the USSR had its own Commissariat of Public Health. In the RSFSR, Narkomzdrav was in charge and it monitored the activities of oblast, city and district public health departments. In this book we are referring largely, but not exclusively, to the city health system which was staffed by experienced, committed specialists who were quick to publicise and devise policies in response to the changes in health conditions outlined in earlier discussions. We have highlighted the medical personnel and facilities available in previous tables but given the demographic and political changes, the level of medical care had clearly increased in some areas and declined or become no more than moderate in others.

Given the tight financial and political constraints, it was impossible for the health service to maintain high quality health and sanitation across the board from 1928–40 and so against this background the main priority areas were curative measures (hospital aid, out-patients and non-hospital provision); health care for women and children and combating social diseases, such as TB. Next came wages (as a result of the need to retain old and attract new staff), followed by new construction and capital repairs, and finally anti-epidemic measures and the provision of additional staff.[255] Financial crises throughout the First to Third FYPs led to a reduction in quantitative indicators of medical care and undermined many of these priority programmes. Hospital repairs and the building of new facilities lagged behind the population increase and developments in the local economy. Moreover, insufficient capital investment meant that medical equipment was not serviced. Other restraints meant medical staff could not be hired. Thus, the number of pharmacists, vaccination staff, surgical beds, maternity beds, hospitals and children's consultation clinics all declined between 1930–37.[256] To add to these difficulties, patient treatment was sometimes of poor quality, there was little improvement in the standard of the average diet and water supply and sewage programmes made no demonstrably positive impact on the likelihood of infection.

'Planning' was used in the Soviet economy as a whole to gave a clear idea of government priorities and served as a means of mobilising resources to achieve specific objectives. Given the all-pervasive shortages, resources, and finance. were allocated on an order of priority basis. Heavy industry received the lion's share at the expense of other socio-cultural sectors, such as public health and housing. Such a situation prevailed not only at national but also at a local level. There were a range of priority sectors in Leningrad from 1928–40 but public health was not one of them, it was a low priority sector.

Having to work and operate under the pressure of the plan and the fear of not meeting its objectives, especially as Stalin's Great and Mass Terrors occurred between 1934–37, members of the Leningrad medical profession, did their best to adapt. The situation became particularly complicated for Tsarist trained staff, during the Cultural Revolution and the purges, which we will now consider.

Medical disorder, class war and the health service under attack

The local Party leadership was not surprisingly becoming greatly concerned about public health and sanitation. This was partly a reaction to growing working-class discontent regarding access to health facilities. Surveys of Soviet emigres coming to the West have revealed overwhelming approval for the Soviet medical system[257] but events in Leningrad during the mid-late 1920s show a different picture. Ewing argues that at several district insurance conferences held in Leningrad in 1925–26, workers gave an endless list of complaints: long waiting times for treatment; poor quality care by unqualified doctors; and, in some cases, a total lack of staff altogether.[258] At one such meeting in Vasilevskii district, a factory representative noted that many workers were going blind because of a shortage of spectacles whereas others were having difficulties eating because false teeth were not being supplied fast enough.[259] The consequence of this was a lack of satisfaction with both the health service and the insurance organs.

Under Stalinism, nothing changed. In February 1929, the newspaper *Krasnaia Gazeta* noted that in the Moscow-Narva district of the city excessive bureaucracy was preventing workers from receiving treatment resulting in senior insurance doctors having to intervene on their behalf.[260] The Party used these frustrations to mobilise support for a shake-up of the Leningrad health service and at the same time it sought to remove those undermining industrialisation. In the mid-1920s, the Party through NKZ tried to implement a 'dispensarization' policy geared to the needs of industry, as we saw in Chapter 3. This strategy was extended in 1928 and a proletarian class line in medicine was also introduced at this time.[261]

In 1929, a more factory orientated health programme was started, in which the emphasis was firmly placed on health provision for the industrial proletariat.[262] One indication of the priority assigned to this was the rapid expansion in the number of enterprise-based health points and the increase in medical staff running them.[263] Of course, the aim was to increase labour productivity. The Party reasoned therefore that in furnishing medical aid they could either prevent illness or enable the incapacitated worker to regain their health in the shortest possible time.[264]

A December 1929 decree led to the restructuring of Republican, city and district health departments to bring them in line with the government's industrialisation drive.[265] Health service leaders in Leningrad, like many of their counterparts in other cities, resisted calls for adjustments in health plan targets and health policy but given the political climate prevailing, such resistance was interpreted as an expression of 'Right opposition' and as a challenge to central authority.[266] For Barsukov and Zhuk, 'wrecking' was allegedly responsible for the fact that public health service efforts lagged 'behind the general tempo of socialist reconstruction.[267] Increased Party vigilance was, therefore, deemed necessary in order to eradicate these tendencies.[268] Allegedly physicians had begun to directly challenge the validity of Stalinist policies by arguing that 'the high tempo of industrialisation was leading to a growth in morbidity and the level of industrial injuries among the proletariat'.[269] Despite these accusations, of anti-Soviet agitation cases considered by the Supreme Court of the RSFSR by September 1935, a mere 0.7% involved doctors.[270] There must therefore be another more important reason why the Party leadership launched the purges of the medical profession. This part of the chapter argues that it was the failure to prevent medical disorder that was used to justify the terror amongst the medical profession and that the Terror in turn increased the level of disorder as key medical personnel were dismissed now killed.

In Leningrad, as we saw in previous chapters, the Party had tried to penetrate the medical profession but without much success. This was not really necessary because the old tsarist medical staff had cooperated with the Soviet regime since the civil war to combat epidemics and other health crises, and they continued to do so during the NEP. The issue was that relatively few health service personnel had become members of the Party and therefore it appeared as that they were not fully committed to building socialism or loyal to the Party. This led to increased suspicion. In any case Sheila Fitzpatrick points out that it was not easy for bourgeois experts to join the Party.[271] Whilst this Party anxiety was nothing new, the political context had fundamentally altered since 1926, and during the First FYP and beyond, criticisms of health service leaders and administrators became more and more frequent due to declining health conditions in the 1930s as detailed earlier on in this chapter.

A practice had developed since the Russian civil war in which the Party credentials, records, reputation of all state employees was checked to eradicate careerism, corruption and counter-revolutionary aims. Post-1921, there was a new recruitment drive into the Party, and new members were admitted at a time, when Stalin was General Secretary. The consequence was a massive expansion in the number of Party members from five million in 1923 to 35 million in 1932. There were also attempts to replace 'old Bolsheviks' and tsarist officials with new Stalinists after Lenin's death in 1924, against the background of the power struggles between Stalin and the Left, Right and United Oppositions. After 1928, there was still growing dissatisfaction with Stalin's policies, his style of leadership, division within the Politburo and criticism of Stalin and his policy and decision making from Syrstov, Laminadze and the Ryutin platform. This was the time of various industrial trials – Shakty in

1928, the Industrial party in 1930, Mensheviks in 1931 and Metro-Vickers in 1933. Also after the Shakty trial in early 1928, it was now acknowledged that Party administrators working alongside bourgeois specialists had not been vigilant enough so new measures were required, this included the eradication of 'counter-revolutionary threats from bourgeois specialists' and new drives took place to recruit working class cadres via the mobilisation of communists into higher education.[272] These purges were driven by a perception of political opposition and due to concerns regarding social instability posed by criminals and other alien or dangerous elements. As the collectivisation and industrialisation campaigns were stepped up, coercion or disciplinary measures were used against perceived opposition. These events and new Stalinist strategies would impact upon the medical profession.

Stalinist ideology with its desire to put in place the new 'class line' in medicine and the circumstances in which this was taking place between 1928–40 (industrialisation, collectivisation, planning and widespread disease), together with the various social, economic, cultural and other factors, all shaped the terror and its impact upon the medical profession and health service.

The terror and suspicion of the medical profession was not the product of a particular agency or event but of a general mindset that developed in the formative civil war years.[273] During 1918–20, epidemics were rife and the regime was at stake (see Chapter 2). What this period (1918–20) and Stalinism (1928–41) have in common is a high level of insecurity and health crises, coupled with a strong feeling of 'anti-Bolshevism',[274] and in terms of this book, the association, not really justified, of the old medical profession with the latter. Sarah Davies argues that under Zinoviev, 'Leningrad became a stronghold of the opposition movement within the Party'.[275] Kirov was sent in to quell the dissent but he was murdered in December 1934. The Terror created an 'Us' (workers, peasants, masses) versus 'Them' (other, enemy, non Party members, bureaucrats, Jews) *mentalité*.[276]

We argue here that the use of terror and Soviet health policy go together. In January 1933 one circular from police and health officials concluded: 'The spread of epidemic disease is caused by mobile and unorganised groups within the population'.[277] As is well-known throughout the late 1920s and 1930s, the Stalinist state sought to generate loyalty by granting access to food, commodities and living space, which were linked to the rank of the institution at which Leningrad citizens were employed, a person's place of residence or importance. As we saw earlier in this chapter, the Soviet regime did not fully succeed in achieving this goal. The regime also categorised, identified and monitored the health and other characteristics of the population using officially ascribed social, occupational or other identities, such as social origins, ethnicity or nationality. Towards the end of 1932, passport and residency laws were used to 'cleanse' the population of Leningrad city and oblast, of so-called 'socially harmful' groups including criminals, the unemployed, beggars, prostitutes, itinerants and orphans. These new passport and associated regulations 'affected where a person could live, work and travel and the privileges and rights to which a person had access'.[278]

As in pre-revolutionary times, seasonal workers (*otkhodniki*), rural inhabitants of Leningrad oblast or other regions of Russia, seeking city jobs on a seasonal or permanent basis, were needed in Leningrad, and travelled to and from the city throughout the period 1928–40. Although it was not possible to guarantee the acceptability of the 'social status' of the otkhodniki, which was a concern to police and security services in the 1930s, Leningrad as a 'regime area' had a high demand for labour. Because of this, Shearer notes that 'local officials tended to enforce residency laws loosely'.[279] People who broke the passport or residency laws (by falsifying passport information or migrating illegally) were accused of causing the crime and social disorder outlined by David Shearer. The aforementioned 'undesirable populations' were not just causing social and political contamination, they were also causing diseases – infectious and social, and influenza, for instance – to spread in the city and region of Leningrad, as they moved in, around and out of the area. These groups unintentionally, or in the official mindset deliberately, contributed to the deteriorating health situation in the 1930s, as detailed throughout this chapter. This class war against 'socially alien or dangerous elements'[280] in the early–mid-1930s, also indirectly helped health crises occur. Thus, the medical profession was not just attacked in the purges because it had many of the characteristics of the enemy in the 'them' category, it also more importantly failed to prevent medical disorder.

The Stalinist regime could not cope with the massive social and economic dislocation caused by rapid industrialisation, forced collectivisation and central planning, and this also generated medical chaos. All parts of the state were under severe strain, and the police and security services, were thinly stretched (and inefficient, poorly educated and lacking guidance at least at the start) and in carrying out political surveillance of *déclassé* groups and their actions (thefts of state property, train derailments, the black market, crime and hooliganism, sabotage), they were unable to medically secure the railroads, boats and streets. Militsia and OGPU/NKVD staff were so busy checking for criminals or class enemies, and carrying out sweeps of these groups, that the sick and those with infectious diseases and social diseases slipped through the cordon. The police and security services were unsuccessful in both politically and medically sealing off Leningrad, as the local authorities 'did not have the material resources and manpower to keep a constant registry of whom was coming and going in their precincts'.[281]

The Soviet state saw its role as protecting the health of the collective but its policies had an adverse effect upon the health of the population of Leningrad. The Party needed, without pointing the finger at Stalin and the Soviet leadership, to direct the blame elsewhere. In the mid–late-1930s, the Stalinist state cleansed parts of the medical profession. The victims of the terror served as scapegoats for health policy and government failures and its dire consequences as detailed above. As the health crises increased in scope, and hit more and more sections of the collective, the medical purges were seen as means of survival – survival of the Soviet system, as once again infectious disease and other epidemics threatened the state, as under War

Communism, and so called 'class enemies' were also accused of undermining Stalinist welfare principles. The risk from a regime viewpoint was two-fold: the health crises might destabilise the USSR, and quiet sabotage (*tikhii zapoi*)[282] by former zemstvo doctors, convinced the Party that these 'former people' were now a threat to the Stalinist state.

For example, one article published in *Krasnaia Gazeta* in early July 1929 noted that at the end of one such 'purge', 117 members of the Leningrad oblast public health department were removed from their posts because 'of sluggishness in responding to central directives and other reasons'.[283]

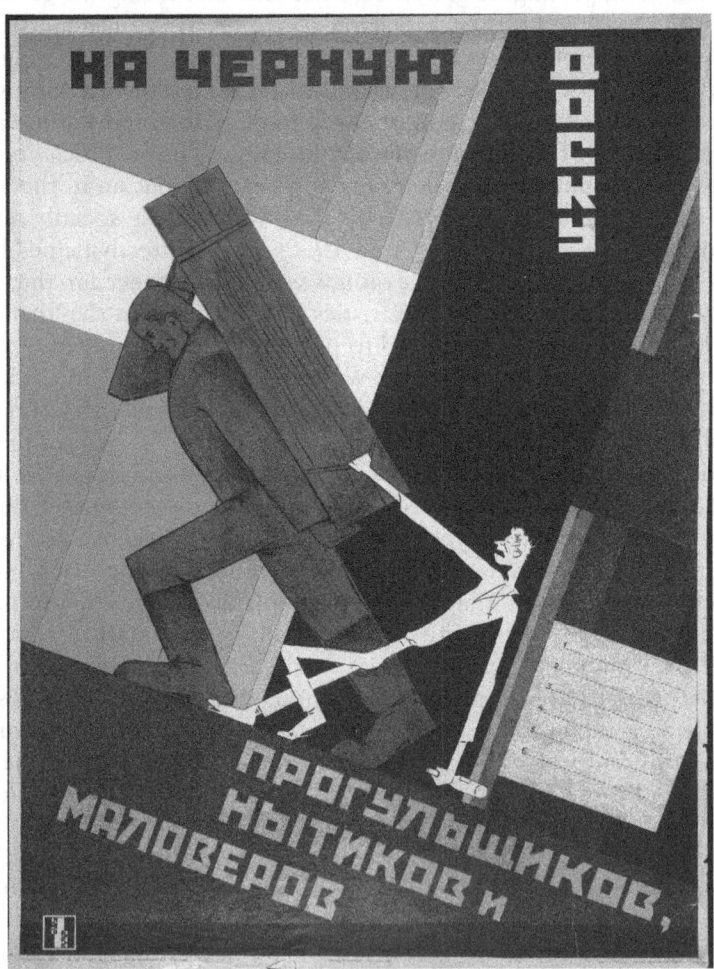

Poster 25 Blacklisting under Stalin

Source: 'On the blacklist – shirkers, whiners and sceptics', Moscow State press
    'Red proletariat' 1930s. Courtesy of Soviet Poster Collection, Swarthmore
    College Peace Collection.

Poster 25 'On the blacklist' criticises those defined as 'shirkers, whiners and sceptics' by the Stalinist regime in the 1930s for not following Party instructions or for criticising government policy. Members of the medical profession were also victims. Archival material now provides more detail on the 'purge' process, the criticisms made, and staff reactions to these accusations. This material reveals the final outcome but not the processes in between. We only possess a summary of the outcomes (dismissal, reprimand) and the grounds for denunciation or complaint, and if the latter was successful or not. There is no indication given on the number of charges that were groundless or if the accusers themselves were punished. We also do not know if these denunciations were examined with great thoroughness or not by the relevant agencies.

The Stalinist regime was able, via the purges, to carry out political and sanitary surveillance at the same time, to create a climate of vigilance, fear and suspicion of the medical profession, to assert its collective power and to protect the health of the collective. The denouncers evoked a Party, trade union and health service response that advanced their interests or highlighted their concerns, such as need for better health care for the insured.

In Leningrad oblast, a major purge was carried out in October 1930 and this hit 300 pharmacists, 118 staff in the mother and infants' department, 123 hospital and 130 non-hospital staff and 123 other staff. In the health sub-departments of the Leningrad regional health system, 70 staff in statistics, 62 in accounting, 51 in planning, 176 in health education, 156 in sanitary-epidemiological work, 131 in first aid and 79 others in personnel and technical observation, were purged.[284] The People's Commissariat of Workers' and Peasants' Inspection (*Rabkin*) review, which was responding to issues raised by the Leningrad branch of TsPS, the Union of Metallurgists and the Leningrad Party about the unsatisfactory care at the Red Putilov and March factories. Denunciations of medical personnel had clearly been sent to the government agency, Rabkin, through the trade unions and Party, who might have been contacted by their members voicing their concern about the provision of medical aid.

Rabkin justified the purge of the Leningrad oblast public health department because of a range of unsatisfactory issues including shortages of key staff such as disinfection brigade personnel, inadequate anti-epidemic measures and a failure to liaise with the Pasteur Bacteriology Institute on inoculations and poor cleanliness and hygiene in urban and especially collectivised rural areas. The 'cleansing' reports criticised staff, especially doctors, for devoting insufficient attention to primary services in enterprises, for not significantly reducing industrial injuries, for not improving conditions of labour in factories, for poor quality preventive and prophylactic work and for failing to abide by the necessary health and safety measures. In addition, food hygiene conditions and other 'sanitary minimums' were not maintained. Particular emphasis was placed on the poor quality of the region's health education work, staff attitude towards labour and failure to change the byt of Leningrad's citizens. Rabkin recommended a structural review, merges to improve efficiency and to ensure that essential sanitary cultural work was carried out in key industrial enterprises, such as the 'Red Putilov' and in factory kitchens.[285] The Rabkin review criticised the quality of medical staff, their qualifications and the lack of specialists, such as X-ray staff and physiotherapists as well as other staff such as dieticians and crèche staff. Some staff were criticised for their inability to adapt to the demands of rapid industrialisation and forced collectivisation not protecting health conditions in the factories and not addressing the new challenges such as epidemics. The quality of first aid offered at enterprises was highlighted as an area of concern and the work of pharmacies, the supply of medicines and dispensary provision for workers in dangerous jobs was criticised. There was also a lack of crèches for factory workers. This also showed the lack of planning and the failure to cater for the medical needs of the insured.[286]

On 1 October 1930, one Leningrad oblast public health department meeting reflected upon the 16th Party Congress resolutions and how well the department was responding to Party policies and goals. It was concluded that there was a failure to protect the standard of living and labour conditions of workers. There was talk of the 'class line' and the need for the regional health service to provide adequate medical aid and meet the needs of workers and peasants. The best way to do this, according to the meeting, was to improve the level of health protection, fight industrial diseases, for health staff to promote a socialist way of life with regards to health and for medical personnel to become a part of building a socialist welfare state. The meeting argued that these changes were needed because the 'apparatus' was inadequate in a number of key respects such as insufficient decision making, not adopting the 'class line', bureaucracy and red tape, lack of rationalisation and a failure to adhere to Party directives. Calls were made following the purge for a 'higher class' of personnel drawn from workers and peasants who were more literate, practically oriented and knowledgeable people.[287]

In 1931, these criticisms of the Leningrad oblast public health department continued amidst discussion of public health and its relationship to socialist construction. At one 1931 meeting concerns about the qualifications of medical staff were highlighted. Criticisms were made of shortages of TB and lungs specialists, physiotherapists and dieticians at enterprises. It was also pointed out that measures against infectious diseases, the hospitalisation of patients and poor public health department liaison with the Zhakty failed to ensure that 'sanitary conditions' in factory crèches (idolised in earlier health posters) were adequate. Health service leaders were criticised for their lack of planning and for the above errors. The purging commission urged greater vigilance and a clearer focus on social diseases (TB), health education, cadres and leadership.[288]

These attacks did not stop at regional level and at the periphery. They also happened at district level. For instance, a meeting was held on 27 October 1930 in the Moscow district public health department in Leningrad, chaired by the President Konovalov and including Party and Medsantrud (trade union) representatives. The meeting highlighted deficiencies in leadership, lack of planning, a failure to follow instructions and a lack of 'labour discipline'. The purge commission stated that sanitary conditions in Moscow district and the level of bureaucracy were 'a cause of concern'. One attendee at the meeting, Bainchikov, acknowledged the shortcomings and blamed them on the deputy head of department who 'sat in their office and had no real knowledge of the workings of the district health service' and so failed to realise that the medical network in Moscow district was in such a 'sorry state'.[289] Other health service workers, such as Viktorov concurred with Bainchikov. Such responses are reminiscent of shop floor disputes. Other unnamed participants shifted the blame from district health service managers and staff onto the trade unions and accused Medsantrud of not protecting its members against purge commission criticisms. Finally, Rumaintsev acknowledged that there were 'organisational problems' and 'medical network issues' which were 'very bad' but the chief doctor was not to blame. They provided strong guidance and leadership. Rumaintsev said that the 'masses' needed to participate in this cleansing process and he also stated that the commission needed to recognise that there are 'abnormal influences affecting the work of medical establishments'. These statements highlight the pressure which Stalin's policies or the medical disorder put on health service managers and staff, and that any problems arising where often beyond their control. Konovalov reached the conclusion after this debate that a 'purge' would not be the most useful tactic in this instance.[290]

District public health department staff were criticised because of the failure to implement the 'face to industry' policy and the relevant medical line towards industry and factories set by the Party and trade unions. Blame was firmly placed upon 'chief doctors' who were criticised for making 'basic mistakes' in their work, for failing to plan their work properly, to follow the rules on health education and to provide the necessary leadership. The purge commission reminded district medical leaders and other personnel that they were required to safeguard the health of workers, combat industrial illnesses and accidents, plan public health work, increase labour productivity and fulfil the goals of the various FYPs. The commission called for greater rationalisation in the utilisation of workers' time and for the reorganisation and reconstruction of public health work to reduce bureaucracy, improve out-patient care and first aid at enterprise medical points, to increase the provision of medical transport facilities and to ensure that doctor's and other staff adopted a more 'personal' approach when treating workers. It was highlighted that doctors must be more easily contactable, more responsive to the sick, able to mobilise resources to the 'right' areas and control the workload of staff and oversee the administrative processes. In line with these changes from 1 January 1931, the commission also advocated the setting up a childrens' committee and maternity department at the Koniashin hospital as in 1930 work was 'unsatisfactory' at this hospital. The commission also criticised the level of food hygiene in Stoloviya No. 22 on International Prospekt No. 41.[291]

In the above reviews, doctors and other medical staff were either labelled 'class enemies' of the state or cleansed in an effort to ensure that health service personnel complied with and followed Party objectives. The implicit accusation made was that a disloyal, unreliable group of 'alien elements' within the health service were responsible for damaging the health of the collective. Whilst purges of the medical profession appeared to be a 'witch hunt' for certain categories of medical staff or as an attempt to eradicate political opposition on the basis of social origins, in reality this strategy was actually geared towards restoring order in certain parts of the health sector during key policy changes. Archival reports paint a picture of the chaos prevailing within the Party, state and health system. The above early 1930s purges were also partly a product of shifting relations with, and within, Leningrad city and region. This analysis allows us to assess the degree of conflicts between the Party and medical profession over health issues under Stalin.

One 1931 report on the Leningrad regional public health department, focused less on the explicit health issues as highlighted earlier, and more on the social composition of the Leningrad oblast health service.[292] In December 1930, when the purge commission reviewed the Leningrad regional health department, it had 240 staff including 47 doctors and five engineers. In terms of social origins: 11.2% were workers; 20.4% peasants; 9% white-collar workers; 17% were petty bourgeois (*meshchanin*); 2% were children of traders; 3.3% were from servant backgrounds; 3.3% were children of clergy; 3.7% were handicraft workers; and the social origins of the remaining 55 people was unknown. As to educational level, 30.8% had primary, 38.4% secondary and 30.8% a higher education. Finally, 20% were Party members, 0.4% candidate members, 2% Komsomol members and 77% (186) non-Party members.[293] In the Party mindset, a correlation was made between the social composition of the Leningrad regional public health department and its failure to plan properly, prevent industrial diseases and injuries, to ensure 'sanitary minimums' were maintained in factory canteens, to monitor the child population and create crèches, to follow the 'class line', to carry out the expected hospital mergers, to organise medical transport and to keep to local budget levels. These failures were said to be hindering progress towards industrialisation and collectivisation in Leningrad oblast.[294]

This review of the social composition of the Leningrad oblast public health department and its relationship to the organisational structure, the degree of economies made, the level of proletarian patronage and of the way in which medical staff were following Party directives in order to improve medical aid to workers and peasants in Leningrad oblast, led to an assessment of certain staff and the purges were used as a way of criticising some medical staff through the well-established 'self criticism' process or to weed out 'alien elements' such as Dmitri Chuzhov, a former officer, who was discontent with Soviet authority and was dismissed on anti-Semitic grounds[295] whilst Mark Brown (Broun), who had worked in the organisation for seven years, was accused of being a weak manager who adopted a 'protectionist attitude', failed to carry out 'mass work' and had not correctly prioritised shock workers, so he was also dismissed.[296]

During the same review, medical personnel in the Leningrad regional health department were also heavily criticised for not adhering to the 'class line' in referring patients to the TB out-patient services (only 40.9% of workers) and for not sending workers to TB sanatoria (only 38%).[297] For instance, A. N. Ivanov, a Leningrad Oblast hospital manager, in relation to the hospitalisation of patients, and Grigorii Besedin, a sanitary or medical inspector, was accused of not understanding the principles of socialist construction of health care. He had failed to consider the 'social class make-up' of hospitalised patients and did not notify the right authorities when a typhoid epidemic broke out. Besedin was reprimanded.[298] Certain members of the Leningrad oblast public health department, such as V. B. Didrikhson who was highly educated, a doctor and a social hygiene specialist, said that accusing his colleagues of disloyalty was like losing a limb ('cutting off one's hand') and that the cleansing process was influencing the effectiveness of health education and other work, though he acknowledged the need for 'cleansing'.[299] Clearly at this point the 'purges' were influencing staff morale and affecting their ability to deal with the health challenges discussed earlier on in this chapter. A good example, is the removal of senior sanitary-epidemiological inspector, Dr. A. A. Filapetov, who had worked from 1918–30 as deputy of the serum-vaccine committee, but was dismissed following this 1930 purge commission review.[300] Filapetov made a statement to the commission defending himself stating that he was professional, well experienced and prepared, had fully planned the logistics of the Leningrad oblast anti-epidemic work and carried out effective anti-epidemic work regarding scarlet fever since 1927 and had acted as an instructor to doctors active in immunization. Scarlet fever was a serious challenge in Leningrad as shown in Table 4.1. Unfortunately for Filapetov, scarlet fever was on the rise by 1930, and had increased by over 6,000 cases between 1928–30. This made him extremely vulnerable to criticism, so he was purged despite his long service and previously valuable work.[301]

Thus, staff were being dismissed or reprimanded for their failure to prevent medical disorder. This review did not just take place midway through the First FYP, it also occurred at a time when epidemics existed, thus there was a smallpox epidemic in 1929–30 and one million people were inoculated, half a million in Leningrad oblast.[302] Having the right staff, in the right place at the right time was essential. From the Party's perspective, those running various parts of the Leningrad oblast public health department were considered 'alien elements' and this flaw was tolerated in earlier periods because the medical profession had proved indispensable to the regime. The value of certain parts of the medical profession was now in doubt in 1930–31. The social backgrounds of medical personnel now became a liability, and this was compounded because of the alleged poor quality of their work in disease prevention, health education work etc. The Party therefore deemed it necessary to remove these 'alien elements' to restore medical order. The Party wanted greater vigilance and regular checks on medical management and staff performance. This was necessary to guarantee their adherence to FYP objectives, to financial plans and to ensure that they carry out adequate health education and sanitary epidemiological work.[303]

Sheila Fitzpatrick argues that

> [d]enunciation as a social practice was greatly encouraged by the regime's decision in the late 1920s to expropriate, deport, and otherwise punish whole categories of class enemies.... 'Bourgeois' (i.e., non-Communist) specialists and 'former people' (members of the old privileged classes) also came under fire at this time. Class enemies, who were prone to conceal their identities, had to be 'unmasked', and denunciation was an important part of this process.[304]

Denunciation was motivated by a denouncers desire to display loyalty to the regime by exposing members of the medical profession who were hiding disreputable pasts or revealing compromising facts such as supporting the Whites in the civil war, links to Opposition to Stalin or the Soviet regime, to foreigners or émigré relatives. Second, such a process was also part of the class war at the time against the old nobility, kulaks, clergy and other class enemies within and finally, denunciations sometimes involved complaints against those abusing power.[305]

A discussion of the 46 denunciation cases in Leningrad regarding medical personnel in 1930–31, 22 of which led to dismissal, will serve to illustrate the point. Examples of those in the first category, 'disreputable pasts', included Nikolai Nikolaev who was sent to prison for speculation in 1919–22,[306] Vlacheslav Nikol'skii who was a White Army doctor,[307] Dimtry Chuzov who was a former Tsarist officer,[308] as was Lev Shamis.[309] Finally, we had Meizr Grodskii whose wife lived in Warsaw and he just allegedly lived off her money.[310] Those in the second category, suspect 'social class', included Iakov Kovarskii and Iser Messel', sons of a trader,[311] Andrei Filapetov whose father was a bank official,[312] Aleksander Rudakov, Mark Broun and Grigorii Gol'dshtein who had merchant backgrounds,[313] Vladimir Abmazov, son of a priest,[314] Vladimir Uglov who came from the gentry and George Beselin who was the son of a landowner.[315] Finally, a few medical staff were accused of abusing their power, such as V. M. Udotov, who had private clients and did so for personal gain.[316]

Thus the 'wrong' past, social class or orientation made medical staff targets and this in addition to a failure to allegedly fulfil their jobs led to the dismissal of staff. These purges of the medical profession were the product the

State's desire to create new medical elite that was 'Red' (Communist) rather than supposedly 'non-Red', that is former tsarist, bourgeois and allegedly unreliable public health and medical experts and to restore medical order. This was part of a deliberate long-term policy geared towards eliminating the 'bourgeois intelligentsia' as a group. This required not just removal but recruiting more medical staff from the working class and peasantry. The Stalinist regime envisaged the gradual replacement of such old tsarist medical personnel with proletarian or working-class cadres. Although the number of students entering the Leningrad medical institute increased from 250 in 1929 to 1,500 by 1931,[317] they were not of the same calibre as earlier intakes and their attitudes and behaviour had also changed. They were no longer in any position to determine precisely how living conditions, the pace of collectivisation and/or industrialisation etc. affected health status or health system development in Leningrad. Growing Party control over this public field had now put an end to any undesired investigations in health-related matters.[318]

The aim was to censor critical thinking. Just as Semashko was replaced in January–February 1930 by Vladimirskii, the Party hack, as the People's Commissar of Public Health for the RSFSR,[319] so Smirnov, who had criticised the second plan variant, was removed from his post as leader of the Leningrad health service. Lamkin took over in early 1931 until his death in August 1932. He was more of a Party technocrat than a medical practitioner. He was a graduate in physics and mathematics, who later took up medicine, and prior to being head of the Leningrad health service he held many military, government and political posts.[320] With the exception of E. Ben, who headed the statistics sub-section of the oblast level public health department, Smirnov's colleagues in other departments also lost their jobs.[321]

In any event, these upwardly mobile working-class medical students, the product of this drive to replace 'bourgeois' medical specialists with 'proletarian' ones, were far more likely to lend their support to the regime 'from below' as they had much to gain in doing so. Medical policy, practice and research would change dramatically in the future as a result.

In 1929, of the 252 graduates from the Leningrad medical institute, 27.4% were of working-class and 21% from peasant backgrounds, the rest came from other backgrounds. This was deemed as unacceptable by the Party. By 1930–31, 52.2% of medical training college (*medtekhnikum*) students were from working-class and 21.8% from peasant backgrounds. The corresponding percentages for higher education medical students were 53.7% and 14.4% respectively, a much greater proportion and more pleasing from a Stalinist regime perspective.[322]

On 1 October 1930, the workers' and peasants' inspectorate (*Rabkin*) carried out one of its periodical reviews of the city of Leningrad health department. The commission, led by Krasnokovskii, justified the move as it was preparing for the Second FYP, and evaluated the composition of the student body in Leningrad medical higher education establishments.

The commission discovered that 80% were of worker and peasant social origins and 52% were members of the Komsomol. Among the 219 post-graduates working for the city of Leningrad health service, 148 (67.5%) were members of Party and 16 (7.3%) Komsomol members but 55 (over a quarter) were still non-Party.[323] It was the non-Party contingent that raised political eyebrows.

Health staff were singled out for criticism for not ensuring that medical student entrants at the Second Medical Institute in Leningrad adhered to government policy, and came from the required social backgrounds. Thus, on 1 December 1930, 35% of them were from the working class and 17% of peasant social origins with the rest coming from white collar workers and handicraft backgrounds. Medical student material circumstances were deemed 'inadequate', many were said to be 'badly trained' and shortages of staff – nine within the regional services and 114 in its periphery organisations had not been filled. Hence existing staff were accused of poor staff management and planning.[324]

During the Second FYP period, another review of the political orientation of teachers and students of medical training college (*medtekhnikum*) was carried out in 1933 to see how much progress had been made. The total number of students was 699 and on entry 44 were Party and 75 Komsomol members, whereas of the 144 evening course students, five were Party and 15 Komsomol members.[325] The number of medical technical college students who were Party or Komsomol members varied according to college from as low as one Party member and two Komsomol members out of 315 students at the Leningrad pharmaceutical college; five Party members out of 210 students at the Fourth Leningrad medical technical college to 43 Komsomol members out of 572 students at the Karl Marx medical technical college. Thus, the state was still struggling to get its new recruits to join the party, which suggests that medical students were rather conservative and more interested in practising medicine than political participation.[326]

The Party might have wanted to remove socially harmful elements – alcoholics, prostitutes, back street abortionists, pimps and drug dealers – and to medically and socially quarantine Leningrad via the passport and residence registration (*propiska*) system to control not just public but medical disorder but the evidence suggests that it was unable to do so for reasons explained above. Blame was placed on the medical profession. This led to sweeps of urban areas such as the city of Leningrad, as well as its more rural parts in Leningrad oblast. This process produced checks on the social backgrounds of medical staff and led to dismissals not for 'political crimes' but because of the failure to deliver the right quality services and to prevent epidemics. Old tsarist doctors and other medical professionals who had cooperated with the Soviet state since the Russian civil war were now purged, sometimes for actual medical reasons and sometimes simply due to their social origins. Both were connected in the Stalinist mindset with medical disorder. This led to the desire to remove these 'bourgeois' medical specialists and to replace them with proletarian cadres. This was part of the late 1920s and onwards mobilisation campaigns to fill the gap in medical students possessing the necessary political and class-conscious skills. As the above analysis shows it was not easy to replace the purged members of the medical profession and so instead of preventing medical disorder, the purges in Leningrad generated further medical disorder and chaos. A new medical elite over time did emerge, but despite these 1929–33 purges and harassment of the medical profession, some of the older tsarist members of the medical profession survived after 1934, and subsequently became victims of the Great and mass terrors between 1934–37, which is the subject of ongoing research.[327] This merely compounded the earlier purges and meant that the health situation declined still further because the newly trained medical students did not have the high quality training and skills to combat the serious health crises, as they experienced rapid promotion during the Great and mass terror, but could not master the seriously deteriorating medical circumstances on the eve of or during the outbreak of war with Finland. This left Leningrad in an increasingly difficult situation prior to the siege.

Conclusion

This chapter has examined the impact which new challenges such as industrialisation, collectivisation and central planning had on the medical system and health conditions in Leningrad between 1928–41. It is clear that the above policies led to the mass influx of workers demanding food, housing, hygiene and health services. The Communist Party responded by urging Narkomzdrav to introduce the First and subsequently two more five-year plans. These FYPs set increasingly ambitious targets. Although some advances in quantitative indicators occurred, many health targets were not fulfilled and this resulted in a dramatic fall in the quality of medical care and standards of living. In Leningrad, too, the first variant of the First FYP for health tended to be modest while the second set targets which were unrealistic and far too ambitious given resource availability. As a result, developments in the health service failed to keep pace with those in the rest of the Leningrad economy. Given the widespread financial constraints operating, a series of priority sectors emerged and health care was still assigned low status in government policies, with planning being used as a means of mobilising resources to fit specific objectives such as the provision of medical care for insured, industrial proletariat, women and children. The demands of industrialisation and collectivisation served only to increase morbidity and mortality, with the introduction of health planning, increasingly based on political aspirations rather than economic realism, exacerbating things still further. Demand for health care exceeded supply and medical facilities; manpower and supplies all failed to expand rapidly enough to keep pace with the population explosion. The Leningrad health system and local authorities responded to these adverse changes by formulating appropriate strategies but their hands were tied by lack of resources, which stemmed from insufficient finance, and ultimately led to the underdevelopment of parts of the medical infrastructure. These problems were further compounded by inefficiency. Serious underfunding whilst still an issue, was overshadowed after the 'great turning point' by the growing subordination of welfare objectives, staff and resources to the political and economic goals of the Stalinist State. For failing to adhere to central policy directives, Semashko was purged from his post as head of Narkomzdrav, and mirroring these events at a local level, Smirnov lost his position as head of the Leningrad Health Service. These top-level purges then occurred at district, city and regional level in Leningrad as health service leaders, administrators and other medical staff started to lose their jobs for failing to prevent medical disorder and in some cases for their disreputable pasts or suspect social origins. As the public health crisis deepened in the mid–late 1930s, so the scope of those deemed 'socially harmful' or 'social dangerous' widened. As a consequence, many medical staff in Leningrad perished in the Great and mass terror of 1934–37. This terrible loss of life led to further public and medical disorder. So the Soviet state and its policies far from protecting the health of the collective actually put it in increasing danger after 1928, and into the 1930s, so the hope of participants in the October Revolution for improved health conditions and care had still not been met by 1941 as war broke out with Nazi Germany and the siege of Leningrad followed.

Acknowledgments

Earlier versions of parts of this chapter have been published in 'The Revolution from above in Soviet medicine, Leningrad 1928–32', *Journal of Urban History,* 20 (4), August 1994, 512–540 and in 'The Modernisation of Russian health care: Challenges, policy, constraints' in J. R. Smith and M. Kangaspuro (eds), *Modernisation in Russia Since 1900* (SKS Helsinki, Studia Fennica Historia, 12, 2006), 206–220.

Notes

1   On this concept see R. C. Tucker, 'Stalinism as Revolution from above', in R. C. Tucker, *Stalinism: Essays in Historical interpretation* (New York 1977) and S. Fitzpatrick, *The Russian Revolution, 1917–32* (Oxford University Press, 1986), Chapter 5.
2   GARF f. A-482 op. 24, d. 952, list 11.
3   GARF f. A-482, op 10, d. 1689, list 1; GARF f. A-482, op. 29, d. 18 list 11; GARF f. A-482, op 47, d. 6164, list 72; TSGAIPD f. 25, op 2, d. 80, list 63–66; *XV let diktatory proletariata: Ekonomiko-statisticheskii sbornik po gor. Leningradu i Leningradskoi oblasti* (Leningrad 1932), 135, 143; *Ves Leningrad: adresnaia i spravochnia kniga 1935* (Leningrad 1935), 2; *Iubilienyi statisticheskii sbornik Sankt-Peterburg 1703–2003,* Vypusk 1 (St. Petersburg 2001), p. 47; N. Cherepenina, 'The demographic situation and health care on the eve of war' in J. Barber and A. Dzeniskevich (ed.), *Life and death in besieged Leningrad, 1941–44* (Palgrave, London 2005), 14, 16.

4 *Iubilienyi statisticheskii sbornik Sankt-Peterburg 1703–2003*, Vypusk 1 (St. Petersburg 2001), 48.
5 *Iubilienyi statisticheskii sbornik Sankt-Peterburg*, 49.
6 Cherepenina, 'The demographic situation and health care', 14.
7 For more discussion see J. Barber, 'The composition of the Soviet working class, 1928–41', CREES, University of Birmingham, SIPS Discussion Paper No. 16, 1978.
8 *XV let diktatory proletariata*, 146.
9 Cherepenina, 'The demographic situation and health care', 15.
10 Ibid., 15.
11 GARF f. A-482, op. 47, d. 6164, list 72.
12 *Okhrana zdorov'ia trudaishchikhsia Leningrada (K vyboram v mestnye sovety deputatov trudaishchikhsia)* (Leningrad Soveta 1939), 10.
13 Catriona Kelly, *Children's World: Growing Up in Russia, 1890–1990* (New Haven and London: Yale University Press, 2007), 1.
14 'Dvizhenie ostrov-zaraznoi zabolevaemosti v Leningrade' *Zdravookhranenie* 1928, No. 2, February, 156; *Zdravookhranenie* 1929, No. 4, 124; *Zdravookhranenie* 1929, No. 7–8, 216; *Zdravookhranenie* 1929, No. 10, 121; *Sotsialisticheskoe zdravookhranenie* February 1931, No. 2, 75; 'Vserossiskoe obshchestvo sotsial'noi i eksperimental'noi gigieny (Leningradskoi otdel)', *Sotsialisticheskoe zdravookhranenie* 1932, No. 10–11, November-December, 62; I. Ia. Vol'fson, 'Organizatsiia bor'by so skarletinoi v Leningrade v 1934/35 godu', *Sovetskia vrachebnaia gazeta* No. 19, 15 October 1935, 1522 and *XV let diktatory proletariata: Ekonomiko-statisticheskii sbornik po gor. Leningradu i Leningradskoi oblasti* (Leningrad 1932), 135.
15 'Dvizhenie' 1928, 156; *Zdravookhranenie* 1929, No. 4, 124; 1929, No. 7–8, 216; 1929, No. 10, 121; *Sotsialisticheskoe zdravookhranenie* February 1931, No. 2, 75; 'Vserossiskoe' 1932,, 62; Vol'fson, 'Organizatsiia bor'by'1935, 1522 and *XV let diktatory proletariata* 1932, 135.
16 F. I. Krasnik, 'Epidemiologicheskaia effektivnost' protivodifteriinykh privivok v Leningrade', *Sovetskii Vrachednyi Zhurnal* No. 1, ianvar' 1941, 58.
17 M. I. Rozanova, 'Organizatsiia protivodifteriinykh privivok v Leningrade', *Sovetskii Vrachednyi Zhurnal* No. 1, ianvar' 1941, 63.
18 Krasnik, 'Epidemiologicheskaia', 58–59.
19 A. F. 'Smertnost' i dozhivaemosti grudnykh i mal'nykh detei v Leningrade', *Sotsialisticheskoe Zdravoohranenie* No. 6–7, June–July 1930, 109.
20 See G. N. Speranskii, 'Gosudarstvennyi nauchnyi institut okhrany materinstva i mladenchestva', *Zhurnal po izucheniyu rannego detskogo vozrasta* No. 3–4 1923, 122 and GARF f. A-482, op. 47, d. 6164, list 72
21 Elizabeth Waters, 'The modernisation of Russian motherhood, 1917–1937', *Soviet Studies* Vol. 44, No. 1, 1992, 123–135.
22 Waters, 'Modernisation of Russian motherhood', 132.
23 J. Berent, 'Causes of fertility decline in Eastern Europe and the Soviet Union', *Population* Studies Volume 24, 1970, 35–58, 247–92; Ch. Blayo and P. Festy, 'La fecondite a l'est et l'ouest de l'Europe', population 1975, 855–888 and R. Andorka, *Determinants of fertility in advanced societies* (London, Methuen 1978).
24 N. V. Lebina, *Povsednevnaia zhizn' sovetskogo naroda: Normy i anomalii. 1920–1930 gody* (St. Petersburg Zhurnal 'Neva' and 'Letnii sad' Izd 1999), 273.
25 By 1 January 1935, women constituted 44.3% of all workers in all branches of labour in Leningrad. 25.7% worked in the metal and electrical industries, 55% in the chemical industry, 78.5% in textiles, 83.8% in the sewing industry and 66.6% in the food industry. Many women entered these occupations during the First five-year plan. Numbers continued to rise so that by 1937, the height of Stalin's

purges, 49.6% of Leningrad blue-collar workers, 21.4% of engineering-technical workers and 66.1% of white-collar employees were women. By 1940, after the introduction of military conscription for men, women constituted almost 60% of the factory labour force (Sarah Davies, 'A Mother's Cares': Women Workers and Popular Opinion in Stalin's Russia, 1934–41' in Melanie Ilic (ed.), *Women in the Stalin Era* (Palgrave, Houndsmills 2001), 90).

26 See A. V. Shakmet, 'Deiatel'nost' Zhenotedlov Leningrade po okhrane materin-stva i detstva (1926–1929)', *Sovetskoe zdravookhranenie* 1980, No. 4, 64–67.
27 *XV let diktatory proletariata*, 143.
28 Lebina, *Povsednevnaia zhizn' sovetskogo naroda*, 272.
29 Ibid., 273.
30 *Statisticheskii spravochnik po gor. Leningrady 1930* (Izd. Leningradskogo ispolkoma 1930), 39 and W. Berelowitch, 'L'evolution de la fécondite légiti-mite a Saint-Petersbourg-Petrograd-Leningrad (1860 – 1926)', *Annales de Demographique historique*, Paris 1982, 261.
31 Wendy Z. Goldman, '"Free Union" and working women: Marriage and mate-rial life in Russia, 1917–1928', paper presented to the American Historical Association New York, December 1985.
32 See Christopher Williams, 'Demographic trends and health conditions in pre- and post-revolutionary Russia: the case of St. Petersburg/Petrograd/Leningrad, 1897–1927', paper presented to the Wellcome unit for the history of medicine, University of Oxford, 24 May 1988, 28–30.
33 GARF f. A-482, op 24, d. 13, list 2.
34 Alice W. Field, *Protection of Women and children in Soviet Russia* (Gollancz, London 1932), chapter 4; F. W. Halle, *Women in Soviet Russia* (Routledge, London 1933), 139 and A. Newsholme and J. A. Kingsbury, *Red Medicine: Socialised health in Soviet Russia* (Heinemann, London 1934), 180–187.
35 GARF f. A-482, op 24, d. 13, lists 2–3.
36 GARF f. A-482, op 24, d. 13, list 2.
37 GARF f. A-482, op 24, d. 13, list 4.
38 'Aborty za platu', *Gigiena i zdorov'e rabochei sem'i* No.8, April 1927, 16.
39 'Aborty v Leningrade', *Gigiena i zdorov'e rabochei sem'i* No.23, December 1930, 16.
40 TsGA SPb f. 7384 op. 2, d. 52, lists 12–13 cited in N. B. Lebina, '"V obstanovke sovetskikh bolnits" (Novye dokumenty o sovetskoi abortnoi politike pervoi poloviny 1930-kh-gg)', *Noveishnaia istoriia* No. 2, 2014, 175–177.
41 *Pravda* 28 May 1936.
42 Ibid.
43 'O zapreshchenii abortov, uvelichenii material'noi pomoshchi rozhenitsam, ustanovlenii gosudarstvennoi pomoshchi mnogosemeinym, rasshirenii seti rodil'nykh domov, detskikh iaslei i detskikh sadov, usilenii ugolovnogo naka-zaniia za neplatezh alimentov i o nekotorykh izmeneniiakh v zakonodatel'stve o razvodakh. Postanovlenie TsIK i SNK SSSR 27 iiunia 1936 goda', *Kodeks zakonov o brake, sem'e i opeke* (Moscow: Yuridicheskoe izdatel'stvo NKIu SSSR, 1937), 86–95.
44 Davies, 'A Mother's Cares', 62.
45 GARF f. A-482, op. 29, d. 20, lists 17, 19.
46 Lebina, *Povsednevnaia zhizn'*, 289.
47 Ibid.
48 See Lebina, *Povsednevnaia zhizn'* 1999, 289–290 for an example of one such 23-year-old from Borovich district in Leningrad oblast in April 1941.
49 'Tezisy doklada zadachi zdravookhraneniia v tret'ei piatiletke' (1938) in GARF f. A-482, op. 24, d. 1128, lists 2–3.

50 'Tezisy doklada zadachi zdravookhraneniia v tret'ei piatiletke' (1938) in GARF f. A-482, op. 24, d. 1128, lists 3–4.

51 'Ob'iansnitel'naia zapiska k materialam po III-mu piatiletnemy planu zdravookhraneniia RSFSR 1038–1942gg' (1938) in GARF f. A-482, op. 24, d. 1112, list 2.

52 See N.S. Nazarova, *Iasel'noe stroitel'stvo: Printsipy planirovki i elementy iaslei* (Moscow, Leningrad, 1934, 32

53 GARF f. A-482, op. 10, d. 2839, list 115.

54 Natalia.Chernyaeva, 'Childcare manuals and construction of motherhood in Russia, 1890–1990', unpublished PhD in Women's Studies, University of Iowa 2009, 147.

55 Chernyaeva, 'Childcare manuals', 147.

56 Michael Z. David, 'Vaccination against TB with BCG: A study of innovation in Soviet public health, 1925–41' in Frances L. Bernstein, Christopher Burton and Dan Healey (ed.), *Soviet Medicine: Culture, practice and science* (Northern Illinois University Press, Dekalb Illinois 2010), 134.

57 David, 'Vaccination against TB with BCG', 138.

58 Dr Nesline, 'The fight against tuberculosis in the RSFSR' in *La Lutte contre de la tuberculose dans la RSFSR* (Moscow-Leningrad 1934), 5–6.

59 *VKP (b) o sotsial'nom strakhovanii* (Moscow 1940), 42–46.

60 'Kurorty, sanatoria, doma otdyakha v pervim cohered vedushchim ostrasliam proizvodstva', *Voprosy strakhovanie* 1931, No. 14, 10.

61 D. Antoshkin (ed.), *VKP(b) i profsoiuzy o sotsial'nom strakhovanii* (Moscow 1934), 36. For a discussion of Sochi as a health resort see Johanna Conferio, 'Inventing the subtropics: An environmental history of Sochi, 1929–36', *Kritika: Explorations in Russian and Eurasian History* Volume 16, No. 1, Winter 2015 (New series), 91–120.

62 Jack Minkoff, 'The Soviet Social Insurance system since 1921', PhD Dissertation, Faculty of Political Science, Columbia University, 1960, 295–296.

63 Minkoff, 'Soviet social Insurance system since 1921', 296.

64 Ibid., 292.

65 David, 'Vaccination against TB with BCG', 139.

66 Ibid., 140–141.

67 Ibid., footnote 61,141.

68 Ye. E. Ben et al, 'Tuberkuleznaia zabolevaemost' i smertnost' sredi batsilliarnykh kontaktov v Leningrade' in Ye. E. Ben et al, *Voprosy sotsial'noi gigieny tuberkuleza* (Izd. Kargosizdata Leningrad 1939), 15.

69 Ben et al, 'Tuberkuleznaia zabolevaemost' i smertnost', 18, 29–30.

70 Ibid., 31, 34.

71 Ibid., 40.

72 Ibid., 41.

73 See Stephen Kotkin, *Magnetic Mountain: Stalinism as a Civilization* (University of California Press, Berkeley, 1995), 204 on protection of workers in Magnetogorsk.

74 For an example of conflicts during Stakhanovist period in Magnitogorsk see Kotkin, *Magnetic Mountain* 1995, 214. For a useful discussion of this issue before 1917 see S. A. Smith, 'Workers against foremen in St. Petersburg, 1905–197' in L. H. Siegelbaul and R. G. Suny (ed.), *Making workers Soviet: Power, class and identity* (Cornell University Press, Ithaca and London 1994), 113–137.

75 Kotkin, *Magnetic Mountain*, 319.

76 Laura L. Phillips, *Bolsheviks and the Bottle: Drink and worker culture in St. Petersburg, 1900–1929* (Northern Illinois University Press: Dekalb 2000), 19–20.

77 'Bor'ba s alkogolizmom', *Gigiena i zdorov'e rabochei sem'i* No.13, July 1930, 1.

78 Ibid.

79 Phillips, *Bolsheviks and the Bottle*, 20.
80 Ye. D. Tverdikova, '"O pivnom uklone i torgashchevskikh izrashcheniiakh": torgovliia alkogolem v Leningrade 1930-kh-gg', *Noveishaia istoriia Rossii* No.2, 2012, 89.
81 'Novye zakony protiv alkogolizma', *Gigiena i zdorov'e rabochei sem'i* No. 10, May 1929, 12.
82 B. Sigal, 'Pervye itogi antialkogol'noi bor'by', *Gigiena i zdorov'e rabochei sem'i* No. 3, February 1930, 2.
83 'Protiv starogo vraga', *Gigiena i zdorov'e rabochei sem'i* No. 24, December 1929, 7and Sigal, 'Pervye itogi antialkogol'noi bor'by', 2.
84 Tverdikova, '"O pivnom uklone"', 89–90.
85 Ibid., 91–93.
86 A survey of 223,000 enterprises found that in one month alone in 1928, 22,000 days were lost due to absenteeism caused by drinking and in 1928, this cost the economy 225 million roubles. (I. Sazhin, 'Vypivka i proguly', *Gigiena i zdorov'e rabochei sem'i* No. 14, June 1929, 2).
87 83 A. Mendel'son, 'Dekret protiv p'ianstvo', *Gigiena i zdorov'e rabochei sem'i* No. 24, December 1928, 12 and 'Na alkogol'nom fronte;', *Gigiena i zdorov'e rabochei sem'i* No. 1, January 1929, 3.
88 Phillips, *Bolsheviks and the Bottle*, 22, footnote 34.
89 Ibid., 23.
90 See 'Kto prichaet detei k spiritnym napitkam' poster 1930 Hoover Institution Archives poster no. RU/SU 613 available at http//www.politicalposters.hoover.org/poster/rusu-613 (accessed 28.09.2016) . A study of 6,641 questionnaires from school pupils in Moscow-Narva district of Leningrad in 1931 showed for example that 3,014 (or 47.5% of pupils) abstained from drinking whilst 3,325 (or 52.5%) drank alcohol. Of this sample, 37.6% of children's parents both drank; in 55.9% of cases only the father drank; in 6% only the mother drank and in 0.5% of cases their relatives drank alcohol (S, 'Deti i alkogolizm', *Gigiena i zdorov'e rabochei sem'i* No. 10, April 1931, 11). As regards to who introduced them to drink as young as 4 years old, it was acquaintances (30.5%), elders (12.2%), both parents (5.4%), father (14%), mother (3.8%), friends (10.1%) and ironically the doctor (1.5%) (S, 'Deti i alkogolizm', *Gigiena i zdorov'e rabochei sem'i* No. 10, April 1931, 11).
91 See 'Doloi tserkovye prazdniki!' (Down with religious holidays) 1929 poster which depicts two drunken workers, one with a cross around their neck, and discouraging celebrating religious holidays by heavy drinking. It implies that church holidays led to hooliganism, fights and drunkenness. It was part of Soviet atheism but also served the anti-alcohol purpose detailed here. See Hoover Institution Archives poster no. RU/SU 1674 available at http//www.politicalposters.hoover.org/poster/rusu-1674 (accessed 28.09.2016).
92 Mendel'son, 'Dekret protiv p'ianstva', 1928, 12.
93 'Na alkogol'nom fronte;' January 1929, 3.
94 Ibid.
95 'Novye zakony protiv alkogolizma;', *Gigiena i zdorov'e rabochei sem'i* No. 10, May 1929, 12.
96 Statisticheskii spravochnik po Leningradu 1930g (Leningrad 1930), 36 and B. Sigal, 'Pervye itogi antialkogol'noi bor'by', 1930, 2.
97 Phillips, *Bolsheviks and the Bottle*, 26.
98 Ibid., 36, 60.
99 Lebina, *Povsednevnaia zhizn' sovetskogo naroda* 1999, 36 and Tverdikova, '"O pivnom uklone"', 2012, 96
100 Tricia Starks, *The Body Soviet: Propaganda, Hygiene and the Revolutionary State* (Madison: University of Wisconsin Press, 2009), 5.

101 Starks, *The Body Soviet*, 187.
102 Ibid., 210.
103 T. Sosnovy, *The housing problem in the Soviet Union* (Research Program on the USSR, New York 1954), 50–52.
104 'Housing space' in Soviet parlance excludes kitchens, bathrooms, toilets etc (A. Block, 'Soviet housing – the historical aspect', *Soviet Studies*, Volume V, January 1954, 247, footnote 2.
105 Sosnovy, *The housing problem in the Soviet Union* 1954, 107 and *XV let diktatory proletariat* 1932, 170.
106 District dwelling space figures in m² varied as follows:

District	Year				
	1928	*1929*	*1930*	*1931*	*1932*
Vasileostrovskii	8.9	8.6	7.9	7.1	5.9
Volodarskii	7.2	6.9	6.4	5.6	4.7
Vyborg	8.1	7.8	7.2	5.8	4.8
Moscow	6.2	6.0	5.6	5.4	4.5
Narva	5.9	5.6	5.5	5.3	4.4
October	8.7	8.3	7.7	6.6	5.7
Petrograd side	9.6	9.1	8.5	7.5	6.3
Smol'nyi	10.2	9.8	9.1	7.7	6.4

(*XV let diktatory proletariat* 1932, 170)

107 There was a shortage of skilled and experienced housing construction workers as early as May 1928 (Stroitel'nye nedochety', *Krasnaia Gazeta* 12 May 1928, 3) and as late as July 1931, houses were started by not completed due to a lack of cement ('Zhilishnaia stroika, zhdet novaykh stroii materialov', *Krasnaia Gazeta* 23 July 1931, 4). On bureaucracy and supply problems see 'Vysokami tempami – k sotsializmu', *Krasnaia gazeta* 14 January 1928, 3 and ('Zhilishnaia stroika vse eshche bez oburudovaniia', *Krasnaia Gazeta* 20 February 1932, 4).
108 The First FYP for housing was only fulfilled by 55.4% which impacted on all cities including Leningrad (T. Sosnovy, 'The Soviet housing situation today', *Soviet Studies* Volume XI, No. 1, July 1959, 2).
109 A. Block, 'Soviet housing – the historical aspect: Some notes on problems of policy – II', *Soviet Studies*, Volume III, January 1952, 245. As early as 1928, the housing lease cooperative societies (*Zhakty*) were giving priority in house building and allocation to workers in the metalworking industry (see 'Premii; "Kr. Gazeta" prisuzhdeny', *Krasnaia Gazeta* 10 January 1928, 4).
110 On this see 'kvartiry demobilizanovym', *Krasnaia Gazeta* 17 August 1928, 4 and 'Rabota i kvartiry demobilizannym krasnoarmeitsam' *Krasnaia Gazeta* 29 September 1928, 3.
111 *XV let diktatory proletariata*, 166.
112 *Ekonomiko-statisticheskii sbornik po gor. Leningradu i Leningradskoi oblasti* 1932), 166.
113 S. Moiseev, 'Ob eksploatsii i korenom perestroika suschet vuiushchikh vodoprodov i kanalizatsii i proektirovanii novykh', *Zdravookhranenie* No. 1, January 1929, 44–60.
114 *XV let diktatory proletariata*, 121.
115 'Vse mery za bor'by s zhilishchnym krizisom' *Krasnaia Gazeta* 4 January 1928, 3.

116 See for instance 'Kachestvo zhilishcnoi stroiki ne na vysote', *Krasnaia Gazeta* 23 February 1932, 4.

117 'Chto obnarzhili chleny soveta' *Krasnaia Gazeta* 7 April 1928, 3. At a Leningrad council meeting in June 1928, it was necessary to slow construction of the new Vasileostrovskii sewerage system down because of shortage of money, labour and serious faults in work already completed (Rudakov, 'Obledenie vasileostrovskoi kanalizatsii', *Krasnaia Gazeta* 6 June 1928, 7).

118 V. Belusov, 'Novyi zakon o kvartiroplate', *Krasnaia gazeta* 30 October 1928, 3.

119 '"kulak" v zhilishchnom khozyiastve', *Krasnaia Gazeta* 20 February 1930, 4 and 'Vyiasleno 129 tysiach kv. Metrov zhiloi ploshchadi', *Krasnaia Gazeta* 7 March 1930, 4.

120 Thus only 2,500 out of the 30–40,000 Red Army personnel and local residents were allocated their housing between July 1928-January 1929 despite availability (A. L. 'Desiatki vysiach kv. Metrov zhiloploshchadi ne ispol'zuitsia', *Krasnaia Gazeta* 15 October 1929, 3).

121 M. Baliashnikov and D. Fillipenok, 'Edinym frontam na bor'bu za sotsialisticheskie zhilishcha', *Krasnaia Gazeta* 19 June 1931, 4.

122 'Zhilstroi ne spravliaetsia s zadaniem', *Krasnaia Gazeta* 10 March 1932, 4 and 'Novoe pravlenie obzhilishchsoiuza', *Krasnaia Gazeta* 21 June 1931, 4.

123 'Pervaia obshchegorodskaia konferentsiia po kachestvu zhilostroi', *Krasnaia Gazeta* 11 June 1932, 4 and 122; 'Raizhiloiuzy ne spravilis' s remontov domov', *Krasnaia Gazeta* 29 August 1932, 4.

124 'Olga P. Filipova' in M. Vitukhovskaia (ed.), *Na korme vremeni: inter'viu s Leningradtsami 1930-kh godov* (St. Petersburg: Zhurnal 'Neva' 2000), 230–231.

125 G. E. Al', 'Zhilishchnye usloviia tuberkuleznykh vatsillovydeletelei v Leningrade' in Ye. E. Ben et al, *Voprosy sotsial'noi gigieny tuberkuleza* (Izd. Kargosizdata Leningrad 1939), 58, 60.

126 Ibid., 62–63.

127 Ibid., 72–75.

128 Ibid., 77.

129 Sosnovy, *The housing problem in the Soviet Union*, 66.

130 Ibid., 83.

131 *Trud v SSSR: Statisticheskii spravochnik 1936* (Moscow 1936), 376.

132 'Lilian A. Issakian' in M. Vitukhovskaia (ed.), *Na korme vremeni: inter'viu s Leningradtsami 1930-kh godov* (St. Petersburg: Zhurnal 'Neva' 2000), 249.

133 Minkoff, 'Soviet social Insurance system since 1921', 13.

134 *Okhrana zdorov'ia trudaishchikhsia Leningrada (K vyboram v mestnye sovety deputatov trudaishchikhsia)* Leningrad Soveta, 1939, 9.

135 GARF f. A-482, op. 26, d, 37, list 94.

136 *Analiz sanitarnykh meropriatii po RSFSR az 2-go piatiletku i perspektivy za 3-iu piatiletku tom 1-i (1937)'* in GARF f. A-482, op 24. D. 952, list 17 and '*Plan 3-i piatiletka po zdravookhraneniiu 1938–1942gg tom 2'* in GARF f. A-482 op. 26, d. 37, list 94.

137 TsGAIPD SPb f. 25, op 2v, d. 4282, list 12.

138 TsGAIPD SPb f. 25, op 2v, d. 4282, list 12, 15.

139 TsGAIPD SPb f. 25, op 2v, d. 4282, list 15.

140 TsGAIPD SPb f. 25, op 2v, d. 4282, list 127–128.

141 For example, Lositskii's mass food surveys were discontinued by the late 1920s (See S. G. Wheatcroft, 'Statistics and economic decision-making in the USSR under Stalin', CREES, University of Birmingham Discussion Paper 1979, 6–13).

142 A. A. Barsov, *Balans stoimostnykh obmenov mezdu gorodom i derevnei* (Moscow 1969), 90.

143 M. Lewin, 'The immediate background to Soviet collectivisation', *Soviet Studies* Volume 17, No. 2, 1965–66, 184.

144 A. Erlich, 'Development strategy and planning: The Soviet experience' in M. Millikan (ed.), *National economic planning* (Columbia University Press, 1967), 267.

145 Arvind Vyas, *Consumption in a Socialist economy: The Soviet industrialisation experience, 1929–37* (People's Publishing House, New Delhi 1978), 119–20,159. For more detail see Chapter 8.

146 John Barber, 'The standard of living of Soviet industrial workers, 1928–41' in *L'industrialisation de l'URSS dans les annees trente. Actes de la table Ronde organises par le Centre d'etudes des Modes Industrialisaton de l'ecole des Hautes Etudes en sciences sociales* (Paris 1982), 116.

147 S. G. Wheatcroft, 'Famine and factors affecting mortality in the USSR: The demographic crises of 1914–22 and 1930–33: Appendices', University of Birmingham SIPS Discussion Paper No. 20, 1981, 25.

148 Lesley A. Rimmel, 'Another kind of fear: The Kirov murder and the end of Rationing in Leningrad', *Slavic Review* Volume 56, No. 3, Autumn 1997, 483 and O. Khlevniuk and R. W. Davies, 'The end of rationing in the Soviet Union, 1934–35', *Europe-Asia Studies* Volume 51, No. 4, 1999, 559. 158 On the four rationing categories prevailing see 'Novyi poriadok snabzheniia naseleniia produktami',*Krasnaia Gazeta* 26 October 1929, 4.

149 Khlevniuk and Davies, 'The end of rationing' 1999, 562.

150 Barber, 'The standard of living', 1982, 111; Khlevniuk and Davies, 'The end of rationing' 1999, 560.

151 Khlevniuk and Davies, 'The end of rationing', 562.

152 Ibid.

153 Barber, 'The standard of living', 111.

154 'Olga P. Filipova' in M. Vitukhovskaia (ed.), *Na korme vremeni: inter'viu s Leningradtsami 1930-kh godov* (St. Petersburg: Zhurnal 'Neva' 2000), 229, 232–233.

155 Sarah Davies, *Popular opinion in Stalin's Russia: Terror, propaganda and dissent, 1934–1941* (Cambridge University Press, 1997), 27.

156 Rimmel, 'Another kind of fear', 1997, 484, 487 and 493–494 (Korodev's view is from TsGAIPD f. 25, op. 5, d. 45, list 105).

157 Rimmel, 'Another kind of fear', 496–497.

158 Davies, *Popular opinion in Stalin's Russia*, 28–29.

159 Ibid., 29.

160 The city needed 28 tons of flour but only 13 tons arrived in January and levels fell to eight tons by February 1935 (TsGAIPD f. 24 op 2v, d. 1188, lists 141–142 cited in Rimmel, 'Another kind of fear', 1997, footnote 86, 497)

161 Davies, *Popular opinion in Stalin's Russia*, 29.

162 Khlevniuk and Davies, 'The end of rationing' 1999, 558, 576 and S. G. Wheatcroft, 'Famine and factors' 1981, 20–23.

163 Davies, *Popular opinion in Stalin's Russia*, 35.

164 Barber, 'The standard of living', 113.

165 Davies, *Popular opinion in Stalin's Russia*, 24–25.

166 TsGAIPD SPb f. 25 op. 5, d. 25, lists 2–3.

167 Davies, *Popular opinion in Stalin's Russia*, 40–42.

168 M. I. Kunkite, 'Izmeneniia biudzheta vremeni i deneg Leningradtsev v 1940 godu: Rasskepechenie materialy TsGAPID SPb' in M. I. Kinkite (ed.), *Seminary Peterburgskogo istorika Marii Kunkite 'Istoricheskii kontekst: pravilo bez iskliuchenii'* (St. Petersburg 2013), 13–14. I am grateful to Yury Basilov, European University St. Petersburg for supplying this source.

169 Davies, *Popular opinion in Stalin's Russia*, 42.

170 Kunkite, 'Izmeneniia biudzheta', 16.

171 Ibid.

172 D. Filtzer, *The Soviet workers and Stalinist industrialisation: The formation of modern Soviet production relations, 1928–1941* (Pluto Press, London 1986), 7.

173 See Stephen Kotkin, *Magnetic Mountain: Stalinism as a Civilization* (University of California Press, Berkeley, 1995) for a case study of Magnitogorsk which picks up similar themes to those highlighted here including living in filthy, over-crowded housing, the pressures of working in a planned economy, bureaucracy, a blame culture, fears about the 'peasantization' of urban life etc showing that Leningrad had some things in common with other industrial cities as well as its own distinctiveness.

174 Named after Aleksei Stakhanov, the Donbass miner who mined a record 102 tons of coal in a single shift on 30 August 1935.

175 Competition led to declining quality. For instance, bakers in Leningrad put water in bread to meet competition agreement targets (*Trud* 26 June 1929 cited in Filtzer, *The Soviet workers and Stalinist industrialisation* 1986, 75).

176 D. Filtzer, 'Labor discipline, the use of work time and the decline of the Soviet system, 1928–1991', *International Labor and working class history* No. 50, Fall 1996, 15.

177 H. Kuromiya, *Stalin's Industrial Revolution: Politics and Workers, 1928–1932* (Cambridge University Press 1988), 92–93.

178 Filtzer, 'Labor discipline', 22.

179 For example, in Spring 1929 and dock workers in 1930 see Filtzer, *The Soviet workers and Stalinist industrialisation* 1986), 82–83.

180 George M. Price MD, *Labour Protection in Soviet Russia* (London, Modern Books Limited 1929), 61, 63, 68–70, 78–80, 83.

181 Price, *Labour Protection in Soviet Russia*, 83–93.

182 N. A. Vigdorchik, *Piat let raboty Leningradskogo institute po izucheniiu professional'nykh zabolevanii* (Moscow-Leningrad 1929), 8–12.

183 Melanie Ilic, 'Soviet protective labour legislation and female workers in the 1920s and 1930s', in Marianne Liljerstrom, Eila Mantysaari and Arja Rosenholm (eds), *Gender restructuring in Russian Studies* (Slavica Tamperensia II, Tampere 1993), 127–138.

184 Lewis H. Siegelbaum, 'Okhrana Truda: Industrial hygiene, psychotechnics, and industrialisation in the USSR', in Susan Gross Solomon and John F. Hutchinson (eds), *Health and Society in Revolutionary Russia* (Indiana University Press, Bloomington and Indianapolis, 1990), 228.

185 On average, the industrial worker changed jobs every eight months in 1930; every nine months in 1932; every 14 months in 1936–37; every 17 months in 1938 and every 13 months in 1939 (Filtzer, *The Soviet workers and Stalinist industrialisation*, 135).

186 In 1934–35, Leningrad heavy industry factories had an average of 100 cases of lateness per month officially but Filtzer argues this underestimates the real situation as there was a 15-minute leeway and even if workers were more than 15 minutes late, this was not recorded (Filtzer, *The Soviet workers and Stalinist industrialisation*, 135).

187 Thus 630 doctors' notes were issued in July 1940 alone in the Karl Marx Engineering factory so that workers absences could become official and work-ers did not get dismissed (*Trud* 13 September 1940 cited in Filtzer, *The Soviet workers and Stalinist industrialisation*, 241).

188 These were the subject of health campaigns see "Bor'ba s iadami' poster 1927 Hoover Institution Archives poster no. RU/SU 1567 available at http//www.politicalposters.hoover.org/poster/rusu-1567 (accessed 13.10.2016) which illustrates the safety measures and legislation in industrial enterprises dealing with poisonous substances and 'Promyshlennye lady i profess. Otraveleniia' poster 1927 Hoover Institution Archives Poster no. RU/SU 1566 available at

http//www.politicalposters.hoover.org/poster/rusu-1566 (accessed 13.10.2016), which shows the causes and results of industrial poisonings to Soviet workers at the end of NEP, on eve of Stalin era.

189 TsGAIPD SPb f. 24, op 2v, d. 4412, list 28.
190 Siegelbaum, 'Okhrana Truda', 229.
191 I. Vol'fson, Byt rabochikh 'Krasnogo Putilovtsa' (Po materialam dispansernogo obsledovaniia), *Voprosy Zdravookhraneniia* 1929, No. 12, 56–60.
192 Ia. Davidovich, 'Rabota Leningradskoi trudsessii', *Voprosy Truda* 1929, No. 5, 88.
193 TsGAIPD SPb f. 24, op 2v, d. 4412, list 28.
194 '14,000 bol'nichnykh otrazov: kak rabotaet zdravotdel v Narvskom raione', *Leningradskaia Pravda* 25 March 1931, 4.
195 *Sotsialisticheskoe stroitel'stvo SSSR: Statisticheskii ezhegodnik* (Moscow 1935), 540.
196 V. I. Barbarin, 'Glaznoi travmatizm po zavodu "Znamia Truda" No. 1', *Gigiena bezopasnosti i patologiia truda* 1931, No. 12, 88.
197 S. Shmerling and R. Zaks, 'O vlianii tekuchesti rabochei bor'by s nei', *Stsialisticheskoe Zdravookhranenie* 1931, No. 6, 10, 12.
198 N. Sternin, 'Puti snizheniia zabolevaemosti', *Gigiena i zdorov'e rabochei sem'i* No. 19–20, July 1932, 9. An October 1930 law made it possible to confiscate ration cards and to evict workers from factory housing and a15 November 1932 law made absentees, without good reason, liable to immediate dismissal (Filtzer, *The Soviet workers and Stalinist industrialisation* 1986, 112), but labour shortages made management in Leningrad reluctant to adhere to such rules (see *Trud* 17 December 1932) and if anyone was fired they were taken on in another workshop in the same factory (see the example for Kirov engineering and metallurgical workers in Leningrad in July 1936 in Filtzer, *The Soviet workers and Stalinist industrialisation* 1986, 137).
199 'Luchshiiu meditsinskiiu pomoshch' rabochim promyshlennykh raionov', *Gigiena i zdorov'e rabochei sem'i* No. 21, July 1931, 1.
200 *XV let diktatory proletariata*, 114.
201 Ye. Ye. Grigor'ev and N. A. Vigdorchik (ed.), *Trudy iubileinoi nauchnoi sessii institute (15–19 iiunia 1939g)* (Izd. Instituta gigieny truda i profzabolevanii Lengorzdravotela Leningrad 1940), 22–23.
202 'Bol'nye bez nadzora', *Krasnaia Gazeta* 2 November 1928, 4.
203 Ye. Poliakov, M. Khaiutin and P. El'manovich, 'O roli polikliniki v bor'be za snizhenie zabolevaemosti na promyshlennom predpriiatii', *Sovetskii Vrachebnyi Zhurnal* 1937, No. 11, 847, 849.
204 N. A. Vigdorchik, *Statisticheskii analiz dannykh o rabote Leningradskikh VTEK-ov va poslednie gody* (Leningrad 1941), 4.
205 Vigdorchik, *Statisticheskii analiz VTEK*, 9.
206 Ibid., 23.
207 Grigor'ev and Vigdorchik, *Trudy iubileinoi*, 27.
208 Christopher M. Davis, Economic problems of the RSFSR Health system, 1921–30', CREES, University of Birmingham SIPS Discussion Paper No. 19, 1978, 46–48.
209 See Christopher M. Davis, 'Economics of Soviet public health, 1928–1932: Development strategy. Resource constraints and health plans' in Susan Gross Solomon and John F. Hutchinson (ed.), *Health and Society in Revolutionary Russia* (Indiana University Press, Bloomington and Indianapolis, 1990), 128–128, 164–165
210 Cited in Davis, 'Economics of Soviet public health', 150.
211 Davis, 'Economic problems of the RSFSR Health system', 47, 53.
212 Ibid., 56.
213 Ibid., 60.
214 Ibid., 61.

215 For instance, planned increases in hospitals, medical facilities and medical personnel were all more marked in the second as compared to the first variant of the FYP for health (Christopher M. Davis, 'The Soviet medical system during 1928–32: Development strategy. Resource constraints and health plans' revised version of a paper presented to conference on Russian and Soviet public health, University of Toronto, 31 May 1987).

216 *Finansovoi plan organov zdravookhraneniia na 2-e piatiletie (1-i tur) 1933–37gg t. 1'* in GARF f. A-482 op 26, d. 26, list 25.

217 '*Analiz vypolneniia plana i piatiletiia v oblasti bor'by s epidemiami t. 2* (1937) in GARF f. A-482, op. 24, d. 953, lists 2–3.

218 '*Analiz vypolneniia plana i piatiletiia v oblasti bor'by s epidemiami t. 2* (1937) in GARF f. A-482, op. 24, d. 953, lists 7–9.

219 '*Analiz vypolneniia plana i piatiletiia v oblasti bor'by s epidemiami t. 2* (1937) in GARF f. A-482, op. 24, d. 953, lists 10–11.

220 '*Analiz vypolneniia plana i piatiletiia v oblasti bor'by s epidemiami t. 2* (1937) in GARF f. A-482, op. 24, d. 953, lists 17–22.

221 '*Analiz vypolneniia plana i piatiletiia v oblasti bor'by s epidemiami t. 2* (1937) in GARF f. A-482, op. 24, d. 953, lists 22–25.

222 '*Analiz vypolneniia plana i piatiletiia v oblasti bor'by s epidemiami t. 2* (1937) in GARF f. A-482, op. 24, d. 953, list 31.

223 '*Analiz vypolneniia plana i piatiletiia v oblasti bor'by s epidemiami t. 2* (1937) in GARF f. A-482, op. 24, d. 953, list 34–37.

224 '*Analiz vypolneniia plana i piatiletiia v oblasti bor'by s epidemiami t. 2* (1937) in GARF f. A-482, op. 24, d. 953, list 47–48.

225 '*Analiz vypolneniia plana i piatiletiia v oblasti bor'by s epidemiami t. 2* (1937) in GARF f. A-482, op. 24, d. 953, list 59–61.

226 *Plan 3-i piatiletka po zdravookhraneniiu 1938–1942gg tom 1* in GARF f. A-482 op. 26, d. 36, lists 1–2.

227 *Plan 3-i piatiletka po zdravookhraneniiu 1938–1942gg tom 1* in GARF f. A-482 op. 26, d. 36, lists 23–26.

228 *Plan 3-i piatiletka po zdravookhraneniiu 1938–1942gg tom 1* in GARF f. A-482 op. 26, d. 36, lists 6–15.

229 *Plan zdravookhraneniiu po RSFSR na 1939 god* in GARF f. A-482 op. 10, d. 3085, lists 1–6.

230 M. Donskoi, 'Ocherednye zadachi planirovaniia zdravookhraneniia', *Voporosy zdravookhranenie* 1928, No. 1, 11

231 Donskoi, 'Ocherednye zadachi', 1928, 11.

232 V. Smirnov, 'Osnovy 5-letnogo perspektivnogo plana zdravookhraneniia Leningradskoi oblasti', *Zdravookhranenie* 1929, No. 1, January, 3.

233 Smirnov, 'Osnovy 5-letnogo' 1929, 3.

234 GARF f. A-482, op 26, d. 22 list 45.

235 GARF f. A-482, op 24, d. 7 lists 4–5.

236 GARF f. A-482, op 26, d. 22 list 12.

237 GARF f. A-482, op 10, d. 1689 lists 6, 8.

238 GARF f. A-482, op 10, d. 1689 list 15.

239 A. P. Ivanov, 'Osnovye pokazateli ratsional'nogo ispol'zovaniia koechnoi seti Leningrada i perspektivy planirovaniia ee na 1932g', *Sotsialisticheskoe zdravookhranenie* 1932, No. 1, January, 11.

240 *Raionnoe planirovanie: Materialy* (Leningradskaia oblastnaia planovaia komissia, Leningrad 1933), 5, 22.

241 *Raionnoe planirovanie*, 33.

242 GARF f. A-482, op 24, d. 113, list 56.

243 *Plan 3-i piatiletka po zdravookhraneniiu 1938–1942gg tom 2* in GARF f. A-482 op. 26, d. 37, lists 111–115.

244 *Obiashitel'naia zapiska k planu zdravookhraneniia na 3-go piatletku i materialy k planu (1938)* in GARF f. A-482, op. 24, d. 1113, list 56.

245 *Obiashitel'naia zapiska k planu zdravookhraneniia na 3-go piatletku i materialy k planu (1938)* in GARF f. A-482, op. 24, d. 1113, list 76.

246 *Finansovoi plan organov zdravookhraneniia na 2-e piatiletie (1-i tur) 1933–37gg tom. 1* in GARF f. A-482 op 26, d. 26, list 25.

247 Sarah Davies, "'Us against Them": Social Identity in Soviet Russia, 1934–41', *Russian Review*, Volume 56, No. 1 (Jan. 1997), 88.

248 R. W. Davies, *The Development of the Soviet budgetary* system (Cambridge University Press, 1958), 78.

249 M. Donskoi, 'Kontrol'nye tsifry zdravookhraneniia RSFSR na 1929–1930gg', *Voporosy zdravookhranenie* 1929, No. 23, 27.

250 G. R. Mitchison, 'The Russian Worker' in M. I. Cole (ed.), *Twelve Studies in Soviet Russia* (Gollancz, London 1933), 88.

251 Calvin B. Hoover, *The Economic life of Soviet Russia* (Macmillan, London 1931), 285.

252 *XV let diktatory proletariata* 1932, 116–117 and *Statisticheskii spravochnik po gor. Leningrady 1930* (Izd. Leningradskogo ispolkoma 1930), 211.

253 *XV let diktatory proletariata*, 118–119.

254 Donskoi, 'Kontrol'nye tsifry', 29.

255 V. I. Smirnov, 'Kontrol'nye tsifry buidzhet na 1929–30 god po zdravookhraneniiu Leningradskoi oblasti', *Zdravookhranenie* 1929, No. 9, September, 8.

256 GARF f. A-482, op 10, d. 1915 lists 13–14, 19, 22, 24, 26, 28, 30, 32, 34, 36–37, 40; GARF f. A-482, op 10, d. 2523 lists 1, 1ob, 2, 2ob, 3, 3ob, 4, 4ob; GARF f. A-482, op 10, d. 2839 lists 97, 97ob, 98, 98ob, 99, 99ob, 100

257 See for instance James R. Millar and Elizabeth Clayton, 'Quality of life: Subjective measures of relative satisfaction' in J. R. Millar (ed.), *Politics, work and daily life: A study of former Soviet citizens* (Cambridge University Press, New York 1987), 49–51.

258 Sally E Ewing, 'Social insurance in Russia and the Soviet Union, 1912–33: A study of legal form and administrative practice', unpublished PhD dissertation, Princeton University, June 1984, 277.

259 Ewing, 'Social insurance in Russia and the Soviet Union, 1912–33', 277–278.

260 'Ne slushkom li shedro vydaiutsa bol'nichnye listki', *Krasnaia Gazeta* 21 February 1929, 4.

261 On these changes see V. Chernikov, 'Klassovaia politika vrachego Kritskogo', *Krasnaia Gazeta* 13 July 1929, 4 and 'Lechebno-profilakticheskie ob"edineniia', *Leningradskaia Pravda* 27 November 1929, 5.

262 I. Vol'fson, 'Zapiski putilovskogo vracha', *Leningradskaia Pravda* 9 April 1929, 3 and 'Pervyi plenum sektsii zdravookhraneniia', *Leningradskaia Pravda* 10 March 1931, 4.

263 Thus, the number of medical points in Leningrad increased from 240 in 1928 to 346 in 1932 while doctors staffing them rose from 232 to 314 over the same period (*XV let diktatory proletariat* 1932, 167).

264 Zabelin and Ia Eudin, *Promyshlennost' i sotsial'noe strakhovanie* (Moscow 1928), 7–10. To this end, the system of invalidity classification was revised on 29 February 1932. The first and second groups (i.e. those who required constant care or who were totally unfit for work) were retained but the fourth-sixth groups were abolished and a new third group created. The latter were defined as persons who were unable, under normal working conditions, to engage in systematic activity in their usual occupation, but who could continue to work either in their own job, but for shorter hours, or irregularly, in another occupation which required less skill (See Minkoff, 'Soviet social insurance system since 1921', 88). At this time also, preferential benefit rates were

introduced for women workers and those in underground and dangerous work or in heavy industry (Minkoff, 'Soviet social insurance system since 1921', 162, 205–206).

265 On this decree and its implications see M. Barsukov and A. Zhuk, *Za sotsialisticheshuiu rekonstruktuiu zdravookhraneniia: Osnovye polozheniia vtorogo piatiletnogo plana zdravookhraneniia* (Moscow 1932), 15–16 and Davis, 'The Soviet medical system', 25–26.

266 The Leningrad health service was not exceptional. In the Autumn of 1929–30, there was the Syrtsov-Laminadze affair and in the Summer of 1930, Vesenkha, Gosplan and other organisations were attacked for being 'bourgeois' and 'Menshevik' (see R. W. Davies, 'The Syrtsov-Lominadze affair', *Soviet Studies* January 1981, 29–47 and Kuromiya, *Stalin's Industrial Revolution* 1988, 161–71).

267 Barsukov and Zhuk, *Za sotsialistichesuiu rekonstruktuiu zdravookhraneniia* 1932, 14–16. Regulations on the payment of sickness benefit were also tightened to combat 'malingerers'. By 1930, benefits were not set at full earnings level as this was thought to encourage absenteeism for dubious reasons which threatened labour productivity and hence plan fulfilment. (see V. Kotov, 'Sotsialisticheskoe stroitel'stvo trebuet chetkosti v dele sotsial'nogo strakhovaniia', *Voprosy strakhovaniia* 1929, No.44, 2 and V. Kotov, 'Litsom v proizvodstvu! Sotsstrakhovanie na novykh putiakh', *Voprosy strakhovaniia* 1930, No.31, 13).

268 Barsukov and Zhuk, *Za sotsialistichesuiu rekonstruktuiu zdravookhraneniia*, 16.

269 M. I. Barsukov, *Ocherki istorii zdravookhraneniia SSSR* (Moscow 'Medgiz' 1951), 230.

270 GARF, f. 9474 op. 16 d. 97, list 114 cited in Sarah Davies, 'The Crime of "Anti-Soviet Agitation" in the Soviet Union in the 1930's' *Cahiers du Monde russe*, Vol. 39, No. 1/2, Les années 30: Nouvelles directions de la recherche (January-June 1998), 160.

271 S. Fitzpatrick, 'Stalin and the making of a new elite, 1928–1939', *Slavic Review* Volume 38, No. 3 (Sep. 1979), 379.

272 Ibid., 380–384.

273 Iain Lauchlan, 'Chekist *mentalité* and the origins of the Great Terror' in James Harris (ed.), *The Anatomy of Terror: political violence under Stalin* (Oxford University Press 2013), 13.

274 Epitomised by 'Anti-Stalinism' from 1928 onwards.

275 Davies, *Popular opinion in Stalin's Russia*, 18–19.

276 Ibid., 125.

277 GARF f. 9145 op 3, d. 6, list 1 cited in D. Shearer, 'Elements near and alien: Passportization, policing and identity in the Stalinist state, 1932–1952', *Journal of Modern History* Volume 76, No. 4 (December 2004), 850.

278 Shearer, 'Elements near and alien', 858.

279 Ibid., 855.

280 These include former kulaks, members of anti-Soviet parties, White Guards, returned émigrés, church/religious people, former tsarist government officials etc.

281 Shearer, 'Social disorder', 522.

282 This notion is taken from D. R. Shearer, 'Social disorder, mass repression and the NKVD during the 1930s', *Cahiers du Monde Russe* volume 42, No. 2/4 La Police politique on Union Sovietique 1918–1953 (April-December 2000), 508.

283 'Zakonchilas' chistka v oblzdravotedele', *Krasnaia Gazeta* 6 July 1929, 4.

284 TsGA SPb f. 9156, op. 4, d. 1, list 110.

285 TsGA SPb f. 9156, op. 4, d. 1, list 114–115 ob.

286 TsGA SPb f. 9156, op. 4, d. 1, list 121–123.

287 TsGA SPb f. 9156, op. 4, d. 1, list 126–128.
288 TsGA SPb f. 9156, op. 4, d. 1, list 124–125.
289 TsGA SPb f. 9156, op. 4, d. 1, list 129.
290 TsGA SPb f. 9156, op. 4, d. 1, list 129–130.
291 TsGA SPb f. 9156, op. 4, d. 1, list 119–120.
292 '*Itogi i vyvody po chistke apparata Oblizdravodela 1931g*' in TsGA SPb f. 9156, op. 4, d. 2, list 1.
293 '*Itogi i vyvody po chistke apparata Oblizdravodela 1931g*' in TsGA SPb f. 9156, op. 4, d. 2, list 1.
294 '*Itogi i vyvody po chistke apparata Oblizdravodela 1931g*' in TsGA SPb f. 9156, op. 4, d. 2, lists 1–2.
295 '*Itogi i vyvody po chistke apparata Oblizdravodela 1931g*' in TsGA SPb f. 9156, op. 4, d. 2, lists 12.
296 '*Itogi i vyvody po chistke apparata Oblizdravodela 1931g*' in TsGA SPb f. 9156, op. 4, d. 2, lists 13.
297 '*Itogi i vyvody po chistke apparata Oblizdravodela 1931g*' in TsGA SPb f. 9156, op. 4, d. 2, list 2.
298 '*Itogi i vyvody po chistke apparata Oblizdravodela 1931g*' in TsGA SPb f. 9156, op. 4, d. 2, lists 15–16.
299 '*Itogi i vyvody po chistke apparata Oblizdravodela 1931g*' in TsGA SPb f. 9156, op. 4, d. 2, list 20.
300 '*Itogi i vyvody po chistke apparata Oblizdravodela 1931g*' in TsGA SPb f. 9156, op. 4, d. 2, lists 23–24.
301 TsGA SPb f. 9156, op. 4, d. 2, list 23.
302 '*Itogi i vyvody po chistke apparata Oblizdravodela 1931g*' in TsGA SPb f. 9156, op. 4, d. 2, list 58.
303 '*Itogi i vyvody po chistke apparata Oblizdravodela 1931g*' in TsGA SPb f. 9156, op. 4, d. 2, lists 60, 95, 95ob.
304 Sheila Fitzpatrick, 'Signals from Below: Soviet Letters of Denunciation of the 1930s', *The Journal of Modern History*, Vol. 68, No. 4, Practices of Denunciation in Modern European History, 1789–1989 (Dec., 1996), 833.
305 Fitzpatrick, 'Signals from Below' 1996, 837–845.
306 TsGA SPb f. 9156, op. 4, d. 2, list 9.
307 TsGA SPb f. 9156, op. 4, d. 2, list 11.
308 TsGA SPb f. 9156, op. 4, d. 2, list 12.
309 TsGA SPb f. 9156, op. 4, d. 2, list 14.
310 TsGA SPb f. 9156, op. 4, d. 2, list 17.
311 TsGA SPb f. 9156, op. 4, d. 2, lists 10, 12.
312 TsGA SPb f. 9156, op. 4, d. 2, list 11.
313 TsGA SPb f. 9156, op. 4, d. 2, lists 13–14.
314 TsGA SPb f. 9156, op. 4, d. 2, list 14.
315 TsGA SPb f. 9156, op. 4, d. 2, list 18.
316 TsGA SPb f. 9156, op. 4, d. 2, list 16.
317 'Rabochnaia i kolkhoznaia molodezh' idite v medvuzy i medtekhnikumy', *Gigiena i zdorov'e rabochei sem'i* No. 24, August 1932, 2.
318 For example, Vigdorchik of the Leningrad Institute of Occupational diseases wanted to investigate the impact of shockwork and socialist competition on workers' health and was criticised for suggesting such investigations (see Siegelbaum, 'Okhrana Truda', 1990, 235).
319 On this see Davis, 'The Soviet medical system', 63–64.
320 I. I. Lamkin', *Sotsialisticheskoe Zdravookhraneniia* No. 8–9, August-September 1932, 2–4.
321 *Ves Leningrad na 1931 god* (Leningrad 1932), 107.

322 'Vypusk vrachei L.M. I'., *Gigiena i zdorov'e rabochei sem'i* No. 9, May 1930, 15 and 'Sotsial'nyi sostav slushatelei Leningradskikh medvuzov', *Gigiena i zdorov'e rabochei sem'i* No. 13–14, May 1931, 22.
323 TsGA SPb f. 9156, op. 4, d. 2, list 12.
324 TsGA SPb f. 9156, op. 4, d. 1, list 27.
325 GARF f. A-482, op. 10, d. 2433 lists 28–29.
326 GARF f. A-482, op. 10, d. 2433 lists 30–38.
327 For preliminary findings see Christopher Williams, 'The forgotten victims in Stalin's purges, 1930–38' Inaugural Professorial lecture, Liverpool Hope University, 4 March 2015.

Conclusion

This book has explored public health and medicine in one city – St. Petersburg/
Petrograd/Leningrad from 1900 until 1941. Tsarist St. Petersburg was an
extremely unhealthy environment, with one of the highest death rates in
Europe before 1917. There was no centralised health system and from the
Bolsheviks perspective, the 'body Russian' (industrial workers and poor
peasants) was not properly protected or medically provided for. Whilst the
medical profession was valued, it was not professionalised. Doctors were
employed by the state (zemstvo medicine) and medical care was available
but at a limited level. Some health enlightenment and medical advice was
also given to combat disease.

Prior to 1917, a strong sense of serving the community on the part of
doctors and other members of the medical profession developed and the
case study of social insurance showed that the Bolsheviks wanted to prioritise the health of the industrial working class and poor peasantry. The
causes of ill health were poverty, poor housing, low levels of hygiene and
environmental pollution. Public health was also poorly funded and budgets
badly managed. This book has highlighted the incompetence of the city's
authorities and their inertia in dealing with the public health challenges.

The Bolsheviks primarily blamed the Tsarist government, industrialists
and incompetent local authorities for failing to improve and safeguard the
health of industrial workers and poor peasants. There was a debate over
the need for a Ministry of Health to coordinate medical activity, but this
was cut short by the outbreak of the First World War. Before 1917 Tsarist
doctors were divided on the need for a Ministry and by their politics. Some
conservative doctors in St. Petersburg were in favour of the state, whereas
other more radical doctors were opposed to it and closer to the Bolsheviks.

The Bolsheviks had no blueprint for health care. They first formulated
a detailed programme on public health matters at the Second Congress of
the RSDLP held in 1903. They were acutely aware of the poor health conditions in which workers lived and continually pressured the government and
other groups to take action. It was not until June 1912 that social insurance legislation was finally passed, largely in response to rising social unrest.

Dissatisfied with the nature and scope of the new laws, the Bolsheviks launched an Insurance Campaign in an attempt to protect the interests of the Petersburg working-class.

After 1917, the Soviet government took responsibility for the welfare of the masses. Socialist health care was seen as an 'advance' and tsarist/zemstvo medicine seen as a 'retreat'. The task was an enormous one as there was no State health system and a civil war broke out. Throughout the period, 1918–20, food and fuel were in short supply and public health epidemics were rife. Former zemstvo doctors significantly helped Lenin defeat disease at this time. Lenin took a more co-operative attitude towards the medical intelligentsia at this point. The aim was to create a health service capable of alleviating the sufferings of the workers and one which was run on 'socialist' principles including the provision of comprehensive, universal, free health care for all.

The implementation of these principles was initially hampered by the civil war, and later under the NEP, by financial constraints, political conflicts and Ministerial rivalry over who should have responsibility for medical care for the insured. The insured workers in Leningrad had priority access to State medical facilities in the 1920s and class became a key determinant of eligibility.

The desire in the 1920s was to eradicate private medicine, offer specialised medical care, develop the health service in accordance with a scientifically based plan, eliminate inequality in access to health care between social groups and regions, to bring about a significant improvement in health conditions, to improve insurance medicine and to expand the health service.

Under War Communism and the NEP a pragmatic approach was taken by the state towards the medical intelligentsia, one that was quasi liberal, granting doctors greater freedom and autonomy to fulfil state goals. However, political and economic constraints during the NEP prevented many government objectives from being realised. Private medicine continued to thrive and the elite and the insured benefitted most from the health care available. Stalin and others viewed the NEP and its treatment of the medical profession as a retreat.

In overall terms, the demand for health care far exceeded supply. Health care was not a priority under the NEP and this trend continued under Stalin. There were constant shortages of finance, resources and although some advances in quantitative health indicators occurred, many five-year plan health targets in Leningrad were not fulfilled and this resulted in a decline in the quality of medical care for some groups. The main problem was that while the first variant of the First five-year plan was modest; the second set targets which were unrealistic and far too ambitious especially at a time of rapid industrialisation and forced collectivisation. In the Stalinist era, a more conservative approach was adopted. Greater medical privileges were available to the loyal, economically productive groups and there was discrimination against potential enemies and the persecution of alleged 'class aliens' as developments in the health sector failed to keep pace with those in the rest of the economy. The Leningrad health service's ineffectiveness in dealing with adverse changes in living standards and health conditions especially in the 1930s became a cause of concern and this led to cleansing campaigns and seeing some parts of the medical profession as a 'class enemy'. The Party wanted to provide the best medical care for industrial workers, women, babies and children. This is why industrial hygiene and occupational diseases became a priority, abortion was banned in 1936, divorce made tougher and why there was a temperance campaign under Stalin.

Soviet public health discourses amongst the Party and medical profession, as shown by archival material, official documents, the press, medical journals and health education literature, demonstrates Lenin's desire to eradicate the tsarist legacy and modernise health and welfare so that the health of industrial workers and peasants improved. All this was done in the name of socialism and in the interests of protecting the kollektiv both of which shaped Soviet health policy. This book has analysed how the Soviet state sought to intervene in public health affairs, regulate health behaviour and to implement and construct a 'collectivist lifestyle' among the inhabitants of Petrograd and Leningrad. The goal was to eradicate individualist attitudes towards health and health practice among the population, to reframe public health values and attitudes, and to refashion individual health behaviour so that a new modern, progressive Soviet person emerged within a collectivist setting. The desire was to overcome the backwardness of Tsarist health care detailed in Chapter 1 and to remove threats to the 'body Soviet' in the broadest sense. The goal was to move towards a more modern, advanced health care system which was part of the transformational nature of Bolshevism and Stalinism.[1]

Building a socialist health service required a transition to socialism, a move away from capitalism, the use of health and other forms of surveillance of the population, an emphasis on unity and a move away from individualism to socialist collectivist forms of health care organisation and beliefs. Soviet health education discourses from the civil war onwards were also closely connected with the production of knowledge of and power over health matters and Leninist and Stalinist governments sought to control the population.[2] The aim was the development of a new Soviet self and collective identities and key to this was expert medical advice to a range of social groups in Leningrad. This was not a uniform process due to all the changes occurring under War Communism, the NEP and under Stalinism and more than one model existed. The goal was to modernise all areas, motherhood for instance, and to create perfect mothers and other citizens. This produced conflicts between the materialist versus emancipatory discourses around women during the 1920s and 30s. Thus health, progress and modernity featured in Soviet health education literature.

This desire to protect the health of the collective was used by Lenin and Stalin, and their medical professions, in order to justify sanitary surveillance of the population and to carry out health education campaigns. The aim in health propaganda was to provide advice, improve knowledge, and guarantee greater health security for the citizens of Petrograd and Leningrad. This approach led to the gradual medicalisation of health behaviour and to defining certain actions and health values as 'deviant', if they threatened the collective. In this context, Lenin and Stalin, but the latter in particular, became concerned about the influence of bearers of alien or dangerous/hostile ideas about health care or about potential bourgeois influences such as individualism or scepticism about Soviet socialism.

These public health policies and changes were not the product of socialist ideology alone, they were also shaped by revolution, civil war, the mixed economy of the NEP and the rise of Stalin. This book also argues that the Tsarist medical profession played a major part at least prior to the Great and mass terrors, 1934–38. Thus, continuity of medical staff, approaches and certain values from zemstvo to Soviet medicine contributed to this process of transformation and modernisation, influenced the way the Petrograd/Leningrad service was run and most of all, enabled Tsarist and Soviet doctors to work together to combat diseases and to seek to instil the new norms regarding hygiene, sexual behaviour, drinking, child rearing etc amongst the population. The majority of those who initially headed public health departments in Petrograd were educated and trained in the Tsarist era, and now practiced under Soviet rule.

The conventional view as advanced by Nancy Frieden is that the Tsarist medical profession primarily aimed at professionalization,[3] and some Soviet scholars have argued that the Bolsheviks inherited a well-established medical profession which was hostile to socialism and their aims namely to build a socialist health service. This book challenges both these assumptions arguing that, in Saint Petersburg, some senior members, and many rank and file members, such as junior physicians or medical students, actively participated in political activity and the revolutionary movement from the 1860s onwards. This activity culminated in their involvement in both the 1905 and February and October 1917 Revolutions. These medical radicals often allied themselves with the Bolsheviks.

This activity was not just motivated by professionalisation but by a shared view that Tsarism was responsible for causing damage to the 'body Russian' and so some tsarist doctors shared the Bolsheviks views on the need for political change.

The post-1917 period witnessed the emergence of the Petrograd/Leningrad medical establishment and former Tsarist trained doctors, cooperated with the new Soviet regime to deal with public health crises in the Russian civil war and afterwards. These zemstvo doctors did so because they shared many medical values with the Bolsheviks. The majority of bourgeois medical specialists therefore willingly helped the Bolsheviks define the 'body Soviet', determine health policies and practices and to also defend the health of the community and collective in Petrograd/Leningrad. In the civil war, they demonstrated their loyalty by fighting epidemics, and were rewarded by state-sponsored medical science, research and networks, though like everyone else they faced isolation, food shortages and hunger. This cooperation proved significant, with both sides recognising the need to combat a common enemy – the epidemics of infectious and other diseases. During the NEP, doctors in Petrograd before 1924, and Leningrad 1924–27, carried on working productively with the Soviet state and maintaining valuable links with the West, most notably with colleagues in Germany.[4] They became well acquainted with Western medical practices and devised strategies of their own to suit medical conditions in Petrograd/Leningrad. Medical staff also carried out extensive research into health conditions in the city and region in order to determine the pattern of disease and ill-health. New Soviet and old Tsarist medical practitioners collaborated together and firmly believed that the causes of illness were mainly social rather than biological. The local and central government also played a key role by promoting the emergence of 'social hygiene' as a discipline, and former Tsarist doctors were at the forefront of the new Soviet social or community medicine. This approach allowed all parties – different sections of the medical profession and the state – to construct a health collective and target an audience for its modernisation policies and thinking.

Behind this new health mission was a common desire to eradicate backwardness in attitudes to health and hygiene and the goal was to civilise various social groups by imagining, through health posters, a new way of life and how life should be as well as by making collectivism a central value of the new Soviet order and its health and welfare policies. The aim was to make homes, factories and Leningraders more healthy, hygienic, clean and well ordered. The posters used in this book were part of the Leninist and Stalinist health education campaigns launched from the civil war onwards. These were geared towards enlightening the masses and creating more cultured and health conscious Leningrad workers and peasants. Such posters and accompanying lectures and debates around them provided various medical models for the population to follow. The health of the citizens of Petrograd and Leningrad was now no longer just an individual, private matter, as people were part of a public arena, and of the collective. Thus, the private-public health sphere became increasingly blurred. As David Hoffman notes, '[p]arty propagandists sought to teach peasants and workers to sacrifice personal interests for the sake of the collective'.[5]

The aim was to build a new Soviet welfare state, of which health care was a key element. The masses were encouraged to support the state and join the collective and in exchange the Soviet state promised to provide better living and working conditions through communal housing, dining rooms, crèches, female emancipation, a stable family and a modern, advanced health service. The Party defined who was included in the collective and with regards to public health, the medical profession helped the Party decide, on the basis of their knowledge and expertise, who posed a medical threat. The Party and the medical profession both sought to prevent immoral behaviour, venereal diseases, drunkenness, prostitution and abortion, to name but a few areas of concern to the Soviet state. These 'deviant' individuals and their behaviour were stigmatised and culturally constructed as being medically as inferior in comparison to those with more progressive and conscious health values. The production of certain imagery of who or what was 'good' and what was 'bad' behaviour (as shown by the before and after depictions in health propaganda) was part of the Soviet conception of the environment and how it produced disease and illness, as well as evidence of an urban/rural divide, a hierarchy within Soviet health poster iconography and a fear of the remnants of Capitalism. The aim was to persuade the population to replace any old pre-revolutionary or bourgeois backward ways of life, seen as a 'retreat' with new, Soviet scientifically based viewpoints viewed as an 'advance' as depicted in Soviet health imagery and through Soviet health policies. The challenge that the Bolsheviks in Petrograd and Leningrad faced was to change workers' and peasants' health norms, to eradicate the adverse effects of the capitalist past and traditionalism and to overcome any resistance to the modernisation of health values and attitudes. This was not always a success and there was, as this book shows, a gap between health propaganda and policies and the reality under Lenin and Stalin. Victoria Bonnell points out that visual propaganda acted as 'a powerful tool in the reconstruction of the individual, his ideology, his way of life, his economic activity'.[6] As a result, some Soviet males and females were portrayed as heroic role models in the messages of health posters, whereas those with 'deviant' behaviour became demonised. We have used examples of both throughout this book.

During War Communism and the NEP there were disagreements over whether bourgeois members of the Petrograd/Leningrad medical profession were a threat or an asset to the Soviet regime and its health service goals. Out of necessity, the Leninist regime tolerated potentially anti-socialist bourgeois members of the medical profession and the latter in turn utilised patronage networks to their advantage to gain professionalisation. Lenin might have wanted to destroy old state structures or build new ones but he did not have the resources to implement or fulfil all of his desired policies. As a result, health care strategies and policies show a zigzag pattern.

During the civil war and War Communism, there was a desire to maintain legitimacy, for centralisation as well as to create a socialist health service, however the fight for regime survival and against epidemics forced the Leninist regime to make a pragmatic retreat but the new Soviet government still enforced discipline in society and among medical staff. Although critical of the bourgeoisie, Lenin needed bourgeois members of the medical profession for their experience, knowledge and to co-run the health service. The new health service was based upon a hierarchical command centre led by Pervukhin in Petrograd and when appropriate the government used certain incentives to combat public health crises. We were not yet at the stage of socialism and the new regime had to build a socialist health service from scratch.

In Petrograd's case we see a mix of centralisation and local initiatives being used to deal with public health challenges. It was not just a question of the difference between 'coercion' and 'persuasion' as many members of the zemstvo medicine shared certain public health beliefs with the new regime, so no persuasion was needed and little coercion was required in Petrograd's case. Nevertheless, some within the Party, including Stalin, saw bourgeois medical specialists as a threat.

The question under the NEP was: could this pragmatic retreat with the medical profession be continued after the civil war ended? The Party was still divided, the health service was run by Bolshevik and tsarist medical personnel and worry was voiced about the impact of the market on health care, such as fees, inequality of access and building a socialist health service on an economic basis. There was also Party concern that the NEP had allowed the socialist principles of health and welfare to be watered down and private medicine, on a narrow scale, to survive. In the 1920s, the aim was to improve medical care for the insured but this did not fully occur so discontent amongst industrial workers, the Party and trade unions increased. The 1922 health reform and the 'regime of economy' policy of 1926 led to cost cutting and this generated serious challenges. Although shortages of money were mainly to blame, bourgeois and other staff resisting central pressure to make health savings, were blamed for any resulting failures. Although there was now less repression and less direct Party and security police interference with the medical profession, at the same time there were demands for the proletarianisation of Leningrad medicine, that is to increase the proportion of working class and peasant members in the local health service. This trend was also part of a desire to improve relations between health service workers and managers and demonstrate to the population that it was responding to their needs and concerns.

This book argues that there was a continuity of earlier War Communism policies evident under the NEP. Under early NEP (1921–24), there was a symbiotic relationship between doctors and government, which allowed the medical profession limited autonomy and greater professionalization. The shared values, material rewards (such as better wages, improved working conditions), a key role in decision and policy making and the placement of former zemstvo doctors in important positions, meant that bourgeois medical specialists were able to take up posts in the local health system in Petrograd and Ministry of Health (Narkomzdrav) in Moscow. Members of the old medical profession were becoming integrated into the new social and political order.

In late NEP (1925–27), however, central government and health policy shifted, and there was now a desire to replace bourgeois members with new proletarian medical cadres. This was due to the former zemstvo doctors' lack of willingness to join the Party and hence their perceived lack of loyalty to the communist regime. Social background/class origin was used as the main indicator of trustworthiness. Over time political and other loyalties to the Soviet regime became of increasing significance. This was part of Stalin's commitment to what Stephen Kotkin calls progressive modernity, in which health and welfare were crucial.[7]

After 1928, Stalin's aim was to use health care as a facilitator of socialist construction and to make the great leap forward. His aim was to eliminate the market in health care and to overcome backwardness. He was fully committed to advancing/civilising health care and health service values. The anti-retreat stance was evident during early Stalinism (the late 1920s and early 1930s), as senior Party officials expressed great concern over the dominant role which Tsarist specialists now had in public health affairs. Party penetration of the health service was deemed to be not as high as officially desired. This was not really necessary in Leningrad as conflict was very low, but the numbers of proletarian 'Red' medical cadres still steadily increased nevertheless. The change in economic strategy, which brought about centrally-planned rapid industrialisation and forced collectivisation, also put increased pressure on the bourgeois members of the health service. Medical staff social origins were investigated and loyalties questioned, as health conditions and living standards gradually declined, once the five-year plans (FYPs) were implemented. As the level of medical disorder rose, so did the Stalinist state desire to control medical staff. The Stalinist regime started to believe that bourgeois members of the medical profession were sabotaging socialist health care goals. The FYP was used to increase state control over the medical profession and health service leaders. Medical professionals were also required to exercise greater control over the Body Soviet, the family, sex, children and to eradicate the problem of 'bourgeois individualism' that had emerged under NEP and helped in official eyes to spread venereal disease, prostitution and abortion.

Stalin's policies of industrialisation and collectivisation led to discontent within the Party and broader society. 1928–30 was a time of self-criticism of leaders and medical staff. Stalin possibly tapped in traditional attitudes towards the medical profession in his criticism of bureaucratism. The latter did not just refer to red tape but to a person's commitment to Marxist ideology on health care. Following David Priestland's interpretation of Stalinism, it is possible to argue that Stalin was trying to transform leadership style and behaviour in the Leningrad health service by reducing arrogance, increasing comradely behaviour and to improve relations between the masses and health service leaders.[8] This necessitated a struggle against bourgeois culture in Soviet medicine. The Stalinist government's aim was to transform the psychology and health behaviour of the population, using the posters contained in this book, as well as the ideas of health service officials. In the Stalinist era, there was a belief that a socialist health care system could only be constructed if the working class was behind it and if bourgeois attitudes were eradicated.

For certain parts of the Leningrad medical profession this meant that they were seen as the cause of bureaucratism or as officials of bourgeois social origins. Although Stalin promoted the idea of a more prosperous future, Chapter 4 showed that in Leningrad public health policies were chaotic, at times incoherent and very ambitious. Many targets were not fulfilled so there were shortages of housing, food, a falling standard of living and uneven access to health care, followed by a ban on abortion in 1936 (and restrictions on women's ability to control their own bodies) and increasing sanitary and other types of surveillance of the population in the 1930s.

This Stalinist change in policy had a negative impact on the work of medical professionals. For example, the ability of senior doctors, such as Professor Vigdorchik, Director of the Leningrad Institute of Occupational Disease, to determine precisely how the level of industrial or economic development in Leningrad city or gubernia affected health status was hampered by Party criticism of his work, as discussed earlier. The same applied to those medical staff investigating living conditions, environmental pollution, the pace of modernisation etc and their impact on health conditions.

There were also tensions within the Party over the USSR's direction and Stalin's rule, as well as between the Party and medical profession due to the impact of Stalin's Revolution on the health of the collective in Leningrad. This climate produced a fear that the medical profession pretended to be loyal but, in reality, was actually anti-socialist and guilty of 'wrecking' in the health service sphere. The desire between 1928–41 was to eradicate bureaucratism and bourgeois habits, methods and morals in the Leningrad health service. The question was how? Various means were tried including mass promotion (*vydvizhenie*) of proletarians, the eradication of old tsarist bureaucrats and blaming the bourgeoisie or class aliens for health service failures. The approach taken was to either criticise communists allegedly behaving in bourgeois ways and/or to cleanse (purge) those alien or hostile to the Party and its health policies. In the Leningrad health service, a purge took place. Smirnov was replaced by the Party technocrat Lamkin as head in early 1931 and the editorial staff of the Leningrad medical journal was also changed. So, as part of the 'class struggle', bourgeois medical specialists in Leningrad were now under attack. This strategy was portrayed as evidence of Stalin and the Party's attempts to increase working class influence over the public health apparatus; as a way of protecting the health of the collective; ensuring fulfilment of socialist plans for the economy and health service; to increase support for industrialisation and collectivisation and the FYPs and to increase Party control over public health appointments.

There were many reasons for non-fulfilment of FYP health service goals including: a lack of unity and discipline (Tsarist medical officials allegedly undermining Soviet ones); insufficient resources (capital, staff, materials); and the use of the carrot and stick. There was a strong expectation of loyalty to the state and Party and also an expectation that medical personnel would obey the rules and perform their health service duties well and efficiently.

Disloyal enemies in the Leningrad health service were criticised on various grounds including class, attitude to nation, social background and political consciousness. This book shows that it was not just the latter but more importantly medical disorder that led to calls for vigilance and the checking of the Party credentials of all health service staff. This disorder was caused by Stalinist policies.

Creating a new Soviet person with different health norms and values and internalising the desired new collectivist principles was hindered by shortages of money, staff, political division and by so-called 'wreckers', namely bourgeois elements within the medical profession who allegedly undermined or rejected the official public health policies and norms. Those who failed to conform to the new health norms or policies were labelled as 'deviant', uncultured or classified as politically unreliable, 'class enemies'. These individuals were deemed to be a threat to the 'body Soviet' or the collective in the broadest sense.

The Party decided that the source of this contagion or corruption of the health of the Leningrad population and the nation as a whole needed to be eradicated. In the process, medical disorder, moral degeneration and Stalinist politics all became interconnected during the 1930s. This meant that political and health surveillance of the population of Leningrad also became closely linked. Former zemstvo doctors and other members of the intelligentsia who had been monitored by the Cheka in the civil war, were now monitored again by the Stalinist secret police departments in factories, universities, hospitals, where doctors worked or trained future generations of medical personnel.[9] Thus the lack of Marxist credentials on the part of Tsarist medical staff was questioned from the late 1920s onwards and the new Red doctors trained under the Soviet regime were now expected to take better control and exercise more diligence in order to successfully instil new socialist health values and to deal with the public health crises that emerged in the 1930s. The problem was that the new medical staff, who had undertaken accelerated courses, sometimes lacked the necessary medical skills, knowledge and experience to achieve the goal of prioritising medical care for the insured and especially industrial workers in the city as well as rural workers in collectivised agricultural regions of Leningrad oblast.

This book advances the view that it was the Tsarist medical professions perceived lack of enthusiasm and active participation in building a Stalinist health service that gave cause for concern. Bourgeois medical personnel in Leningrad assumed that simply following policy guidelines was enough, but this was not the case. The purge commissions of the late 1920s and early 1930s discovered discontent among the population concerning the quality of medical care offered in Leningrad and these popular denunciations led to criticism of health staff for bureaucratism, negligence and for failing to combat a lack of discipline, absenteeism and all the diseases mentioned earlier. Such denunciations of health service staff played on the officially promoted fear of anti-Soviet bourgeois elements, which in turn led to further criticism, more discontent about health care and resulted in expanded medical surveillance of bourgeois elements. Thus, staff at all levels of the health system in Leningrad – district, city and region – suffered from criticism. This led to the removal of experienced bourgeois medical staff. Some were reprimanded, others sacked prior to 1934. This situation coupled with the rise of alien, socially dangerous elements and major public order issues, was perceived by the Party as threatening not just the health of the population but the very survival of the Stalinist state, its legitimacy and its unity. So, under Stalinism the struggle was between proletarian and bourgeois elements in the medical profession and this was essential in facilitating a retreat away from capitalist health care of the NEP and a transition to a more advanced socialist one under Stalin.

In 1935, the slogan of the day was that 'cadres decide everything'. Stalin believed that public health bosses and cadres in Leningrad were failing to obey the central authorities and that this was part of a continued resistance to his leadership style and policies. His desire was to root out those who disagreed or failed to believe in socialist health principles and so he wanted to mobilise public health staff in order to create a greater level of medical order. This was necessary because his public health policies were chaotic and diverse. Sometimes he was cautious, at other times chaotic. The purges were required to eradicate the survivals of zemstvo medicine left by the NEP and to gain the loyalty of key sections of the population at a time of major economic change. The purges which were extremely disruptive and violent targeted former people (*byushie liudi*) hiding in the Leningrad health service who were seen as 'class aliens' or simply as 'enemies'. Many of those targeted by the NKVD were former political opponents with rightist or bourgeois attitudes such as White Guardists, kulaks or Trotskyists. Some health service staff lost their jobs and apartments, others their lives. We argue here that the purges of the Leningrad health service led to the unjust persecution of 'passives' who had naturally concealed their class origins under the circumstances (many having put their past behind them) and had been discovered during the checking of Party credentials in the 1930s.

It was medical staff inability to prevent medical disorder, as signified by the significant decline in health conditions (a falling birth rate, increasing alcoholism, prostitution, venereal disease, TB and infectious disease) by 1936 which the Party believed put the collective in danger in Leningrad and this led to the medical purges. In the mid–late 1930s, the goal of the Stalinist state was to remove criminals and social deviants in order to protect the health of the population of Leningrad and to guarantee the purity of the city. This was done through passport and residence permit controls, both of which were part of Stalinist policing and purging. These socially harmful groups included the 'unhealthy' (alcoholics, the homeless, prostitutes, those with venereal diseases and backstreet abortionists) as well as the usual suspects – thieves, convicts, kulaks and former nepmen in Leningrad. However, as population movement increased and the situation became more and more chaotic, state violence increased. The sweeps of marginals and class enemies at this point stretched and drained the Leningrad police and security forces, and left less money and resources to deal with medical disorder. Stalin was unable to control the impact of this purge process and its adverse impact on health service staff and health conditions.

In this context, David Hoffman concludes that Party leaders 'used state economic controls, public health measures, surveillance and excisionary violence to shape their vision of a productive healthy society minus the 'harmful elements of the old order'.[10] The medical disorder of the mid–late 1930s depicted in this book was blamed on bourgeois medical specialists in Leningrad rather than on the flaws of Stalinist policies. Ironically, to get the medical disorder under control, achieve and protect socialism, as well as the health of key members of the collective, many long standing former tsarist members of the medical profession were arrested and executed during the mass operations of 1937–1938.[11] Stalin and his government might have wanted to remove threats but his policies actually undermined the medical stability of the USSR and caused widespread medical chaos in Leningrad. We advance the view here that Stalin's purge campaigns against the medical profession weakened and so achieved its desired goal of eradicating a significant proportion of bourgeois medical specialists. However, this only made matters worse. Far from reinvigorating the Leningrad health service and restoring the city's revolutionary spirit, the Great and mass terrors of 1934–38 substantially damaged the Leningrad health service due to the loss of core tsarist staff who had served it well and many had made self-sacrifices since 1917. This meant that the medical disorder worsened and the public health crisis deepened after 1936.

One of the major contradictions evident in Stalinist public health policies was its aggressive attacks on medical personnel due to pressure from above and denunciations from below. This undermined the ability of the Leningrad medical profession to deal with major health challenges at a time of fear of war (which materialised with Finland in 1939–40 and Nazi Germany in 1941) and to combat mounting social disorder. The Stalinist leadership, in putting great pressure on the Leningrad Party and security services to root out enemies and avoid medical wrecking, was primarily concerned with loyalty and medical security. Both were now closely linked but the state targeted the 'wrong people'. Leningrad medical staff were in fact loyal and many shared the same desire as the Moscow Party leadership to combat the arising public health crises, but their political passivity brought their loyalty into question in the context of a perception of Leningrad as a major terrorist centre.

Stalin may have wished to replace tsarist zemstvo staff with capable and loyal party cadres among the medical profession, to restore medical order, reverse the NEP retreat away from the original socialist principles on which the Petrograd health service was founded and to provide medical security for the population and state, but, in reality, his government's coercive policies seeking to build socialism and a socialist welfare state actually backfired. The promise of improved health and health care fought for during the October Revolution was not fulfilled by Stalin, and, if anything, Stalinism left the health of the collective in Leningrad in an extremely precarious position as the Nazi invasion began in June 1941. This interpretation of the current evidence suggests that the health of the population of Leningrad was already significantly weakened by budget cuts and constraints and by the zigzag pattern of Stalinist health and other policies prior to the siege of Leningrad. This made the local population more susceptible to illness and disease once the latter came and without the necessary staff in place to combat such a situation many more people would suffer after 1941 and the outbreak of the Great Patriotic War.

Notes

1 This follows David Hoffman's notion of both as 'transformational ideologies' see D. L. Hoffman, *Cultivating the Masses: Modern state practices and Soviet socialism, 1914–1939* (Cornell University Press, 2011), 3.
2 M. Foucault, *History of Sexuality: The will to knowledge,* Volume 1 (Penguin 1988), 139.
3 See Nancy Frieden, *Russian physicians in an era of Reform and Revolution, 1856–1905* (Princeton University Press 1981).
4 See Susan Gross Solomon, *Doing medicine together: Germany and Russia between the wars* (University of Toronto Press, 2006).
5 Hoffman, *Cultivating the Masses,* 228.
6 Victoria E. Bonnell, 'Iconography of the workers in Soviet political art', in L. H. Siegelbaum and R. G. Suny (ed.), *Making Workers Soviet: Power, class, identity* (Cornell University Press, 1994), 363.
7 Stephen K. Kotkin, *Magnetic Mountain: Stalinism as a Civilization* (University of California Press, Berkeley 1997), 20.
8 David Priestland, *Stalinism and the Politics of mobilisation: Ideas, power and terror in inter-war Russia* (Oxford University Press, Oxford 2007), 208.
9 Hoffman, *Cultivating the Masses,* 204.
10 Ibid., 13.
11 For preliminary findings see Christopher Williams, 'The forgotten victims in Stalin's purges, 1930–38' Inaugural Professorial lecture, Liverpool Hope University, 4 March 2015.

Index